T0259519

Infant and Early Childhood Mental Health

Guest Editors

MARY MARGARET GLEASON, MD
DANIEL S. SCHECHTER, MD

CHILD AND ADOLESCENT PSYCHIATRIC CLINICS OF NORTH AMERICA

www.childpsych.theclinics.com

Consulting Editor
HARSH K. TRIVEDI, MD

July 2009 • Volume 18 • Number 3

SAUNDERS an imprint of ELSEVIER, Inc.

W.B. SAUNDERS COMPANY
A Division of Elsevier Inc.

Elsevier Inc. ● 1600 John F. Kennedy Boulevard ● Suite 1800 ● Philadelphia, Pennsylvania 19103-2899

http://www.childpsych.theclinics.com

CHILD AND ADOLESCENT PSYCHIATRIC CLINICS OF NORTH AMERICA Volume 18, Number 3
July 2009 ISSN 1056–4993, ISBN-13: 978-1-4377-1199-8, ISBN-10: 1-4377-1199-5

Editor: Sarah E. Barth
Developmental Editor: Donald Mumford

Child and Adolescent Psychiatric Clinics of North America (ISSN 1056-4993) is published quarterly by Elsevier Inc., 360 Park Avenue South, New York, NY 10010-1710. Months of issue are January, April, July, and October. Business and Editorial Offices: 1600 John F. Kennedy Boulevard, Suite 1800, Philadelphia, PA 19103-2899. Customer Service Offices: 6277 Sea Harbor Drive, Orlando, FL 32887-4800. Periodicals postage paid at New York, NY and additional mailing offices. Subscription prices are $238.00 per year (US individuals), $378.00 per year (US institutions), $122.00 per year (US students), $270.00 per year (Canadian individuals), $456.00 per year (Canadian institutions), $156.00 per year (Canadian students), $321.00 per year (international individuals), $456.00 per year (international institutions), and $156.00 per year (international students). International air speed delivery is included in all Clinics subscription prices. All prices are subject to change without notice. **POSTMASTER:** Send address changes to Child and Adolescent Psychiatric Clinics of North America, Elsevier Periodicals Customer Service, 11830 Westline Industrial Drive, St. Louis, MO 63146. **Customer Service: 1-800-654-2452 (US). From outside the United States, call 1-314-453-7041. Fax: 1-314-453-5170. E-mail: JournalsCustomerService-usa@elsevier.com (for print support) or journalsonlinesupport-usa@ elsevier.com (for online support).**

Reprints. For copies of 100 or more of articles in this publication, please contact the Commercial Reprints Department, Elsevier Inc., 360 Park Avenue South, New York, New York 10010-1710 Tel.: (212) 633-3812; Fax: (212) 462-1935, e-mail: reprints@elsevier.com.

Child and Adolescent Psychiatric Clinics of North America is covered in *MEDLINE/PubMed (Index Medicus), ISI, SSCI, Research Alert, Social Search, Current Contents,* and *EMBASE/Excerpta Medica.*

Printed and bound by CPI Group (UK) Ltd, Croydon, CR0 4YY
Transferred to Digital Print 2011

Contributors

CONSULTING EDITOR

HARSH K. TRIVEDI, MD
Site Training Director and Director of Adolescent Services, E.P. Bradley Hospital;
Assistant Professor of Psychiatry and Human Behavior (Clinical), Brown Medical School;
President, Rhode Island Council for Child and Adolescent Psychiatry, East Providence,
Rhode Island

CONSULTING EDITOR EMERITUS

ANDRÉS MARTIN, MD, MPH

FOUNDING CONSULTING EDITOR

MELVIN LEWIS, MBBS, FRCPSYCH, DCH

GUEST EDITORS

MARY MARGARET GLEASON, MD
Assistant Professor, Departments of Psychiatry & Neurology, and Pediatrics, Tulane
University School of Medicine, New Orleans, Louisiana

DANIEL S. SCHECHTER, MA, MD
Chief of Consult-Liaison and Parent-Infant Research Units, Division of Child and
Adolescent Psychiatry, University Hospitals of Geneva, Switzerland; and Adjunct
Assistant Professor of Psychiatry, Columbia University College of Physicians & Surgeons,
New York, New York

AUTHORS

LETIA O. BAILEY, MSW
Instructor of Clinical Psychiatry, Tulane University School of Medicine, and Institute
of Infant and Early Childhood Mental Health, New Orleans, Louisiana

SUSAN BERRY, MD, MPH
Associate Professor of Clinical Pediatrics, Louisiana State University Health Sciences
Center, New Orleans, Louisiana

NADIA BRUSCHWEILER-STERN, MD
Pediatrician, Child Psychiatrist and Director of the Swiss Brazelton Centre, Geneva,
Switzerland

EMMA CARDELI, AB
Department of Psychiatry, Washington University School of Medicine, St. Louis, Missouri

ALICE S. CARTER, PhD
Professor and Director, Graduate Clinical Psychology Program, Department of Psychology, University of Massachusetts, Boston, Massachusetts

ANIL CHACKO, PhD
Assistant Professor of Psychology, Department of Psychology, Queens College, City University of New York, Flushing, New York

SUSAN COATES, PhD
Clinical Professor of Psychology in Psychiatry, College of Physicians and Surgeons, Columbia University, New York, New York

BARBARA DANIS, PhD
Department of Psychiatry, Institute for Juvenile Research, University of Illinois at Chicago, Chicago, Illinois

SUSAN DICKSTEIN, PhD
Associate Professor, The Warren Alpert Medical School of Brown University; and Director, Early Childhood Clinical Research Center, Bradley/Hasbro Children's Research Center, Providence, Rhode Island

HELEN LINK EGGER, MD
Assistant Professor, Department of Psychiatry and Behavioral Sciences, Center for Developmental Epidemiology, Duke University Medical Center, Durham, North Carolina

KIMBERLY ANDREWS ESPY, PhD
Associate Vice Chancellor for Research, Professor, Department of Psychology, University of Nebraska-Lincoln, Lincoln, Nebraska

JOHN FANTON, MD
Assistant Professor, Department of Psychiatry, Tufts University School of Medicine, Western Campus at Baystate Medical Center, Springfield, Massachusetts

MARGARITA FORCADA-GUEX, PhD
Division of Neonatology, Department of Pediatrics, University Hospital Lausanne, Lausanne, Switzerland

NATHAN A. FOX, PhD
Distinguished University Professor, Department of Human Development, University of Maryland, College Park, Maryland

THEODORE J. GAENSBAUER, MD
Clinical Professor of Psychiatry, University of Colorado Health Sciences Center, Denver, Colorado

MARY MARGARET GLEASON, MD
Assistant Professor, Departments of Psychiatry & Neurology, and Pediatrics, Tulane University School of Medicine, New Orleans, Louisiana

CARRI HILL, PhD
Assistant Professor of Psychiatry, Department of Psychiatry, Institute for Juvenile Research, University of Illinois at Chicago, Chicago, Illinois

ALICIA F. LIEBERMAN, PhD
Irving B. Harris Endowed Chair in Infant Mental Health and Professor, Department of Psychiatry, University of California San Francisco; and Child Trauma Research Program, San Francisco General Hospital, San Francisco, California

JOAN LUBY, MD
Department of Psychiatry, Washington University School of Medicine, St. Louis, Missouri

FRANCES DE L. MARTÍNEZ-PEDRAZA, BA
Graduate Student, Graduate Clinical Psychology Program, Psychology Department, University of Massachusetts, Boston, Massachusetts

SUSAN C. McDONOUGH, PhD
Associate Research Professor of Social Work and Associate Research Scientist, Center for Human Growth and Development, University of Michigan, Ann Arbor, Michigan

CAROLE MULLER-NIX, MD
Department of Child and Adolescent Psychiatry, University Hospital Lausanne, Hôpital Nestlé, Lausanne, Switzerland

CHARLES A. NELSON III, PhD
Professor of Pediatrics and Neuroscience, Harvard Medical School; and Richard David Scott Chair in Pediatric Development Medicine Research, Children's Hospital Boston, DMC Lab of Cognitive Neuroscience, Boston, Massachusetts

ANA SANCHO ROSSIGNOL, FSP
Service of Child and Adolescent Psychiatry, Department of Child and Adolescent Medicine, University Hospitals of Geneva and University of Geneva, Geneva, Switzerland

SANDRA RUSCONI-SERPA, FSP
Service of Child and Adolescent Psychiatry, Department of Child and Adolescent Medicine, University Hospitals of Geneva and University of Geneva, Geneva, Switzerland

DANIEL S. SCHECHTER, MA, MD
Chief of Consult-Liaison and Parent-Infant Research Units, Division of Child and Adolescent Psychiatry, University Hospitals of Geneva, Switzerland; and Adjunct Assistant Professor of Psychiatry, Columbia University College of Physicians & Surgeons, New York, New York

STEPHANIE A. SHEPARD, PhD
Assistant Professor, The Warren Alpert Medical School of Brown University; and Staff Psychologist, Early Childhood Clinical Research Center, Bradley/Hasbro Children's Research Center, Providence, Rhode Island

ANNA T. SMYKE, PhD
Associate Professor of Clinical Psychiatry, Department of Psychiatry and Neurology, Tulane University School of Medicine, New Orleans, Louisiana

MINI TANDON, DO
Department of Psychiatry, Washington University School of Medicine, St. Louis, Missouri

PATRICIA VAN HORN, PhD, JD
Associate Professor, Department of Psychiatry, University of California San Francisco; Child Trauma Research Program, San Francisco General Hospital, San Francisco, California

LAUREN WAKSCHLAG, PhD
Associate Professor of Psychiatry, Department of Psychiatry, Institute for Juvenile Research, University of Illinois at Chicago, Chicago, Illinois

ERICA WILLHEIM, PhD
Instructor in Clinical Psychology, Department of Psychiatry, Columbia University College of Physicians & Surgeons, New York Center for Child Development; and Parent-Infant Psychotherapy Training Program, Columbia University Center for Psychoanalytic Training and Research, Early Childhood Mental Health Consultation and Treatment Program, New York Center for Child Development, New York, New York

CHARLES H. ZEANAH, JR, MD
Sellars Polchow Professor, Department of Psychiatry and Neurology, Tulane University School of Medicine, New Orleans, Louisiana

PAULA D. ZEANAH, PhD, MSN
Professor of Clinical Psychiatry and Pediatrics, Tulane University School of Medicine and Institute of Infant and Early Childhood Mental Health; and Clinical Director, Louisiana Nurse Family Partnership, New Orleans, Louisiana

Contents

Foreword   xv

Harsh K. Trivedi

Preface   xvii

Mary Margaret Gleason and Daniel S. Schechter

Section I: Assessment

The Neonatal Moment of Meeting—Building the Dialogue, Strengthening the Bond   533

Nadia Bruschweiler-Stern

It is proposed that in the early neonatal period there are moments of meeting between parent and infant, such as mutual gaze, in which parents realize that their baby is a true interlocutor with meaningful behavior who is ready to engage in interactions. These events significantly strengthen the attachment and are foundational for the beginning of intersubjectivity. The use of the Newborn Behavioral Assessment Scale is described in scaffolding these neonatal moments of meeting.

**Perinatal Assessment of Infant, Parents, and Parent-Infant Relationship:
Prematurity as an Example**   545

Carole Muller-Nix and Margarita Forcada-Geux

This article reviews the stresses for parents, infants, and other caregivers during the period surrounding the birth of the premature infant. Principles of assessment of infant discomfort, parental stress, the parent-infant relationship, and the match of the medical caregiving environment to the individual infant's needs are discussed. Relevant tools to aide in these aspects of assessment are reviewed. The role of early assessment as preventive intervention and the indication for subsequent intervention in complicated cases of premature infants and their parents are further discussed. The article offers detailed clinical examples to illustrate these and other points throughout.

Psychiatric Assessment of Young Children   559

Helen Link Egger

In this article, the author reviews the characteristics of developmentally appropriate criteria for the identification of early childhood mental health symptoms and disorders and the key components of a comprehensive, empirically based, psychiatric assessment of young children and their families. In the first section, the author discusses the infant/early childhood mental health field's perspectives on mental health and mental health problems in infants, toddlers, and preschoolers. The author then provides an overview of the objections to diagnosis of psychiatric disorders in young children and different approaches to the definition of early childhood psychopathology, including descriptive, dimensional, and categorical approaches. In the second section, the author describes the six essential components of a comprehensive mental health assessment of young children: (1) multiple sessions (2) multiple informants (3) a multidisciplinary approach (4) a multicultural perspective (5) multiple modes of assessment, and (6) a multiaxial diagnostic formulation and treatment plan. The author ends with a discussion of the challenges of diagnosing and assessing mental health symptoms and disorders in children younger than 2 years.

Relationship Assessment in Clinical Practice   581

Mary Margaret Gleason

Early childhood mental health and psychopathology occur within the primary context of the parent-child relationship. Thus, any comprehensive mental health assessment must include attention to the qualities of that relationship that may impact the clinical presentation, influence the history provided, or guide treatment choices. This article introduces the rationale for parent-child relationship assessments and presents clinically useful informal and formal approaches to understanding the behavioral and psychological components of the parent child relationship.

Section II: Disorders

**Internalizing Disorders in Early Childhood: A Review of Depressive
and Anxiety Disorders**   593

Mini Tandon, Emma Cardeli, and Joan Luby

This article reviews the use of the broad category of internalizing disorders and data on young children using this definition. It also reviews the emerging support for more specific internalizing diagnoses in very young children. The current empiric database on nosology and treatment of mood and anxiety disorders in young children is examined, and a clinical case example is included. Identification of recent advances in the understanding and treatment of anxiety disorders in young children and areas in which future studies are needed also are explored.

Event Trauma in Early Childhood: Symptoms, Assessment, Intervention   611

Susan Coates and Theodore J. Gaensbauer

Expanding research over the last two decades has documented that very young children's responses to an event trauma will involve the same three basic categories of posttraumatic symptomatology observed in older children and adults that is, reexperiencing, numbing/avoidance, and hyperarousal. The ways in which these three symptom clusters will be manifested in very young children and recent progress in the establishment of developmentally sensitive and reliable criteria for the diagnosis of posttraumatic stress disorder (PTSD) in this age group are described. In addition to PTSD symptomatology, three additional factors that differentiate young children's responses to a trauma from those of older children and adults—their cognitive immaturity, their developmental vulnerability, and the relational context of early trauma given young children's dependence on caregivers—also are discussed. Principles of assessment and treatment are then described. These discussions emphasize the importance of normalizing traumatic responses, supporting the parent-child relationship and restoring trust, desensitizing the child's distress to traumatic reminders, helping the child and parents to process and develop a meaningful narrative of the traumatic event through expressive therapeutic techniques, and promoting effective strategies of restoration and repair.

Viewing Preschool Disruptive Behavior Disorders and Attention-Deficit/Hyperactivity Disorder Through a Developmental Lens: What We Know and What We Need to Know   627

Anil Chacko, Lauren Wakschlag, Carri Hill, Barbara Danis, and Kimberly Andrews Espy

Empirical investigation into disruptive behavior disorders (DBDs) and attention deficit/hyperactivity disorder (ADHD) in early childhood has expanded considerably during the past decade. Although there have been considerable gains in the understanding of the presentation and course of these psychiatric disorders in early childhood, the lack of a developmental framework to guide nosologic issues likely impedes progress in this area. The authors propose that enhanced developmental sensitivity in defining symptoms of DBDs and ADHD may shed light on outstanding issues in the field. In particular, developmental specification may enhance specificity, sensitivity, and stability of DBDs and ADHD symptoms as well as inform our understanding of which type of treatment works best for whom. This article provides an overview of these critical issues.

Autism Spectrum Disorders in Young Children   645

Frances de L. Martínez-Pedraza and Alice S. Carter

Retrospective research studies, videotape analyses of children later diagnosed with autism spectrum disorders (ASD), and recent studies on younger siblings of children diagnosed with ASD, at high-risk of ASD, provide evidence of the early signs of ASD in children as young as 12 months. This article provides a review of early identification, diagnostic assessment, and treatment for young children (0–5 years old) with ASD. Several screening tools as well as comprehensive assessment measures are described. The authors also discuss how the family context is affected by the diagnosis, in terms of adaptation to the diagnosis and to treatment. Finally, the authors present a brief review of interventions for young children with ASD.

Disturbances of Attachment and Parental Psychopathology in Early Childhood   665

Daniel S. Schechter and Erica Willheim

As the field of attachment has expanded over the past four decades, the perturbations in the relational context which give rise to disturbances of attachment are increasingly, though by no means conclusively, understood. In Part I, this article reviews the historical and current state of research regarding normative attachment classification, the diagnosis of Reactive Attachment Disorder, and the proposed categories of Secure Base Distortions and Disrupted Attachment Disorder. In Part II, the article explores the role of parental psychopathology and the manner in which disturbed caregiver self-regulation leads to disturbances in the mutual regulation between caregiver and infant. The question of the relationship between particular types of maternal pathology and particular forms of attachment disturbance is examined through recent research on the association between maternal posttraumatic stress disorder (PTSD), Atypical Maternal Behavior, and child scores on the Disturbances of Attachment Interview (DAI). The authors present original research findings to support that the presence and severity of maternal violence-related PTSD were significantly associated with secure base distortion in a community pediatrics sample of 76 mothers and preschool-age children. Clinical implications and recommendations for treatment of attachment disturbances conclude the article.

Section III: Treatment

Preventive Intervention for Early Childhood Behavioral Problems: An Ecological Perspective   687

Stephanie A. Shepard and Susan Dickstein

The purpose of this article is to highlight the importance of preventive interventions targeting parents when addressing early childhood behavior problems. The authors briefly review evidence-based parent management training programs, focusing on one particular program, the Incredible Years (IY) Series. Next, the authors discuss the barriers to embedding evidence-based practice such as IY in community contexts and demonstrate how early childhood mental health consultation can be used to enhance community capacity to adopt evidence-based practice and improve outcomes for the large number of young children and their families in need.

Giving Voice to the Unsayable: Repairing the Effects of Trauma in Infancy and Early Childhood   707

Alicia F. Lieberman and Patricia Van Horn

The research on early trauma establishes conclusively that, although there are marked individual differences in how children in the first five years of life respond to and recover from trauma, they consistently show negative biological, emotional, social, and cognitive sequelae after enduring traumatic events. This evidence lends particular urgency to the development, evaluation and implementation of approaches to prevention and treatment that are both empirically supported and can be effectively adapted to mental health community programs and other service systems that serve traumatized children and their families. This article describes the clinical applications and community dissemination of child-parent psychotherapy (CPP), a relationship-based trauma treatment for young children and their families that has substantial empirical evidence of efficacy in decreasing symptoms of traumatic stress and restoring young children's normative developmental trajectories. Clinical illustrations are provided to demonstrate how this intervention is conducted and to consider how it might effect therapeutic change.

A New Model of Foster Care for Young Children: The Bucharest
Early Intervention Project   721

Anna T. Smyke, Charles H. Zeanah, Jr, Nathan A. Fox,
and Charles A. Nelson III

> The Bucharest Early Intervention Project is a randomized controlled trial of
> foster care as an intervention for young children who have spent most of
> their lives in institutions in Bucharest, Romania. The authors implemented
> an attachment-based model of child-centered foster care there, and
> a team of three Romanian social workers trained and supported foster par-
> ents in managing the complex challenges of caring for postinstitutionalized
> infants and toddlers. They received regular weekly consultation from
> US-based clinicians designed to guide their work with foster parents
> and children. From language development to toilet training to encouraging
> the development of the young child's ability to trust, foster parents re-
> ceived ongoing support to help these young children transition to family
> life. Developmental outcomes so far indicate significantly better outcomes
> for young children in this foster care program than children who remained
> in institutions. For some domains of development, earlier placement was
> associated with better outcomes but for others, timing of placement did
> not appear to matter.

Video Feedback in Parent-Infant Treatments   735

Sandra Rusconi-Serpa, Ana Sancho Rossignol, and Susan C. McDonough

> Video feedback has been integrated into several therapeutic approaches
> as a way of engaging parents to focus on interactive behavior to reinforce
> positive interactions and to identify areas of noncontingent behavior. This
> article reviews the technical and theoretical contributions of the most
> important video feedback–based interventions that are currently used
> with families that include young children.

Psychopharmacology and Preschoolers: A Critical Review of Current Conditions   753

John Fanton and Mary Margaret Gleason

> Rates of prescriptions for very young children have increased notably in
> the last 20 years. These changes have occurred in the context of increas-
> ing attention to early childhood mental health, availability of medications
> perceived to be safer than older medications, application of the medical
> model to the mental health care of young children, as well as other cultural
> shifts. Psychopharmacological treatment for any patient, but especially
> very young children, requires consideration of central nervous system
> (CNS) and metabolic development and issues of diagnostic validity and
> should be guided by an empirical literature. In young children, this litera-
> ture is quite limited. In this article, the authors review developmental issues
> involved in psychopharmacological treatment and present existing litera-
> ture and practical guidelines for common preschool diagnoses, recogniz-
> ing that for some disorders, the extant literature does not support even
> consideration of medications.

Infant Mental Health and the "Real World"-Opportunities for Interface and Impact   773

Paula D. Zeanah, Letia O. Bailey, and Susan Berry

A growing literature highlights established and developing approaches to infant mental health assessment and treatment. Like other evidence-based and theory-based interventions, real world application of these approaches requires an understanding of the theoretical and empirical foundations of infant mental health as well as consideration of cultural, systemic, and logistical factors. In this article, the authors present models of universal and targeted interventions in infant mental health, with attention to the adaptations used to apply evidence-based practice in real world settings.

Index   789

FORTHCOMING ISSUES

October 2009
Sleep in Children and Adolescents
Jess P. Shatkin, MD, MPH,
and Anna Ivanenko, MD, PhD,
Guest Editors

January 2010
Practice Management
Michael Hudson, MD, and
Barry Sarvet, MD, *Guest Editors*

April 2010
Collaborative Care
Harsh K. Trivedi, MD, *Guest Editor*

RECENT ISSUES

April 2009
Bipolar Disorder
Jeffrey I. Hunt, MD, and
Daniel P. Dickstein, MD, *Guest Editors*

January 2009
Eating Disorders and Obesity
Beate Herpertz-Dahlmann, MD, and
Johannes Hebebrand, MD,
Guest Editors

October 2008
Treating Autism Spectrum Disorders
David J. Posey, MD, MS, and
Christopher J. McDougle, MD,
Guest Editors

RELATED INTEREST

October 2008 (Vol. 55, Issue 5)
Developmental Disabilities, Part I
and
December 2008 (Vol. 55, Issue 6)
Developmental Disabilities, Part II
Donald E. Greydanus, MD, FAAP, FSAM, Dilip R. Patel, MD, FAACPDM, FAAP,
FSAM, FACSM, Helen D. Pratt, PhD, *Guest Editors*

THE CLINICS ARE NOW AVAILABLE ONLINE!
Access your subscription at:
www.theclinics.com

Foreword

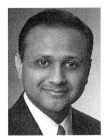

Harsh K. Trivedi, MD
Consulting Editor

Every Monday at noon, I help conduct an interactive seminar for our child and adolescent psychiatry fellows, general psychiatry residents, and medical students. Each week, either a child or an adolescent is interviewed. In an adjoining room a large class of trainees and faculty observe the interview via a live feed through a closed-circuit television system. Through the course of an academic year, our trainees develop fundamental skills and progress in their ability to understand the patient's current status. Some of our interviews involve children as young as 4 years from our children's inpatient unit.

For the trainees, the hardest concept, or rather skill, to develop has been the understanding and formulation of "context." We see a child with dysregulated behaviors. The child is overly familiar with the unfamiliar interviewer. The child exhibits regressed behavior and has delays in speech development. All of this may be true; however, a simple checklist of symptoms does not equate to a true understanding of the child.

Eventually, 10 to 15 minutes before the class ends, comes the dreaded question that makes the best of trainees cringe—"What is your formulation of this case?" How does one put together the story of this child? How does one make sense of what has happened along the way? How does one weigh the multitude of biological, psychological, and psychosocial factors that led the child to sit in front of the interviewer today?

This issue on infant and early childhood mental health is fascinating for many reasons. First, starting with the youngest of children, there is a genuine effort to use a developmental perspective. As opposed to many topics covered in the *Child and Adolescent Psychiatric Clinics of North America* that deal with psychopathology, this is a field that first asks questions with primary prevention in mind. How does one improve the life of this child? How does one prevent any major issues from developing?

Second, in this regard, akin to the child's development, the field of infant and early childhood mental health is also grappling with its own development. There is an inherent tension being played out through this issue. How does one use the diagnostic processes and treatment modalities to help those children who are falling off the curve? To be provocative, how severe do the symptoms need to be or how many interventions need to fail before one decides to prescribe medication for a 3-year-old?

Child Adolesc Psychiatric Clin N Am 18 (2009) xv–xvi
doi:10.1016/j.chc.2009.03.007
childpsych.theclinics.com
1056-4993/09/$ – see front matter © 2009 Elsevier Inc. All rights reserved.

Lastly, there is the matter of "context." How does one understand a 3-year-old without knowing his or her environment, meeting the primary caretakers and observing their interactions with the child? How does one diagnose and treat without having access to a rich developmental history? What happened during the pre-natal course, the in utero period, or the past 1095 days since birth? Developing the ability to understand context with these youth gives a better ability to develop an appropriate "context" when one is treating a 5-year-old, an 11-year-old, or a 17-year-old. Indeed, the same can be said for a 30-year-old or a 92-year-old.

Before I end, let me apologize for the poor use of puns, particularly in this last paragraph. I thank Mary Margaret Gleason and Daniel Schechter for guest editing this issue. They have indeed provided a meaningful "context" from which to understand this developing field. I am also grateful to each of our contributors for sharing their knowledge and expertise. It is fair to say that this field is beyond its infancy and developing quite admirably.

Harsh K. Trivedi, MD
Site Training Director and Director of Adolescent Services
E.P. Bradley Hospital
Assistant Professor of Psychiatry and Human Behavior (Clinical)
Brown Medical School
President, Rhode Island Council for Child and Adolescent Psychiatry
East Providence, RI 02915, USA

E-mail address:
harsh_trivedi@brown.edu

Preface

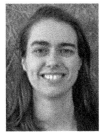 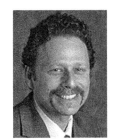

Mary Margaret Gleason, MD   Daniel S. Schechter, MA, MD
Guest Editors

The field of infant and early childhood mental health has been developing a clinical and research knowledge base for more than three decades.[1,2] In 1995, *Child and Adolescent Psychiatry Clinics of North America* devoted an issue to the emotional needs of infants. That issue filled a gap in the literature by providing "empirically based information on infants who show dysfunctional behaviors."[3] In the intervening 14 years since that first issue focused on infant psychiatry, the field has grown and the scope of the empiric work has broadened.

The multidisciplinary field of infant mental health includes clinicians and researchers who interface with young families, including child psychiatrists, pediatricians, developmental and clinical psychologists, speech and language pathologists, occupational and physical therapists, special educators, nurse-practitioners, and many more. These professionals explicitly define their mission as having two components: (1) reduction of current problems and (2) prevention of future adverse outcomes, always with a focus on family relationships and enhancing social-emotional competence during the rapid development of early childhood.[4] To this end, infant mental health providers focus on the developmentally specific emotional needs of infants and very young children, *and* on the complex interactions of young children's mental health with biologic, family, and community factors. An increasing body of research and scholarship has shown the value of this work as benefiting the individual child, the family through generations and the society at large.[5]

The rapid growth of this knowledge base has provided opportunities for professionals who command a wide range of philosophic, cultural, and theoretical backgrounds to shape their clinical and research foci during recent decades. The traditional "Infant Mental Health" field grew out of psychoanalytic, object relations, social learning, attachment, and ethological theory; clinical experiences; and research. Empiric study in infant mental health found fertile ground in the detailed clinical observations by the pioneers of infant mental health during the Second World War and the two following decades—pioneers such as Spitz, Anna Freud, Bowlby, Fraiberg, Provence, Ainsworth, Piaget, Winnicott, and Lebovici.

Child Adolesc Psychiatric Clin N Am 18 (2009) xvii–xix
doi:10.1016/j.chc.2009.03.008   childpsych.theclinics.com
1056-4993/09/$ – see front matter © 2009 Elsevier Inc. All rights reserved.

This multidisciplinary field has expanded its purview from the first 3 years of life to include the first 5–6 years of life, a broader period characterized by rapid development in all domains. Its purview further extends to embrace the complexity of the parent-child relationship and family experiences that emerge beyond the dyadic context and that are so important to the child's mental health and development.

Recently, there has been a downward extension of the medical model of child psychiatry into the preschool years. This pattern is most notable with respect to the controversial use of medications in this population,[6] but it has also been seen as researchers have examined adaptation of the standard diagnostic nosology to identify preschoolers with clinical problems.[7] The best of each of these valuable, and previously nonintersecting, approaches to mental health can be integrated into a stronger, theoretically guided, empirically based research and clinical approach to the assessment and care of very young children and their families.

We chose to name this issue "Infant and Early Childhood Mental Health" in recognition of the important influences that the aforementioned multidisciplinary approaches have had on our current understanding of the emotional experiences of very young children. We have included contributions from an international group of authors who use a broad range of traditional infant mental health as well as early childhood psychiatry and developmental psychopathology approaches. Although it is impossible to review the field of infant and early childhood mental health in a single issue, this issue is intended to provide an overview for practicing clinicians, with attention to assessment, clinical syndromes, and treatment approaches.

This issue begins with Bruschweiler-Stern's discussion of clinical approaches to understanding the very early infant-parent relationship in typical development and Mueller-Nix and Forcada-Geux's presentation of assessment and intervention when development goes awry in the situation of prematurity. Next, Egger provides a thorough review of the current state of early childhood assessment including challenges of integrating traditional infant mental health approaches with the medical model of child psychiatry. Gleason's review of parent-child relationship assessment further contributes to the wider "multiperson psychological lens" through which the infant mental health specialist is accustomed to viewing families with infants and young children in terms of both behavior and their inner representational worlds.

In the following section, each author presents the current state of understanding of early childhood psychopathology in mood and anxiety disorders (Tandon and colleagues), trauma-related disorders (Coates and Gaensbauer), externalizing (Chacko and colleagues), autism spectrum disorders (Martinez-Pedraza and Carter), and parental psychopathology (Schechter and Wilheim). In the third section, authors present examples of evidence-based, clinically useful treatment for psychosocial approaches to early childhood mental health problems including parent management training (Shepard and Dickstein), child–parent psychotherapy (Lieberman and Van Horn), quality foster care for children who are institutionalized (Smyke and colleagues), and the use of video in dyadic and triadic intervention (Rusconi-Serpa and colleagues). No discussion of early childhood is complete without considering the role that psychopharmacological agents play in early childhood mental health treatment (Fanton and Gleason). Finally, the issue closes with a discussion and presentation of the application of the assessment and treatment principles in "real-world" settings including detailed discussion of two programs that are currently addressing the needs of high-risk families with infants and young children in the state of Louisiana (Zeanah and colleagues).

As active clinicians with clinical research interests, we are aware of the important gaps between theory and practice, between efficacy and effectiveness research in child psychiatry, especially in early childhood mental health. Authors in this issue provide the most clinically salient information, and link that information to research findings and clinical vignettes that serve to illustrate particular theoretic frameworks and point to areas in which further empiric research is necessary.

This overview shares some continuity with the first Infant Psychiatry issue in *Child and Adolescent Clinics of North America*, to which Drs. Alicia Lieberman and Charles Zeanah contributed. However, this issue reflects the inspiring expansion of the field, with its more inclusive age range and ever broadening theoretical and empiric base, with contributions from attachment theory, psychiatric epidemiology, psychodynamic principles, developmental psychopathology, biologic contributions, and an eclectic practical perspective.

We are grateful for the opportunities provided to us by the rich clinical experiences we share with the families with whom we work and grateful to our colleagues in this multidisciplinary field, especially in the vibrant professional community of Zero to Three, which has supported our development in this field. In addition, we are grateful to the authors for their dedication to present their topics with attention to the needs of practicing clinicians and we look forward to the ongoing growth of this field.

Mary Margaret Gleason, MD
Departments of Psychiatry & Neurology and of Pediatrics
Tulane University School of Medicine
1440 Canal Street, TB 52
New Orleans, LA 70112, USA

Daniel S. Schechter, MA, MD
Consult-Liaison and Parent-Infant Research Units
Division of Child and Adolescent Psychiatry
University Hospitals of Geneva
51 Boulevard de la Cluse, 2nd Floor Geneva 1205, Switzerland

E-mail addresses:
mgleason@tulane.edu (M.M. Gleason)
daniel.schechter@hcuge.ch (D.S. Schechter)

REFERENCES

1. Bowlby J. A secure base: parent-child attachment and healthy human development. New York: Basic Books; 1988.
2. Ainsworth MDS, Blehar M, Waters E, et al. Patterns of attachment. Hillsdale (NJ): Erlbaum; 1978.
3. Minde K. Preface. Child Adolesc Psychiatr Clin N Am 1995;4(3):xiii–xv.
4. Zero to Three Infant Mental Health Steering Committee. Definition of infant mental health. Washington, DC: Zero To Three; 2001.
5. Shonkoff JP, Phillips D. From neurons to neighborhoods: the science of early childhood development. Washington, DC: National Academy Press; 2000.
6. Zito JM, Safer DJ, Valluri S, et al. Psychotherapeutic medication prevalence in Medicaid-insured preschoolers. J Child Adolesc Psychopharmacol 2007;17(2): 195–203.
7. Egger HL, Angold A. Common emotional and behavioral disorders in preschool children: presentation, nosology, and epidemiology. J Child Psychol Psychiatry 2006;47(3–4):313–37.

The Neonatal Moment of Meeting—Building the Dialogue, Strengthening the Bond

Nadia Bruschweiler-Stern, MD

KEYWORDS

- Neonatal moment of meeting • Early relationship
- Attachment • Intersubjectivity • Early intervention
- Newborn behavioral assessment scale

The openness and great psychic permeability of mothers that the clinician can observe during the neonatal period are in search for answers to many questions. They reveal the mother's interrogation concerning her new baby, herself in her new role as mother, and the new relationship that they will build at the same time: "This baby who came from me, is he really mine? Who is he? Does he know I am his mother? Does he love me? Shall I love him and understand him? Will I know how to keep him alive? Be a good mother to him?" These are fundamental questions for establishing a harmonious relationship.[1,2]

If deliveries must happen in the therapeutic milieu of a hospital, a mother should not be discharged without the clinicians checking that she is on the path to answering her questions.[3]

A positive response to these questions provides a massive relief. Beginning from this point, the mother can let herself be carried away by a baby who is doing well and by interactions that continue to validate her competencies as a mother and nourish this developing bond in contingent loops of interactions.[4]

When the answers are slow to emerge or do not come, maternal anxiety rises very quickly and impedes her self-confidence. The mother-infant bond suffers, their coregulation derails, the infant does not feel "held," and so-called "functional" troubles begin. Intense crying, colic, feeding problems, failure to thrive, sleeping problems, and anarchic rhythm may appear. This generates tensions and exhaustion for the whole family. The expected happiness becomes transformed into a nightmare. The parent-infant relationship can easily spiral downwards. However, this adverse

The Brazelton Center is a nonprofit organization supported by the Rumsey-Cartier Foundation and the Niarchos Foundation and hosted by the Clinique des Grangettes, Geneva, Switzerland.
Centre Brazelton Suisse, Clinique des Grangettes, 1224 Geneva, Switzerland
E-mail address: nadia.stern@grangettes.ch

Child Adolesc Psychiatric Clin N Am 18 (2009) 533–544
doi:10.1016/j.chc.2009.02.001
1056-4993/09/$ – see front matter © 2009 Elsevier Inc. All rights reserved.

childpsych.theclinics.com

outcome can be prevented or relieved almost as easily as it began when intervention is provided early.[5–7]

The Newborn Behavioral Assessment Scale (NBAS or Brazelton Scale) is a clinically valuable tool for this type of early intervention. After the parents have discovered their baby's behavioral signals and their meaning, there is often a turning point. The baby emits an orienting behavior that is clearly aimed at his mother, and she experiences that he knows her, that he is indeed searching for her and seeking comfort from her. This is the answer she was looking for. This realization washes over her as a wave of fulfillment and reinforces the grounding of her maternal feelings. This is a neonatal moment of meeting.

THE NEONATAL MOMENT OF MEETING

The neonatal moment of meeting (NMM) is one of the steps of the cascade of mother-infant attachment that unfolds after the delivery, which I address in greater detail in a later article. Briefly, this cascade, observed and described in European and American families, consists of four successive steps.[8]

The Four Steps of the Unfolding of the Mother-Infant Attachment Process

1. First, at the very moment of birth, survival of the baby emerges as the mother's first preoccupation. She immediately needs to make sure he is alive at an animal level: to physically experience the weight of his little body on her, his smell, his texture, and to feel him as warm, active, and alive. This is the first theme of the Motherhood Constellation.[1]
2. After that, she wants to know that he is anatomically intact and in good health. She needs to see him naked, see his face, his belly, his genitals, count his toes. The medical examination of the baby also answers this question. It is as if a satisfactory surveying of the infant's physical being gives the mother a "green light" to pursue the attachment process.
3. When she has been reassured on this point, the mother seeks to discover how this new member of her family is related to her and to his father. She wonders: "Is he like us? What do we have in common? How are we related?" She is wide open to perceive who this familiar stranger is, who has been created inside her all this time. She will search to make him hers through physical resemblances such as "He has his father's mouth and chin, but my eyes!" and through his behavioral similarities. She might say "When he cries, you have to be there right away! He is demanding like my father."

   During the neonatal period, a mother is psychologically open to discover her new baby and herself in her new role. This openness makes her particularly sensitive and vulnerable to the attitudes and comments of those surrounding her. Words can have the effect of kind prophecies like those of the good fairies to Aurore in the fairytale Sleeping Beauty. However, words can have a terrible effect when a negative remark, as innocent as can be, corresponds to a mother's fear about her baby or herself. They can be engraved in her mind and strongly influence her future relationship with her baby.

   If all goes well, the first two steps usually unfold very naturally. The third is often introduced by comments of family and relatives around the crib.

   Belonging to his family does not yet make the baby an active social partner in his parent's mind. In their view, he is not yet someone who can grasp what is expressed to him. He is not seen either as someone who is able to express himself in a way that is understandable. He is not seen as a baby who can gather in and respond back to his caregivers. A mutual field of communication and emotional contact has not yet been established. That is the task of the fourth step.

4. The NMM is the exact moment when mother and infant for the very first time make a full contact with each other, with the mother knowing that she is recognized by her baby.[9] It involves mother-directed behaviors followed by a prolonged mutual gaze. This moment reveals a newborn who communicates and who specifically seeks for contact with his mother. He is fully there for this contact that shows the parents that their presence is unique for him. This will strongly ensure the early attachment bond. When parents experience it, they are irreversibly transformed. It may be what Lebovici meant when he said "It is the baby who makes the mother."[10]

   Indeed, newborn behavior has a meaning. Such behavior needs to be seen as communication and its meaning understood. In that process, the mother's fundamental questions will find their answers. This is the path proposed by the neonatal consultation with the NBAS.

How Can a Single Moment Be So Determinant?

There are examples in the literature of "special" moments in development, such as imprinting, determining the future of many behaviors. The evidence for human imprinting during a critical period has not yet been shown. However, there is a current interest in the existence of "innate *gestalts*" or motifs of relating to one another that are ready to encounter their appropriate environmental cues or "releasers." There may be important genetic, environmental, and cultural influences on this process.

The baby responding to the mother's voice and orienting to her face are examples of such *gestalts* that meet her need for feeling connected with him. In turn, she will be more available and attentive to him. This will feed into a "positive spiral" of mutually responsive behaviors. When this happens, maternal instinct can flourish and grow.

The neonate is predisposed to seek contact with his mother from birth. He has learned her voice with her own tone and rhythm in utero. In addition, he seems genetically equipped to search and show interest in a visual structure corresponding to the face with 3 dots figuring the eyes and the mouth.[11] The optimal visual distance and the reflex of raising the gaze when starting to breastfeed illustrate even more this need to learn the maternal face.[12] The familiar face of his mother will be an organizing support for the baby as seen in breastfeeding[13]– and later in social referencing.

This predisposition to orient toward the human voice and face may seem similar to the psychoanalytical idea of "primal fantasies."[14,15] However, they are radically distinct. Original fantasies reside in the mind and are the product of a retrospective theory derived from adult pathology. On the contrary, the infant's preference for face and voice as behaviorally observed gives evidence of a predisposition with a prenatal origin.

The specialness of this moment between mother and baby can also be seen from a different point of view. Chaos and complexity theory make it clear that change, small or dramatic, in the form of emergent properties can alter a system irreversibly. This can be done in an instant at an unpredictable time and in an unpredictable way.

With the Boston Change Process Study Group, we have used this notion of change to account for shifts in implicit knowing about the relationship during adult psychotherapy. In this context, the emergent properties and tensions can bring about a resolution that takes place in a "moment of meeting," which brings about a change in the relationship.[16,17]

The NMMs that are the subject of this paper occur in normative life crises. They are conceptualized in the above light and are viewed as bringing about irreversible changes. The mother-infant dyad is an unstable system open to change. During this time, catalyzing the best outcome is very efficient and fast. Providing a favorable context for these emergent properties will propel change toward a positive direction.

With this in mind, let us turn to the clinical situation.

The Clinical Situation Using the Newborn Behavioral Assessment Scale

Here is a brief description of the Newborn Behavioral Assessment Scale (NBAS).[18,19] The Brazelton Scale provides an opportunity for the parents to discover their newborn's repertoire of behaviors during an interaction with the clinician. In the course of a series of manipulations, the examiner will elicit a wide range of behaviors in providing all the necessary support for the infant to show his best performance. In pursuing this goal, the mother has to remain closely attuned to his signs of self-regulation so he does not become overloaded and loses his availability to relate.

The examination starts with habituation during sleep (ie, showing the infant's capacity to maintain sleep in spite of light or noises), neurologic reflexes (ie, grasping, rooting, sucking); primary reflexes (ie, walking, crawling), self-protective behaviors during the "defensive package" (ie, his reaction to the obstruction of his vision by a cloth on his eyes), and the orientation to objects and to the human face and voice. During the process, all infant behaviors are observed and commented on by the examiner: his signs of fatigue, his self-soothing resources, his threshold for stimulation, his preferred pace, the support he needs to console himself if he cries, and his engagement in the direct interaction.

The procedure aims at allowing the parents to see their infant as a whole person with his own goals, as an active agent in his own regulation and in his interactions, as well as depending on them for many functions, being already oriented toward them, and eager to relate and attach to them. This understanding will help the parents to build positive representations of their baby and leave less room for negative attributions.

Another central goal of the neonatal intervention with the NBAS is to validate parental representations when they match what their infant actually shows. The aim is also to realign the distortions that are based on the parent's fantasies toward the real baby as revealed by the NBAS. It does this while their representations are still attributions and not yet fixed after many cycles of interactions. The whole world of their representations about the baby that takes origin in their past and from the time of the pregnancy is ready to crystallize with any observation or comment made around birth. The NBAS is a unique opportunity for them to discover their "real" baby.[20–24]

At the end of the assessment, the infant is often placed in front of the parents, perpendicularly, and the mother is asked to talk to him. She can then see her baby turning toward her with much more determination than he did with the examiner before. Alternatively, if he is exhausted or half asleep, he will often, despite his fatigue, gather all his energy and make his best effort to organize and turn his face toward her, even with his eyes closed. After the discovery of a communicative human being via the NBAS, a mother's encounter of her infant's gaze often convinces her that her baby has the intention to communicate with her specifically, thus revealing a person who is already able and eager to enter into a real dialogue, even without words.

This experience will shift her feelings and the level of connection between them.

Concerning the father, he experiences this connection indirectly. Yet he will usually be eager to connect with his baby in the same way. He is also a witness to this very special event, which becomes a landmark in their common experience that the couple will be able to refer to.

Two Clinical Examples

Here are two examples.

Louis

Louis full term baby (FT), 11-days old, the parents consulted out of curiosity).

Louis's mother never took care of an infant. She talked about him in quite a distant and detached way with some humor as if he were a little animal; she showed significant difficulty in identifying with him. She did not show much understanding of his behavior or feelings, and she said she did not think that he had any interest in her. When she was asked to describe him, she answered: "I don't know...a big question mark...." (**Fig. 1**A, B). The father also made a face and said: "...He is cute for a baby." (**Fig. 1**C).

The NBAS is performed with the parents next to me (**Fig. 2**).

Although the optimal distance for a neonate's accommodation is about 10 in, Louis needed a little more to remain focused on the ball or the face during the NBAS, which he could then do very well (**Fig. 3**). This preference for a longer distance from the object may explain the previous lack-of-gaze encounter that the mother experienced as disinterest.

After having seen him together with the Scale, I invited his mother to talk to him, and the change was striking. Now she could put herself "into his skin," her voice and whole attitude became much softer, and she commented on Louis's behavior from *his* perspective: "Do you hear me?...You are captivated by the women...what does she do?...She looks at you straight in the eyes?...." At this point the mother came closer, having realized that her baby could see her better if she was not too far (**Fig. 4**A).

Louis became agitated looking around and in the opposite direction from his mother for almost 30 seconds (**Fig. 4**B).

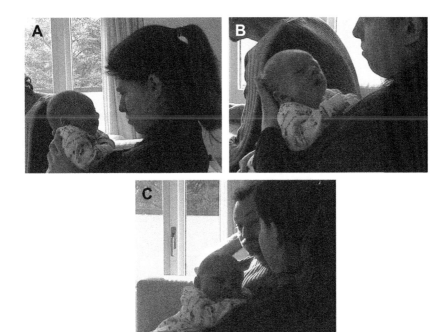

Fig. 1. (*A–C*) "How would you describe Louis?"

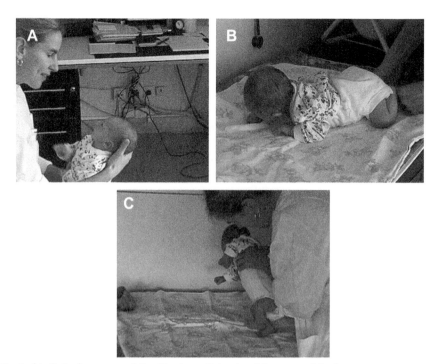

Fig. 2. (*A–C*) Performance of the Newborn Behavioral Assessment Scale.

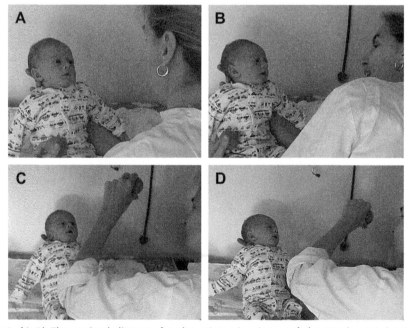

Fig. 3. (*A–D*) The optimal distance for the orientation items of the Newborn Behavioral Assessment Scale.

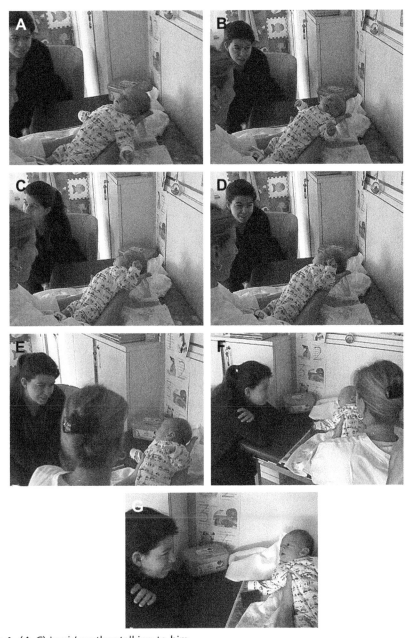

Fig. 4. (*A–G*) Louis' mother talking to him.

It took him a while to organize and orient, but once he found her, he totally quieted down and remained focused on her face, intensely looking at her and listening to her voice for 50 seconds!

The father did not say anything right then, but a little later, when he had his son in his arms, he rubbed his nose against Louis' in a sweet encounter (**Fig. 5**).

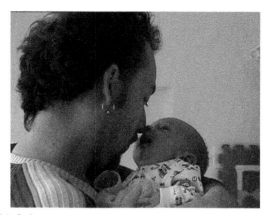

Fig. 5. Louis with his father.

Not only did Louis have behaviors that his mother and father could read and understand, but he clearly showed us that he could recognize his mother and had a great interest in her.

His mother seemed to have discovered that a softer voice and a slower pace worked better to keep him interested. She then experienced right before our eyes, Louis' clear interest in her and his pleasure in hearing her voice and looking at her.

In this NMM, the mother experiences and integrates something new in her understanding of her baby that changes their relationship. In her mind, the infant has a new status: he is changed from an object of care to a person in search of her. They went from a loving and well-intended monologue to a dialogue.

Anton

Anton—The first of two *twins* (birth weight [BW]: 2.1 kg, 7 days old. The parents were filmed for a show on public television).

During the beginning of the examination, Anton's mother moved around, and she was curious and receptive but also quite tense (**Fig. 6**A). She asked "And why does one open his eyes a lot and the other (twin) much less? …Because the other (twin) keeps them open all the time but not him. For instance, when I feed him, Daniel gazes at me all the time, but not Anton."

I wondered if the twins' mother felt recognized by Daniel and closer to him but not by Anton in the same way, and this could contribute to her anxiety.

Right then, Anton heard his mother's voice and just opened his eyes. I seized the opportunity:

"Did you see now? He just opened his eyes too to see where you were!" (**Fig. 6**B).

His mother watched him, bent forward, and began to speak melodiously: "Anton, Anton, hello, hello, darling, are you awake?" (**Fig. 6**C).

Anton opened his eyes again and raised his gaze toward his mother.

He searched for her during almost 10 seconds. Then, he became more animated and raised his head (**Fig. 6**D, E).

I congratulated him. His mother praised him and calmed him down.

"Did you see that?!" Both parents nodded, as Anton began to crawl.

I suggested to the mother: "If you could stand on the other side of the bed, he would come to you." (**Fig. 7**A).

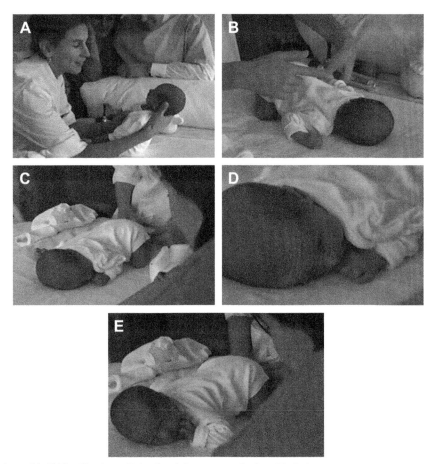

Fig. 6. (A–E) The Newborn Behavioral Assessment Scale with Anton.

His mother went around to the other side and called him. Anton crawled actively toward her and lifted his face toward hers (**Fig. 7**B, C).

She congratulated and kissed him.

I said admiringly: "Look at this! Do you want to take him in your arms?" (**Fig. 8**A).

His mother grabbed him in her arms, lightening up and saying:

"How nice is my baby! My nice baby!" (**Fig. 8**B).

With a hand gesture, the father joined this moment of meeting and admired: "Bravo!"

The mother hugged Anton, kissed him, and talked to him.

His father participated quietly in this intense moment.

I commented": This is a great happiness!" Anton's mother kept her son close in her arms and kissed him again (**Fig. 8**C).

Once this has happened, the mother knows that her son searches for her and that he wants to look at her and be close to her. She knows that he knows her as his mother. The relief and the transformation in this realization are readily seen in her actions: she grabs her son and hugs him with gratefulness for letting her know that he recognizes her. She is then able to feel as a mother to him and to love him the same way she loves his twin Daniel.

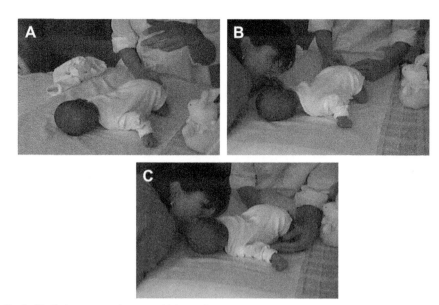

Fig. 7. (*A–C*) Anton crawls toward his mother.

FUNCTIONS OF THE NEONATAL MOMENT OF MEETING: THE DEVELOPMENT OF ATTACHMENT AND THE EMERGENCE OF INTERSUBJECTIVITY

The NMM has two essential functions: the development of attachment and the emergence of intersubjectivity.[25,26]

Orienting behaviors of the baby toward his mother, the rapprochement by crawling, and the molding of her son's warm little body against hers are strong triggers for

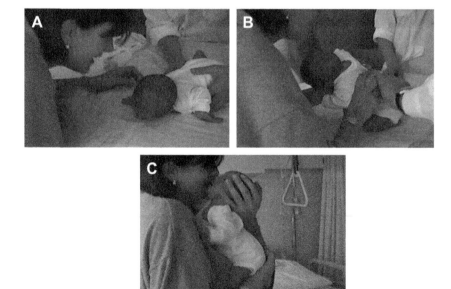

Fig. 8. (*A–C*) Anton held by his mother.

a mother's attachment. These behaviors are also messages that a mother understands at a psychological level: the baby who twists his neck to look at his mother and listens to her with such attention gives her the feeling that he has chosen her and loves her. This answers many of a mother's fundamental questions of the second theme of what Stern and I have called the "Motherhood Constellation,"[1] about being able to bond with her child: "Will he love me? Will I know if he loves me? Will he know that I am his mother? Will I love him? Will I be able to connect with him?" Effectively, when the baby's gaze finds his mother's, this NMM releases a flow of love in the mother. One can feel it. The dialogue can now deepen, the mother can say: "You come toward me, you know me, I am your mother."

Even more, intersubjectivity is beginning. The mother now feels: "I know that you know me." Furthermore, she feels: "I know that you know that I am your mother." Her intersubjectivity is the context for the infant's emerging intersubjectivity.

Without this intervention, the realization by the parents that their infant has intentions and expresses himself in his behavior will come about anyways, but sometimes much later. Until this happens, there will be plenty of room for parents' attributions and projections that can put them on the path of a negative relational spiral. Sometimes negative attributions will be played out in various interactions with the infant; they are the seeds for building negative mental representations of self as parent and of the baby during this sensitive time of early life.

NMMs are the result of the parents' need to connect with their newborn and to make sense of what he does. One might think that they come about naturally. Yet it is not always the case. When the parents are unaware of the infant's competencies or unable to see them, there is a need for an intervention with a professional who scaffolds these moments, witnesses and underlines them, and validates their value. In this sense, the scaffolding of NMM as described here can be a powerful preventive and therapeutic intervention.

NMMs during these first days of life pave the way for a more positive relationship in the future.

REFERENCES

1. Stern DN. The Motherhood Constellation: a unified view of parent-infant psychotherapy. New York: Basic Books (HarperCollins); 1995.
2. Stern DN, Bruschweiler-Stern N. The birth of a mother- how the motherhood experience changes you forever. London: Basic Books, Bloomsbury Publishing; 1998.
3. Bruschweiler-Stern N. Reflections on the process of psychotherapeutic change as applied to medical situations. Infant Mental Health Journal 1998;19.
4. Bowlby J. Attachment. In: Attachment and loss, vol 1. London: Hogarth Press; 1969.
5. Stern-Bruschweiler N, et Stern DN. A model for conceptualizing the role of the mother's representational world in various mother-infant therapies. Infant Ment Health J 1989;10(3):16–25.
6. Bruschweiler-Stern N. Modèle d'intervention préventive au cours de la période néonatale. n 33. Prism 2000;33:126–39 [French].
7. Bruschweiler-Stern N. Neonatal interventions for relationship problems. In: Sameroff AJ, McDonough SC, Rosenblum KL, editors. Treating parent-infant relationship problems: strategies for intervention. New York: Guilford Press; 2003. p. 188–212.
8. Bruschweiler-Stern N. Early emotional care for mother and infants. Pediatrics 1998;102:1278–81.

9. Bruschweiler-Stern N. Moments of meeting: Pivotal moments in mother, infant, father bonding. In: Nugent JK, Petrauskas BJ, Brazelton TB, editors. The newborn as a person. New Jersey: John Wiley & Sons; 2005. p. 70–84.

10. Fraiberg SH, Adelson E, Shapiro U. Ghost in the nursery: a psychoanalytic approach to the problem of impaired infant-mother relationships. J Am Acad Child Psychiatry 1975;14:387–422.

11. Lebovici S. Le nourisson, la mère et le psychanalyste: Les interactions précoces. Paris: Editions du Centurion; 1983 [French].

12. Pascalis O, de Haan M, Nelson CH. Is face processing species-specific during the first year of life? Science 2002;296:1321–3.

13. Klaus M, Kennel J, Klaus Ph. Bonding. Reading, MA: Addison-Wesley Publishing Company, Inc; 1995.

14. Sander L. Living systems, emerging consciousness, and the emerging person. New York: The Snalytic press; 2008. p. 187.

15. Freud S. A case of paranoia running counter to the psychoanalytic theory of the disease (1915f), GW, X, 242; SE, XIV, 269.

16. Klein M. Notes on some schizoid mechanisms. Int J Psychoanal 1946;27:99–110.

17. Boston Change Process Study Group, Stern DN, Sander LW, et al. Non interpretive mechanisms in psychoanalytic therapy. Int J Psychoanal 1998;79:903–21.

18. Lyons-Ruth K. The two-person unconscious: intersubjective dialogue, enactive relational representation, and the emergence of new forms of relational organization. Psychoanalytic Inquiry 1999;19(4):576–617.

19. Brazelton TB. Neonatal behavioral assessment scale. 3rd Edition. Cambridge, MA: Mac Keith Press; 1995.

20. Brazelton TB. Touchpoints. New York: Guilford Press; 1992.

21. Ammaniti M. Maternal representations during pregnancy and early infant-mother interactions. Infant Ment Health J 1991;12(3):246–55.

22. Fava Vizziello GM, Antonioli M, Cocci V, et al. From pregnancy to motherhood: the structure of representative and narrative change. Infant Ment Health J 1993;14(1): 4–16.

23. Bruschweiler-Stern N. The concept of maternal representations: clinical implications for perinatology. Ab Initio 1997;4(1):1–4.

24. Zeanah CH, Keener MA, Stewart L, et al. Prenatal perception of infant personality: a preliminary investigation. J Am Acad Child Psychiatry 1986;24:204–10.

25. Beebe B, Stern D. Engagement-disengagement and early object experiences. In: Communicative structures and psychic structures. New York: Plenum Press; 1977.

26. Trevarthan C. Communication and cooperation in early infancy: a description of primary intersubjectivity. In: Before speech: the beginning of interpersonal communication. New York: Cambridge University Press; 1979.

Perinatal Assessment of Infant, Parents, and Parent-Infant Relationship: Prematurity as an Example

Carole Muller-Nix, MD[a],*, Margarita Forcada-Guex, PhD[b]

KEYWORDS

- Premature infant • Infant assessment
- Parent-infant relationship • Parental posttraumatic stress
- Perinatal care

The perinatal period is a particularly sensitive period for any parent, from pregnancy through the first months of the parents' relationship with their newborn baby. This period has been described as a maturational crisis.[1] It is a dynamic period formed by a continuum between a state of maternal psychological vulnerability during the second-half of pregnancy, which has been termed by Bydlowski as "prenatal psychic transparency"[2] and a state of healthy maternal psychological functioning in the perinatal period and beyond, which has been termed by Winnicott as "primary maternal preoccupation."[3] The baby is the source of a number of emotions, sometimes conflictual emotions related to the parents' own relational history. Parents see themselves in their baby and may also identify themselves with their own parents. These powerful emotional experiences take place already before the baby's birth, as the still unknown child is idealized, yet at the same time can trigger fears of who he might be and might become.[4]

The moment of birth reveals a real baby, who is both unique and limited by his apparent specificities which often contain potentially frightening, imagined representations of the unborn baby. In the first months of life, the baby' specific characteristics

Grants: Swiss National Science Fund. # 32-49712.96 & # 3200B0-104230/1, Fondation pour la Psychiatrie de la Petite Enfance, Lausanne. Fondation Biaggi, Lausanne.

[a] Department of Child and Adolescent Psychiatry, University Hospital Lausanne, Hôpital Neslté, av. P. Decker 5, 1011 Lausanne, Switzerland

[b] Division of Neonatology, Department of Pediatrics, University Hospital Lausanne, Néonatologie, av. P. Decker 2, 1011 Lausanne, Switzerland

* Corresponding author.

E-mail address: carole.muller-nix@chuv.ch (C. Muller-Nix).

Child Adolesc Psychiatric Clin N Am 18 (2009) 545–557
doi:10.1016/j.chc.2009.02.008
1056-4993/09/$ – see front matter © 2009 Elsevier Inc. All rights reserved.

childpsych.theclinics.com

and social capacities play a crucial role in the coconstruction of the parent-infant relationship. The sum of strengths and vulnerabilities the parents' interpretation of and their adaptation to them, are vital for the infant's psychic as well as psychosomatic formation of self-identity over time. Assessment of the parent-infant relationship in the perinatal period thus requires consideration of the infant's characteristics and behavior as well as the parents' characteristics and mental representations,[5] as affecting one another in a mutual and dynamic way over time. This dynamic mutual exchange usually fosters the building of a complex, rich, and rewarding relationship.[6]

Parents who have had a history of painful or unresolved conflictual relationships might have more difficulties in engaging with their infant in the postnatal period. They are at risk to repeat past relational difficulties with their newborn baby. Moreover, if the baby presents with a medical problem at birth, and if his survival, well-being, or outcome are at risk, the distressful, potentially traumatic, parental experience weakens the parents psychologically, creating greater vulnerability for unresolved conflictual affective dimensions to come alive. Parents or infant symptomatic behaviors will then manifest the suffering at stake.

Premature birth is a very special example of a stressful and intense emotional experience for parents in the perinatal period, which carries potentially long-term consequences for parents and premature infants, siblings, and also possibly others members of the family.[7] Assessment of parent-preterm infant dyads in the perinatal period can provide particularly instructive information for clinicians, to appreciate as a model the complexity of early symptoms of both parents and infants in distress or disturbed parent-infant relationships.

The birth of a preterm baby is usually sudden and elicits intense fear for the infant's survival. Preterm babies have left the adaptive environment of the womb too early and are abruptly subject to intrusive medical procedures at birth. Such procedures are often repeated and varied for weeks or months during the course of their hospitalization in the Neonatal Intensive Care Unit (NICU). Parental subjective experience has long been investigated, but only recently has the infant's perspective been more precisely explored. The pain and stress endured by the preterm baby can represent an experience of helplessness for him. Indeed a premature baby is often at risk to be overwhelmed by external and internal (ie, physiologic) stimuli as he is unable to discharge or organize them.[8–10] The premature infant might experience primitive anxieties and react with a range of primitive defenses, such as somnolence, withdrawal, aversion, and somatic disorganization, in the face of distress.[11–13] This realization has led to notable changes in standards of neonatal care and the NICU environment itself. Increased sensitivity to the needs of the premature infant has promoted programs of interventions specifically adapted for premature babies, taking into account their range of weights, gestational ages (GAs), specific vulnerabilities and comorbidities, as well as those babies' parents, and parent-infant relationships.

Research has shown that the period in which premature babies are born, between 26 and 36 weeks of GA, is a critical developmental period for the organization of the human cortex and maturation of the central nervous system. The baby is then particularly dependent and highly sensitive to the quality of his or her environment, including medical care.[14,15] The immaturity of the central nervous system is a crucial aspect of the vulnerability of an immature infant, especially for infants born with a very low birth GA (ie, before 32 weeks GA), very low birth weight (BW) (<1500 g), or with intrauterine growth retardation.[16] A number of specific circumstances can be the source of pain and stress for these infants and need to be acknowledged. During hospitalization, pain- and stress-inducing procedures and insensitively overstimulating surroundings in the NICU (such as excessive noise, overly bright lighting, for example)[17] are particularly challenging for the premature and/or ill infant's abilities to organize himself at a psychosomatic level. These factors challenge that baby's availability for essential social communication and thus pose a risk for emerging early social-emotional development.

ASSESSMENT OF THE PREMATURE INFANT

In general, it is possible to assess a baby regardless of gestational status, from birth on, in particular her individual sensitivity and reactivity to stressors. During the first months of life, the clinician observes somatic, behavioral, and affective signs that are typical of different early infant and toddler psychopathological disturbances. Several authors have described the infant's range of disturbances and psychosomatic symptoms (sleep, feeding, behavior symptoms in particular),[18–20] possible withdrawal reactions (ie, social avoidance, uncommunicativeness),[21] depressive symptoms,[22,23] early defensive symptoms (avoidance, freezing, "fighting"),[12,13] sensori- and psycho-motor organization, and signs of disorganization.[24,25] The Diagnostic Classification: 0-3-Revised attempts to provide a developmentally based description of infant symptoms and disorders (DC: 0-3-R).[26]

To explore the nature and integrative function of early psychic life, mental health professionals classically use minutely detailed observation of babies' behaviors and affective responses, in particular during interaction with their parents. The "Tavistock Model of Infant Observation"[27] is one such useful form of organized observation of the baby in his family during the first 2 years of life, with specific procedures meant to develop the trainee's capacities to appreciate early development as it unfolds and to imagine the infant's perspective and psychic life.

In the perinatal period and up to 2 months of age, the Neonatal Behavior Assessment Scale or "NBAS"[28] (see the article by Bruschweiler-Stern, elsewhere in this issue) is another structured observational tool that has been shown to have predictive value. The NBAS was designed to assess the baby in different functional domains: state of consciousness, sleep-awake state regulation, motor and autonomic organization, attention, orientation abilities, and, most importantly, his responses to interaction and capacities for adaptation to novel stimuli, situations, and relationships.

In the case of a premature baby, besides genetic, medical, and neurologic conditions that can be a source or exacerbating factor of the preterm infant's social-emotional difficulties, postnatal environmental and social conditions also play an essential role in the outcome of such difficulties. In contrast to full-term infants, who benefit most from an environment that is well-adapted to their level of psychophysiologic development, the preterm baby in the NICU is exposed to insufficient, excessive, or developmentally inappropriate stimulation as well as an affectively unfavorable situation, with frequent separations from his parents or lack of proximity and intimacy with them, all of which are potentially stressful. The clinical assessment of the preterm baby in the perinatal period must, therefore, include the quality of his social and emotional presence, such as engagement in human interaction versus aversion or avoidance. It must take into account the premature infant's muscle tone, motor organization, efforts at self-regulation, or tendency to become disorganized. It should also take into account the flexibility of these behaviors during the course of comprehensive neonatal care and in interaction with his parents or caregivers. Assessment measures such as the Assessment of Preterm Infant Behavior[29] and the Observation Sheet of the Newborn Individualized Developmental Care and Assessment Program (NIDCAP)[30] are very helpful guides to structuring in vivo observations of these infants. They examine similar dimensions to those of the NBAS but with a greater clinical precision that is more specifically pitched to the assessment of the often subtle reactions of immature infants.

Reactions to adverse and stressful stimulation can lead to maladaptive behaviors and affective maladjustment by the infant, which can distance him from his parents, medical caregivers, and environment. Early signs of infant suffering are, for example, excessive hyperextension movements (ie, arching of the back), hyper- or hypotonicity, disorganized autonomic reactions, excessive crying or sleeping, or gaze aversion. By contrast, adapted stimulations in the NICU and affective human protective attention and investment of the preterm infant allow him to remain stable, available for social interaction and beneficial exploration of the environment, helping him to foster both his physical and social-emotional development. Careful assessment of the baby improves most importantly an understanding of his needs and helps fashion individualized care in the NICU and later at home. It needs to take into account the baby's specific signs of vulnerability as well as strengths (ie, self-regulatory capacity). The evaluation should be done at repeated intervals, to monitor changes over time and the outcome of therapeutic interventions.

Interestingly, the assessment itself is also a therapeutic tool. In the NICU, joint observations of the baby, parents, mental health practitioner, and caregiver help parents to understand better their infants' reactions and individual characteristics as well as the premature infant's salient limitations with respect to social interaction. The process of joint observation encourages parental attention and preoccupation with the baby. It enables them to overcome often frightening, traumatic images of their infant and to avoid the fixation of inflexible, negative mental representations, which could threaten the development of a harmonious parent-infant relationship. Nurses who participate in joint observation of the baby better appreciate the affective dimensions implicit to each unique parent-infant relationship and tend to adapt themselves better to each individual situation, especially when they feel moved by parents' often ambivalent reactions toward the baby and their new parental role.[31–33]

To evaluate the premature infant's risk to stressful, potentially traumatic situations, it is important to remember that newborn infants are able to feel pain. This is contrary to what was believed in the past. By 24 weeks' gestation, the nervous system elements required for the transmission of painful stimuli are functional. Infant's pain can be considered as a source of stress. Exposure to repetitive painful and stressful procedures may lead to altered neurobehavioral responses to subsequent stressful events, with decreased behavioral responses and increased physiologic responses.[34,35] Pain can be assessed with a number of reliable, validated instruments, for example, the Neonatal Facial Coding System,[36] the Premature Infant Pain Profile,[37] or Behavioral Indicators of Infant Pain scale.[38] Increased facial and bodily activity, increased heart rate, and decreased oxygen saturation have all been recognized as good predictors of preterm infant's pain.[39,40] In a premature infant, pain is known to be felt differently from that in older children; some have suggested that it is experienced in a more diffuse, possibly more acute way.[41,42] There is growing evidence suggesting that repetitive painful, even routine, procedures that elicit discomfort may be stressful for preterm infants.[43]

One important dimension of assessment of the premature infant that may be less familiar to child psychiatrists is that of sensorimotor and tonic balance (ie, muscle tone and axial coordination).[24,25] These elements are fundamental to the early psychic development[44] and allow the infants to construct an accurate, reliable, and coherent mental representation of their own body in space and time and organized toward stimuli. Specialists in this domain assert that infants who can actively engage caregivers, who can exercise exploration of the environment will be less at risk to be overwhelmed or become helpless.[13,45] A good positioning of the baby in the incubator helps coordinated movements.[46] Routine care (ie diaper changes) should be accompanied by a narrative structure and the caregiver emotional support that contributes to a deeper intersubjective experience. Such narration is linked to the capacity for "reverie" as described by Bion.[47] It often supports the caregiver's or parents' developing internal representations of the child.

Clinical Example

Laura's parents admired her vivid presence, active motion, and responsiveness in the course of a joint observation of their baby with the authors in the NICU. They were reassured by Laura who looked at them intensely. The observer noticed that the infant was in fact hypervigilant, agitated, and seemed as if she was trying to contain herself by staying tuned into the stimuli of the surroundings. She appeared unable to modulate or break the intensity of her staring. The parents very anxious had a tendency to overstimulate the baby. The authors interpreted this as the parents being reassured by the baby's movements that represented "life" for them. The therapeutic intervention was aimed at sensitizing the parents to the differences between well-modulated interactive attention by Laura versus disorganized agitation. Another goal was to consider this behavior as a sign of stress and to see how these parents could help Laura by adjusting their level of stimulation to be more in tune with her needs as an immature infant.

ASSESSMENT OF PARENTAL SUBJECTIVE EXPERIENCE

Assessment of the subjective experience of parents is best begun by first approaching them in a more routine clinical interview. One must pay close attention to the parents' narrative content and process as well as affective response to the interviewer, for example, as they describe the circumstances of their infant's birth and relationship with her. Semistructured interviews (eg, to explore parental mental representations by themes, in particular of their baby)[48] as well as specific questionnaires (eg, to examine parental anxiety, depression, or posttraumatic stress) can add precision to the clinical interview, in particular in a research setting. The parents' subjective experience must be understood to appreciate their possible need for psychotherapeutic intervention and to assess particularly problematic symptoms or behaviors. For the parents, a premature birth represents an intrusive, potentially traumatic situation with a sudden interruption of the pregnancy and a succession of too quickly occurring uncontrolled and unexpected events. The baby is at risk for death, and when this existential threat has subsided, uncertainty concerning the infant's outcome often remains present.[49] This sense of uncertainty is one of the most difficult feelings for parents to endure during the weeks or months of hospitalization and even later.

During the perinatal period, parents evolve through different phases that can be described within a psychodynamic frame of reference.[33,50] At first, at the moment of their infant's birth, they often experience a moment of feeling frozen and numb. This dissociative experience can be helped by supporting immediate contact between parents, particularly mothers, and their newborn infant even if this is only briefly possible due to medical urgency. This contact gives the parents a sensory and affective experience that can help to ground them in the reality to what has just happened: they have given birth to an infant that is alive. Following birth, communication about the infant's medical status by the medical team at regular intervals, coupled with the nurses' active availability during the time of mother-infant separation (when the baby is in the NICU for resuscitation procedures and mother is still in the delivery room or at the maternity ward), can greatly help parents with their distress. The medical team's sensitivity to the parents' concrete and emotional needs, as for example, even simply by visiting mother's room and providing support to the mother and updates about the infant can be helpful and soothing.

Clinical Example

Louise's parents recalled in retrospect the moments right after their first infant's birth (GA, 28 weeks). Her father said, "...during delivery something was still moving, but after delivery, it was difficult ...they told me that I could come to see our daughter in an hour in the NICU. It's true it was strange, the baby was gone... there was a void. It was the worst moment for us... the doctors and all the nurses were gone. There was only a janitor cleaning the delivery room... so we looked at him as he was cleaning the room... there was nothing else... I thought they had forgotten about us... there was only this person cleaning the room."

In a second phase, the parents typically experience multiple contradictory emotions in repeated instances. They go from sadness to anger, from anxiety or uncertainty to hope, and idealization of the infant.[33,51] These emotions are part of the affective normal evolution of stressful or traumatic situations, should improve the parental reality testing, and promote emotional stabilization and resolution of the traumatic state. Certain factors can, however, jeopardize this evolution; in particular, reminders of the traumatic birth, such as not only the infant's medical complications in the NICU but also his transfer to another unit or hospital or even his discharge. All can be very stressful for parents in that they again raise the fear of death and trigger separation anxiety as that experienced at birth. These painful emotions can be reinforced when there is a lack of social and family support or when parent's prior emotional conflicts and difficult affective history are reactivated by the premature birth.[52] Consequences of this type of "retraumatization" can be that the parents distance themselves from their child in an effort to avoid further difficult feelings or on the contrary overstimulate their baby in a desperate search for the infant's responses that could reassure them (see the article by Schechter and Willheim, elsewhere in this issue).

Clinical Example

Paul's mother (GA, 31 weeks; BW, 1650 g) had met her premature infant at birth with a fair amount of confidence and little expression of anxiety. A few weeks later, on the day that his discharge from hospital was planned, the infant presented an unexpected medical complication that postponed his return home. His mother was intensely disappointed and became very ambivalent toward her infant. She recalled: "It was unfair to see him again in an incubator, again with an intravenous line. It was really hard for him and us. I was torn between his need for my attention and my need to distance myself from him, because it was too painful. I couldn't see him suffer again and was then obliged to detach myself from him. Since his birth, our links had been getting stronger, despite the lack of intimacy and the disadvantages of the NICU hospitalization. But this complication was like a punishment. I asked myself if it was a punishment because I had not loved him enough?... Or was it perhaps meant to strengthen our bond? Maybe, because it's in the experience of this second separation that feelings between us arose, that I really felt anxious and sad, probably like what a mother should feel, but that I felt then much more deeply than when he was born."

PARENTAL TRAUMATIZATION FOLLOWING PREMATURE BIRTH

Studies have explored parental experience in terms of anxiety, stress, or depression, with instruments such as: the State-Trait Anxiety Inventory, STAI,[53] the Parenting Stress Index, PSI,[54] the Beck Depression Inventory, BDI,[55] or the Edinburgh postnatal depression scale EPDS.[56,57] Recently studies have explored parents' experience from a trauma perspective, indicating parents reporting a high incidence of posttraumatic stress disorder reactions[58] even up to 1 year or 14 months after birth.[59–63] These symptoms have been assessed with different instruments, among them are the Impact of Even Scale, IES[64] and the Perinatal Posttraumatic Questionnaire, PPQ.[65]

In the long run, persistent parental emotional turmoil can jeopardize the normal process of primary maternal (and paternal) preoccupation[3] and the establishment of a harmonious parent-infant relationship[66] and can contribute to the formation of mother-infant attachment difficulties.[67] Parents can continue to feel challenged to assert themselves as parents and to be recognized as such by their family and the social environment.[68] It is in this way important to regularly assess the parent's emotional experience and its evolution in time not only during the NICU hospitalization but also regularly after discharge, at least for the first year or two of the baby's life (ie, during medical pediatric consultations, with additional psychiatric consultation if indicated or desired).

It is important to keep in mind that crisis should not be viewed as leading to an exclusively painful or detrimental course. As difficult to live through as premature birth and perinatal complications are, these experiences can offer parents insight into their own emotional and behavioral responses as parents under stress—they can open doors to reflection upon known repetitive, ill-controlled, or disturbing emotional reactions in the couple's life. Even more, they can stimulate changes in the way stressful situations will be handled further within the couple and in parenting, with the result of the parents' discovering new ways to relate to their baby.

ASSESSMENT OF THE PARENT-INFANT RELATIONSHIP

The quality of parent-infant interactions is directly related to the level of parental distress, parental representations of the baby,[5] as well as to the infant stress (see the article by Gleason, elsewhere in this issue). In healthy babies, as in preterm babies, maternal distress, in particular, when comorbid with depression or anxiety symptoms, is recognized to be associated with less positive mother-infant interactions. Consistently poor parent-infant interaction increases the child's vulnerability to stressful experiences, as parents do not play their role of protection and processing of the baby's primary anxieties and discomfort.[69]

Early investigations have shown preterm infants to be less alert, attentive, active, and responsive than full-term infants in mother-infant interaction and preterm infant's mothers to be more active, stimulating, intrusive, and at the same time more distant than full-term infant's mothers.[70–75] In 2006, one study demonstrated that parents with symptoms of posttraumatic stress have be shown to be at risk for decreased mutuality in the parent-infant relationship, leading to what has been described as a "controlling parent/compliant infant" pattern of interaction that affects the infant's outcome at 18 months.[76]

For a number of parents of premature infants, anxiety regarding the infant's development can remain elevated after discharge from the NICU for months or years. This anxiety can jeopardize their mental representations of their infant and the quality of the parent-infant relationship, as they defensively focus on the infant's competencies, milestone acquisitions, and medical health rather than allowing themselves simply to enjoy being together with their infant and appreciating their infant for who she is. In a paradoxic way, they can have representations of the infant as fragile and vulnerable or at imminent risk of dying or being sick or hurt, and within the same narrative, describe her in an idealized manner, as being particularly strong, resistant, lively, curious, a quick learner, a winner, even a hero who has decided to live and overcome her difficulties.

Clinical Example

John's mother (GA, 32 weeks; BW, 1690 g) described her relationship and feelings toward her son at 18 months (corrected age) in this contrasted way: "I'm frightened all the time...frightened that he could die. On the road it's awful, I'm afraid he could be run over, that he might fall. I see the lake and imagine he could drown. I'm frightened of everything for him. This, I'm sure, is because I've been so afraid he could die, it's still in me, it will stay I'm sure… For me, the fact he was born prematurely made him stronger than others. Of this I'm sure, I can see it very well. He is going to be stronger than others. For me he chose to live, another baby doesn't need to choose. John needed to fight for his life."

A major protective factor for the parent-infant relationship is the parent's active participation in the infant's care, which brings sensorial proximity and intimacy with the infant and that reassures parents of their parental role regarding their infant. The parents' confidence in themselves as parents has to be repeatedly reinforced during hospitalization and reevaluated before discharge. Parents who persist in feeling that they are insecure (or inadequate relative to the NICU staff) once they return home with their infant are more at risk for subsequent relational difficulties with their infant. Such insecure parents often feel helpless and may be unable or too frightened or ashamed to seek out the support and resources they need.

To prevent this type of outcome, supportive interventions targeted at parent-infant interactions that support the parents' emerging sense of competence are very useful (ie, joint attentive observation in the NICU described here). Such preventive intervention in the NICU is not always sufficient for parents facing successive crises and posttraumatic stress reactions during the course of a prolonged infant hospitalization or its aftermath. A more individualized insight-oriented psychotherapeutic intervention may be indicated in these situations, particularly when parents' own conflictual history manifests in continued relational difficulties with their infant, with other family members, or caregivers.[77] A psychotherapeutic approach helps parents to be more aware of the past experiences interfering in the present situation (see the article by Lieberman and van Horn, and Rusconi-Serpa and colleagues, elsewhere in this issue).

Clinical Example

Sarah presented for her first psychiatric consultation regarding her son Matthew, 9 years old, who showed problematic behaviors of strong dependency and emotional inhibition, at home and at school. He had been born prematurely (GA, 32 weeks) and hospitalized for 4 weeks with an uncomplicated outcome. In the hours after delivery, she recalled having felt completely alone, abandoned in her room at the maternity ward, desperate, guilty, and not daring to call the nurses, for fear to learn that her son had died. When she first met her child, she did not feel relieved, but rather, she felt detached from him. She could not feel the connection she had experienced with her other children. This feeling did not improve after discharge. Moreover, she added that nobody seemed to notice. Later, this lack of connectedness changed to a desire to prove to herself and others that the child was doing well and that she had not damaged him. She became very demanding and her child, very obedient. During the consultation, she repeatedly recalled the fear, guilt, and loneliness that she had originally felt at her child's birth.

A few months later in the psychotherapeutic process, a shift occurred, and she started to recall other aspects of her life, in particular that she had been most obedient herself as a child and very protective toward her mother. Her understanding of an intergenerational repetition and a simultaneous growth of empathy for her child's difficulties led gradually to a change in the relationship with her son.

SUMMARY

Assessment of infants, parents, and the infant-family relationship in situations of premature birth is particularly important, because early stress in critical phases of development has been associated with the child's persistent vulnerability and emotional reactivity to subsequent stress later in life[78–81] and with the possible origin for the development of mood and anxiety disorders.[82,83] The goal of thorough assessment and intervention in the perinatal period is to allow for the containment and easing of both the infant's and parents' stress as well as to promote parent-infant relationship and the infant's self-regulatory capacities. Another very important goal is to evaluate and allow articulation of the traumatic conflicts that may affect a parent's relationship with the newborn baby and that may be intensified due to the traumatic stress surrounding premature birth and related medical intervention. This is done through therapeutic work directed at parents, infants, and the parent-infant relationship. In a traumatic situation, it is important not to view the infant's outcome only in terms of potential risk factors. Each situation must be assessed in and of itself, with its unique potential for dynamic transformation, especially if assisted by an appropriate supportive or therapeutic intervention. Recent research has raised the possibility of the reorganization of early infant experiences with new memories that aide in the contextualization of early experience. The brain's neural plasticity and the mobilization of memory traces that come into play via mutative life experiences can well modify the consequences of early threats to survival and their physiologic impact and can offer a reworking of early infant experience.[84,85]

REFERENCES

1. Bydlowski M. A psychotherapy in the perinatal period. In: Missonnier, Golse, Soulé, editors. Pregnancy, virtual child and parenting. Paris: PUF; 2004. p. 285–8 [French].
2. Bydlowski M. Mental transparency of the pregnant woman. Etudes freud 1991;32: 135–42 [French].
3. Winnicott DW. Primary maternal preoccupation. Through paediatrics to psychoanalysis. London: Karnac Books Ed.; 1975.
4. Lebovici S, Stoléru S. The infant, his mother and the psychoanalyst: Early interactions. Paris: Païdos/Bayard Editions; 1994 [French].
5. Zeanah CH. Subjectivity in parent-infant relationships: a discussion of internal working models. Infant Ment Health J 1987;8(3):237–50.
6. Lebovici S. Infant psychiatry and the psychopathology of early interactions. Psychopathology of the baby. Paris: PUF; 1989. p. 317–21 [French].
7. Meyer EC, Kennally KF, Zika-Beres E, et al. Attitudes about sibling visitation in the neonatal intensive care unit. Arch Pediatr Adolesc Med 1996;150(10):1021–6.

8. Freud A. Comments on trauma. In: Furst SS, editor. Psychic trauma. New York: Basic Books; 1967. p. 235–45.
9. Freud S. Inhibitions, symptoms and anxiety. The Standard Edition. London: Hogarth Press; 1959.
10. Freud S. Project for a scientific psychology. Standard edition. London: Hogarth Press; 1959. p. 281–397.
11. Bick E. Further considerations on the function of the skin in early object-relations, findings from infant observation integrated into child and adult analysis. Br J Psychother 1986;2(4):292–9.
12. Fraiberg S. Pathological defenses in infancy. Psychoanal Q 1982;51(4):612–35.
13. Mellier D. Babies in need, intersubjectivity and labor link, a theory of function containing. Paris 2005 [French].
14. Hüppi P, Sizonenko S, Amato M. Lung disease and brain development. Biol Neonate 2006;89:284–97.
15. Inder TE, Warfield SK, Wang H, et al. Abnormal cerebral structure is present at term in premature infants. Pediatrics 2005;115(2):286–94.
16. Huppi PS. Early alteration of structural and functional brain development in premature infants born with intrauterine growth restriction. Pediatr Res 2004;56:132–8.
17. Als H, Lawhon G, Duffy FH, et al. Individualized developmental care for the very low-birth-weight preterm infant: medical and neurofunctional effects. JAMA 1994; 272(11):853–8.
18. Kreisler L, Fain M, Soulé M. The child and his body, Studies on the Psychosomatic Clinic From First Age. Paris: Presses Universitaires de France 1974 [French].
19. Mellier D. The emotion in babies, a link between sociality and corporeality. Champ psychosomatique 2006;41(1):111–27 [French].
20. Szwec G. Self-soothing procedures in psychosomatics and child psychiatry. Neuropsychiatr Enfance Adolesc 2004;52(6):410–3 [French].
21. Guedeney A. Withdrawal behavior and depression in infancy. Infant Ment Health J 2007;28(4):393–408.
22. Bowlby J. Loss: sadness and depression. London: Hogarth Press; 1980.
23. Spitz RA. Anaclitic depression. Psychoanal Study Child 1946;2:313–41.
24. Bullinger A, Goubet N. The premature baby, an actor in its development. Enfance 1999;51(1):27–32 [French].
25. Vergara E, Bigsby R. Developmental and therapeutic interventions in the NICU. Baltimore, Brookes, P.H. 2003.
26. Zero to Three. Diagnostic classification of mental health and developmental disorders of infancy and early childhood. Washington, DC: Revised Edition (DC: 0-3 R) 2005.
27. Bick E. Notes on infant observation in psychoanalytic training. Int J Psychoanal 1964;45:558–66.
28. Brazelton T, Nugent J. Neonatal behavioral assessment scale. London: Mac Keith Press; 1995.
29. Als HA, Lester BM, Tronick EZ, et al. Manual for the assessment of preterm infants' behavior (APIB). In: Fitzgerald HE, Lester BM, Yogman MW, editors. Theory and research in behavioral pediatrics. 1st edition. New York: Plenum Press; 1982. p. 65–132.
30. Als H. A synactive model of neonatal behavioral organization: framework for the assessment of neurobehavioral development in the premature infant and for support of infants and parents in the neonatal intensive care environment. In: Sweeny JK, editor. The high-risk neonate: developmental therapy perspectives. New York: Haworth Press; 1986. p. 3–55.

31. Borghini A, Forcada-Guex M. The joint observation of the premature infant with parents-caregiver and psychotherapist. Psychoscope 2004;5:20–2 [French].
32. Kraemer SB, Steinberg Z. It's rarely cold in the NICU: the permeability of psychic space. Psychoanalytic Dialogues 2008;16:165–79.
33. Borghini A, Muller Nix C. A strange little unknown: Meeting with the premature infant. 1001 BB. Ramonville Saint-Agne (France): Erès Ed; 2008 [French].
34. Anand KJS, Scalzo FM. Can adverse neonatal experiences alter brain development and subsequent behavior? Biol Neonate 2000;77(2):69–82.
35. Grunau RE, Haley DW, Whitfield MF, et al. Altered basal cortisol levels at 3, 6, 8 and 18 months in infants born at extremely low gestational age. J Pediatr 2007; 150(2):151–6.
36. Grunau RE, Craig KD. Pain expression in neonates: facial action and cry. Pain 1987;28(3):395–410.
37. Stevens B, Johnston C, Petryshen P, et al. Premature infant pain profile: development and initial validation. Clin J Pain 1996;12(1):13–22.
38. Holsti L, Grunau RE, Oberlander TF, et al. Is it painful or not? Discriminant validity of the behavioral indicators of infant pain (BIIP) scale. Pain 2008;24(1): 83–8.
39. Grunau RE, Holsti L, Haley DW, et al. Neonatal procedural pain exposure predicts lower cortisol and behavioral reactivity in preterm infants in the NICU. Pain 2005; 113:293–300.
40. Holsti L, Grunau RE, Oberlander TF, et al. Specific newborn individualized developmental care and assessment program movements are associated with acute pain in preterm infants in the neonatal intensive care unit. Pediatrics 2004; 114(1):65–72.
41. Fitzgerald M, Millard C, Macintosh N. Hyperalgesia in premature infants. Lancet 1988;1(8580):292.
42. Hamon I. Anatomical route of pain in premature newborn infants. Archives de pédiatrie 1996;3:1006–12 [French].
43. Holsti L, Grunau RE, Whitfield MF, et al. Behavioral responses to pain are heightened after clustered care in preterm infants born between 30 and 32 weeks gestational age. Clin J Pain 2006;22(9):757–64.
44. Ajuriagerra J. Neuropsychological organization of certain functions: Spontaneous movements of tonico-postural dialog and in the early means of communication. Enfance 1985;2–3:265–77 [French].
45. Bullinger A. The sensory-motor development of the child and its avatars. Ramonville (France): Erès Ed; 2004 [French].
46. Grenier IR, Bigsby R, Vergara ER, et al. Comparison of motor self-regulatory and stress behaviors of preterm infants across body positions. Am J Occup Ther 2003;57(3):289–97.
47. Mellier D. The emotional value of narrative and infant observation. Funzione Gamma Journal, Time and Narration 2005;17.
48. Meyer EC, Zeanah CH, Boukydis Z, et al. A clinical interview for parents of high-risk infants: concept and applications. Infant Ment Health J 1993;14(3): 192–207.
49. Ansermet F. Clinic of the origin, the child between medicine and psychoanalysis. Lausanne (Switzerland): Payot Ed; 1999 [French].
50. Muller Nix C, Ansermet F. Prematurity, risk and protective factors. In: Zeanah CH, editor. Handbook of Infant Mental Health, 3rd Edition. 2009, in press
51. Muller Nix C, Nicole A, Forcada Guex M, et al. Prematurity, parental representations and trauma. Rev Med Suisse Romande 2001;121(3):241–6.

52. Zanardo V, Freato F, Zacchello F. Maternal anxiety upon NICU discharge of high-risk infants. J Reprod Infant Psychol 2003;21(1):69–75.

53. Spielberger CD. Manual for the state trait anxiety inventory (form Y). Palo Alto (CA): Consulting Psychologists Press; 1983.

54. Abidin RR. Parenting stress index. Charlottesville (VA): Pediatric Psychology Press; 1990.

55. Beck AT, Ward CH, Mendelson M, et al. An inventory for measuring depression. Arch Gen Psychiatry 1961;4:561–71.

56. Cox J, Holden J. Perinatal psychiatry. Use and misuse of the Edinburgh post-natal depression scale. London: Gaskill; 1994.

57. Guedeney N, Fermanian J. Validation study of the French version of the Edin-burgh Postnatal Depression Scale (EPDS): new results about use and psycho-metric properties. Eur Psychiatry 1998;13(2):83–9.

58. American psychiatric association. Diagnostic and statistical manual of mental disorders. Washington, DC: American Psychiatric Publishings; 2000.

59. DeMier RL, Hynan MT, Harris HB, et al. Perinatal stressors as predictors of symp-toms of posttraumatic stress in mothers of infants at high risk. J Perinatol 1996;16: 276–80.

60. Holditch-Davis D, Bartlett TR, Blickman AL, et al. Posttraumatic stress symptoms in mothers of premature infants. J Obstet Gynecol Neonatal Nurs 2003;32(2): 161–71.

61. Jotzo M, Poets C. Helping parents cope with trauma of premature birth: an eval-uation of trauma-preventive psychological intervention. Pediatrics 2005;115(4): 915–9.

62. Kersting A, Dorsch M, Wesselmann U, et al. Maternal posttraumatic stress response after birth of a very low-birth-weight infant. J Psychosom Res 2004; 57(5):473–6.

63. Pierrehumbert B, Nicole A, Muller-Nix C, et al. Parental post-traumatic reactions after premature birth: implications for sleeping and eating problems in the infant. Arch Dis Child 2003;88:F400–4.

64. Horowitz MJ, Wilner N, Alvarez W. Impact of event scale: a measure of subjective distress. Psychosom Med 1979;41(3):209–18.

65. DeMier RL, Hynan M, Hatfield R, et al. A measurement model of perinatal stressors: identifying risk for postnatal emotional distress in mothers of high-risk infants. J Clin Psychol 2000;56(1):89–100.

66. Levy-Shiff R, Sharir H, Mogilner MB. Mother- and father-preterm infant relation-ship in the hospital preterm nursery. Child Dev 1989;60:93–102.

67. Minde K, Whitelaw A, Brown J, et al. Effect of neonatal complications in prema-ture infants on early parent-infant interactions. Dev Med Child Neurol 1983; 25(6):763–77.

68. Minde K. Prematurity and serious medical conditions in infancy: implications for development, behavior, and intervention. In: Zeanah CH, editor. Handbook of infant mental health. 2nd edition. New York: Guilford Press; 2000. p. 176–94.

69. Bion WR. Learning from experience. London: Karnac Books; 1962.

70. Barnard KE, Bee HL, Hammond MA. Developmental changes in maternal interac-tions with term and preterm infants. Infant Behav Dev 1984;7:101–13.

71. Chapieski ML, Evankovich KD. Behavioral effects of prematurity. Semin Perinatol 1997;21(3):221–39.

72. Crnic K, Ragozin S, Greenberg M, et al. Social interaction and developmental competence of preterm and full-term infants during the first year of life. Child Dev 1983;54:1199–210.

73. Goldberg S, DiVitto B. Parenting children born preterm. In: Bornstein M, editor. Handbook of parenting. Children and parenting. Mahwah, NJ: Lawrence Erlbaum Associates; 1995. p. 209–31.

74. Minde K, Perrotta M, Marton P. Maternal caretaking and play with full-term and premature infants. J Am Acad Child Psychiatry 1985;26(2):231–44.

75. Muller-Nix C, Forcada-Guex M, Pierrehumbert B, et al. Prematurity, maternal stress and mother-child interactions. Early Hum Dev 2004;79(2):145–58.

76. Forcada-Guex M, Pierrehumbert B, Borghini A, et al. Early dyadic patterns of mother-infant interactions and outcomes of prematurity at 18 months. Pediatrics 2006;118(1):e107–14.

77. Zeanah CH, Canger CI, Jones JD. Clinical approaches to traumatized parents: psychotherapy in the intensive-care nursery. Child Psychiatry Hum Dev 1984; 14(3):158–69.

78. Perry BD, Pollard RA, Blakley TL, et al. Childhood trauma, the neurobiology of adaptation, and "use-dependent" development of the brain: how "states" become "traits". Infant Ment Health J 1995;16(4):271–91.

79. Taddio A, Katz J, Iiersich AL, et al. Effect of neonatal circumcision on pain response during subsequent routine vaccination. Lancet 1997;349:599–603.

80. Taylor A, Fisk NM, Glover V. Mode of delivery and subsequent stress response. Lancet 2000;355:120.

81. Gunnar MR, Porter FL, Wolf CM, et al. Neonatal stress reactivity: predictions to later emotional temperament. Child Dev 1995;66(1):1–13.

82. Heim C, Nemeroff CB. The impact of early adverse experiences on brain systems involved in the pathophysiology of anxiety and affective disorders. Biol Psychiatry 1999;46(11):1509–22.

83. Bhutta A, Cleves M, Casey P, et al. Cognitive and behavioral outcomes of school-aged children who were born preterm: a meta-analysis. JAMA 2002;288(6): 728–37.

84. Ansermet F, Magistretti P. Biology of freedom, neural plasticity, experience and the unconscious. London: Karnac; 2007.

85. Dudai Y. Reconsolidation: the advantage of being refocused. Curr Opin Neurobiol 2006;16:174–8.

Psychiatric Assessment of Young Children

Helen Link Egger, MD

KEYWORDS
- Psychiatric assessment • Infant mental health
- Psychopathology • Nosology • Diagnosis
- Psychiatric classification

During the last decade, the infant and preschool mental health field has made real strides in showing that clinically significant psychiatric symptoms and disorders are already present and highly impairing in early childhood (for a review see[1]). Recent epidemiologic studies have shown that the overall rates of psychiatric disorders in preschoolers (children aged 2 through 5 years) are remarkably similar to the overall rates reported for older children. For example, the rate of "serious emotional disturbance", a psychiatric disorder that is associated with significant impairment,[2] was 12.1% and 9.1% in two different community studies of preschoolers,[1,3] whereas the median rate across community studies of older children and adolescents was 13.2%[4] and 15.6% in adults.[5] Early onset mental health problems impair functioning across multiple domains and are often predictive of psychopathology and impairment later in childhood and in adulthood (for an overview see[1,3,6–10]). Although much less is known about mental health disturbances in children younger than 2 years, the rich literature on the impact of maternal depression and trauma on the social-emotional development of infants and the parent-infant relationship suggests that mental health disturbances can also begin before the age of 2 years (see the article by Schechter and Willheim, elsewhere in this issue).[11,12]

As the infant/early childhood mental health field has made advances in understanding mental health disturbances in infants, toddlers, and preschoolers, there has been growing recognition of the need for reliable and valid criteria for early childhood psychiatric disorders and for evidence-based assessments and treatments. There has also been growing recognition that the mental health needs of young children are not being met.[13] Few clinicians are trained in the assessment and treatment of toddlers and preschool children. Fewer still have clinical experiences with infants. In this article, we provide a brief overview of the diagnostic classification of psychiatric disorders in young children and then review the components of a comprehensive,

Dr. Egger receives funding from the NIMH, NIDA, NARSAD, and Autism Speaks.
Department of Psychiatry and Behavioral Sciences, Center for Developmental Epidemiology, Duke University Medical Center, Box 3454, Durham, NC 27710, USA
E-mail address: helen.egger@duke.edu

Child Adolesc Psychiatric Clin N Am 18 (2009) 559–580
doi:10.1016/j.chc.2009.02.004
1056-4993/09/$ – see front matter © 2009 Published by Elsevier Inc.

empirically based, psychiatric assessment of young children and their families. We conclude with a brief discussion of the challenges in defining and assessing mental health symptoms and disorders in children younger than 2 years.

DEVELOPMENTALLY APPROPRIATE CLASSIFICATION OF EARLY CHILDHOOD PSYCHIATRIC DISORDERS
Objections and Needs

Many researchers, clinicians, and laypeople wonder whether it is possible, or even desirable, to classify psychiatric disorders in early childhood (for a review of these concerns see[14–16]). Objections to the classification of psychiatric disorders arise from several concerns: (1) that the early childhood period involves such rapid physical (including neural), behavioral, emotional, and cognitive development that it is not possible to identify valid symptoms or clusters of symptoms that can be reliably measured, (2) that individual differences in normal development will be inappropriately identified as psychiatric symptoms or disorders, (3) that the dominant psychiatric taxonomy, the Diagnostic and Statistical Manual of Mental Disorders (DSM)/the International Classification of Diseases (ICD) approach, does not account for developmental variation, (4) that young children will be inappropriately "labeled" with "diseases" that will adversely shape the child's perception of him/herself and parents' or other caregivers' perceptions of the child, and (5) that problematic behavior in very young children is not located "in the child" but rather in the relationships between parents and children and the wider environment.

There have been real questions within and without of the infant/early childhood mental health field about whether is it possible to define a developmentally appropriate classification of psychiatric symptoms and disorders in early childhood that stays true to the central tenets of the infant/early childhood mental health approach. The foundation of the infant/early childhood mental health field is the understanding that mental health in young children is defined by healthy social and emotional development: development of capacities to experience and regulate emotions, to form close and secure relationships, and to learn.[17] From this definition of mental health the field focused as much on fostering healthy development and preventing mental health problems as on identifying and treating young children's mental health problems. Having emerged from collaborations among multiple disciplines, the field also encompasses different theoretical and clinical approaches to the definition of early childhood mental health disturbances. Many feel that the medical model of mental health disorders that is reflected in the diagnostic framework that is dominant in the classification of psychiatric disorders later in childhood and in adulthood does not adequately reflect these multidisciplinary approaches nor the developmental, prevention-oriented, and family-centered perspectives that define the infant/early childhood mental health field (for reviews of these concerns see[1,14–16]).

We would like to highlight two perspectives that are central to the infant/early childhood mental health field approach to understanding mental health problems in young children. We examine how objections to diagnostic classification partially arise from the very perspectives that define the field. We then ask whether it is possible to overcome these objections and define a developmentally appropriate psychiatric classification for young children, which preserves the field's perspectives on early childhood mental health.

The first tenet of the infant/early childhood mental health field is that early childhood mental health must be understood from a developmental perspective and include development across multiple domains, including cognitive, physical, neural, social, emotional, behavioral, and linguistic areas.[17] The second tenet is that early childhood mental health must be understood within the context of the child's relationships and environment. The child's emotions and behaviors do not occur in isolation, but rather within relationships, particularly the primary caregiving relationship, and within the child's family and community.[17,18]

The rapidity and scope of the cognitive, physical, behavioral, emotional, and social changes that characterize development from birth until kindergarten have led to 2 of the arguments against the classification of psychiatric disorders in early childhood. The first argument is that putative psychiatric symptoms will undergo similar changes to those seen in other domains and will present in markedly different ways during this early childhood period compared with how they present later in life. The presumption has been that early childhood symptoms are transient and, therefore, unable to be measured reliably. The second argument is that because young children are growing in so many different domains, mental health problems will present as global perturbations, not specific types and subtypes of psychiatric disorders. This concern leads to this question: Is it possible for the explicitly nondevelopmental, dominant psychiatric classifications, the DSM[19] and the ICD,[20] to incorporate a developmental perspective? The DSM/ICD systems were developed with (1) little attention to developmental differences in the presentation of psychiatric disorders and (2) little or no attention to the emotional and behavioral problems of infants, toddlers, and preschoolers. The way to address these objections about the characteristics of mental health symptoms in young children is to empirically whether it is possible to define reliable and valid developmentally-appropriate classifications in this age group. There are two possible approaches: develop either a separate diagnostic classification for young children or modify the current classifications. The two versions of the Diagnostic Classification: 0-3 (DC: 0-3)[21,22] are examples of the first approach. The Research Diagnostic Criteria-Preschool Age (RDC-PA)[23] and advances in the diagnosis of autism and other pervasive developmental disorders (PDDs) in children younger than 2 years of age (see Martinez-Pedraza and Carter, this issue) are examples of the second. This classification work is making it possible to begin to answer the question whether we can define specific types and subtypes of psychiatric disorders in young children, whether they can be reliably measured, whether they are valid syndromes, and whether they are transient or stable, and limited or predictive of future distress and impairment.

As developmentally appropriate criteria have emerged from these two approaches, resistance within the field to diagnostic classification has decreased. The centrality of relationship/environmental contexts in the understanding of early childhood mental health has naturally led to a focus on early childhood relationship disorders and post-traumatic stress disorders. The importance of these disorders cannot be denied; however, the extensive work in these areas, mostly clinical, not community study samples, has led to the perception that these are the most common disorders of early childhood. Recent epidemiological work suggests that emotional disorders, including depression and anxiety disorders, and behavioral disorders, including disruptive disorders and attention-deficit/hyperactivity disorder, are most common, as they are at other points in childhood. It is far from clear what the correct diagnostic criteria for young children are across the majority of mental health disorders. Current prevalence rates are sure to change as the field develops. It is also true that every child and the child's symptoms need to be understood within the context of his or relationships and environment, although one might argue that this applies across the lifespan. Nonetheless, this does not mean that all mental health disorders are located within the child's relationships nor the results of trauma and stress. Examination of the complex interplay between biology and environment, between parent and child, between the child and the community, and between the child's genetic risk and experiences will lead to a better understanding of how and why mental health problems emerge in early childhood. The challenge at this point is how to incorporate the infant/early childhood mental health field's relationship/environmental perspective within a *comprehensive* mental health assessment and diagnostic formulation.

In sum, differences in the infant mental health field's approach to emotional and behavioral problems, as well as meaningful differences between young children and older children, present challenges for the development of a mental health classification system that adequately addresses young children's problems. However, these differences do not obviate the need for valid diagnostic criteria in early childhood, a need that is the same as the need in other stages of life. A shared language is essential for clinical practice and scientific research. Clinicians use diagnostic classifications so that they can organize their observations and findings, communicate with each other, define targets for treatments, and track whether the treatment is working. Resistance to diagnosis often arises from the misperception that diagnoses reduce individuals to "labels" and minimize the complexity of the person and his or her relationships and experiences.[24,25] It is critical to emphasize that the aim of a diagnostic classification is to classify problems as disorders, not to classify children as problems.[26] All of the current diagnostic manuals describe multiaxial systems, which try to cover the range of domains that are necessary for a comprehensive assessment and development of a cohesive clinical formulation and plan. Thus, identification of specific psychiatric disorders within a multiaxial system is one essential part of the assessment and treatment process (most often coded on axis I) but surely not sufficient to understand individual children, their families, and their needs fully.

APPROACHES TO DEFINING MENTAL HEALTH PROBLEMS IN YOUNG CHILDREN

Next, we briefly review, in historical order, three approaches to the classification of mental health problems in young children: descriptive, dimensional, and categorical approaches (for more detailed discussions of these approaches see[1,14,16,27,28]).

Descriptive Approaches

Early works on infant/early childhood mental health used case reports or case series to describe the clinical manifestations of young children's emotional and behavioral problems. These careful clinical observations, along with psychological studies of typical and atypical development in infancy and beyond, are the foundation for more recent attempts to measure and characterize early onset problems as discrete symptoms and syndromes. Studies of anaclitic depression, attachment and its disturbances, and the impact of maternal depression on the social-emotional development of the infant are but a few examples of the seminal works that have described how problems present and develop in the early years of life (eg,[12,29–34]). In this approach, the child's behaviors and emotional responses are often understood as reflective of the nature and quality of the parent-child relationship. This has led to interventions to prevent these responses (eg, not separating children from parents when in the hospital) as well as to identify relationship-based disorders (eg, attachment disorders). From the mental health perspective, the characteristics and qualities of the parent-child relationship are critical to understanding the child and his or her needs. However, not all early onset mental health disorders are relationship disorders, so there is an additional need to identify emotional and behavioral problems within the child.

Dimensional Approaches

Young children's emotional and behavioral problems have also been approached dimensionally. Dimensional approaches emerge from the perspective of normative development. Cutoff points are set to characterize subsets of children at the extreme of the distribution of normative behaviors and emotions (or other phenomena such as temperament traits). From a mental health perspective, values on the scale above a predefined cutoff point represent problematic (eg, atypical, clinically significant) behaviors. Examples of dimensional scales include the Child Behavior Checklist (CBCL),[35] which can be used with children as young as 18 months, and the Infant-Toddler Social Emotional Assessment (ITSEA),[36] which can be used starting at 12 months. Dimensional measures for children younger than 1 year of age are primarily temperament measures with scales of temperament constructs (eg, activity level, soothability),[37] rather than scales of behavioral or emotional problems. Checklist measures are very useful in identifying broad domains of problems and in showing how an individual child's behaviors compare to other children of the same age as reported by parents or other caregivers. They do not have the level of specificity about the intensity, frequency, duration, or onset of specific symptoms that is required in diagnostic classifications such as the DSM. Although they provide good coverage of common problems, they do not include rare, but highly significant, symptoms (eg, suicidality), which must be assessed to identify a number of clinically significant mental health syndromes.

Some researchers in the infant mental health field argue that the dimensional approach to early childhood mental health problems is preferred to the categorical approach to psychopathology, which is dominant in the psychiatric community (for a discussion see[28]). This argument arises (1) from the presumption that there is a dichotomy between categorical and dimensional conceptualizations of mental health syndromes and (2) from the concern that psychiatric diagnoses are "labels" that minimize the importance of the multiple dimensions of a child's problems (and strengths) and complexity of the child's relationships and environment. The debate whether psychopathology is categorical (making diagnoses) or continuous (identifying dimensions of symptoms) is not confined to infant mental health (for a full discussion of these issues see[38,39]). The answer is that psychopathology is *both* categorical and continuous.[39] Most common psychiatric symptoms and syndromes (clusters of symptoms) show continuous distribution, with no clear line setting the boundary between normality and psychopathology. Depending on the clinical context or the scientific question, we can choose to examine either the categorical or dimensional characteristics of a symptom or syndrome (or both).[39] For example, making a categorical diagnosis might help us to make a decision whether or not to recommend treatment for a particular child. We might then use a dimensional scale to assess, over time, whether the child's symptoms are decreasing and whether functioning is improving during the course of treatment. The concern that categorical, but not dimensional, approaches to mental health problems harmfully "label" a child arises from the reality that there is real stigmatization of people of all ages who are mentally ill, but stigma is not a product of the way psychopathology is classified. Assessing mental health problems dimensionally, rather than categorically, will not eliminate stigma. Using empirical evidence about how to characterize and treat early onset disorders (as is being done for young children with autism), education and policy changes will be more effective against stigma than dismissing the utility of diagnostic approaches in understanding and treating mental health problems in young children will ever be.

Diagnostic Approaches

There have been two approaches to the diagnostic classifications of early childhood psychopathology (1) the DSM/ICD nosology, either unmodified or modified (eg, the RDC-PA[23]) to be developmentally appropriate for young children, or (2) the DC: 0-3

(DC: 0-3R), an alternative system for classifying mental health disorders in infant and toddlers.[21,22] Both of these categorical approaches seek to identify clinically significant syndromes, characterized by severity, pervasiveness, persistence, and impairment, that are themselves early-onset "disorders," rather than simply risk factors for later disorders.

The DSM-IV-TR[19] and ICD-10[20] are the dominant psychiatric classification systems used around the world. Because of the similarity between the DSM and ICD systems, most of our discussion of DSM-IV-TR pertains to ICD-10, as well. As noted earlier, the DSM system is largely nondevelopmental and pays scant attention to the emotional and behavioral problems of infants, toddlers, and preschoolers. Despite its lack of developmental specificity, the current DSM classifications have, in fact, been a useful starting point for examining how psychopathology presents in early childhood, at least in children 2 years and older. For example, the DSM-IV diagnostic criteria have worked quite well as a means of advancing our understanding of the presentation and course of autism spectrum disorders, despite their lack of developmentally specific criteria.[40–43] The dual approach of testing the applicability of current diagnostic criteria for identifying autism spectrum disorders in young children, while exploring the validity and clinical utility of developmentally specific criteria and/or diagnostic algorithms for use with young children, provides an exemplary roadmap for examining the validity of other behavioral and emotional disorders in young children. Similar approaches are being taken now in studies of early onset ADHD, anxiety disorders, depression, posttraumatic stress disorder, and disruptive behavior disorders in young children.[44–54]

In 2003, the RDC-PA[23] was published. The purpose of the RDC-PA was to define clearly specified and, where available, empirically derived, developmentally appropriate criteria for preschool psychopathology so as to facilitate further research on the diagnostic validity of psychiatric disorders in preschoolers. This approach was patterned on the development of the research diagnostic criteria published in 1978,[55] which led to the operationalized diagnostic criteria in the DSM-III and research on the reliability and validity of the psychiatric nosology for adults and then for older children and adolescents. The RDC-PA explicitly sought to modify the DSM criteria using the existing empirical base and extensive clinical experience to make the criteria developmentally appropriate, rather than to propose a wholly new classification system.

The DC: 0-3 takes a different approach from the RDC-PA, with a primary goal of classifying disorders in infants and toddlers that are not covered in the DSM.[56] Despite its title, the DC: 0-3 has commonly been used with children from birth through age 5 years. The DC: 0-3R classification systems includes alternative versions of DSM-IV diagnoses (eg for anxiety and depressive disorders), new diagnostic categories (eg regulation disorders of sensory processing), and a revised multiaxial system that places relationship characteristics and disorders on Axis II and the child's "functional emotional developmental level" on Axis V.[21] A revised version of DC: 0-3 (DC: 0-3R) was published in 2005 with a central goal of operationalizing the diagnostic criteria and categories so as to improve diagnostic reliability and facilitate research into the validity of these disorders.[22] DC: 0-3R, like the first version, was intended to supplement, not replace the DSM/ICD nosologies. The DC: 0-3R explicitly provides a place on Axis 1 for coding DSM/ICD diagnoses. The revised version incorporates many of the modifications proposed in the RDC-PA.

WHICH SYSTEM SHOULD A CLINICIAN USE?

At this point, it is quite certain that our current classifications of early childhood psychopathology are imperfect and will be revised and even supplanted as our knowledge grows. For now though, we have fairly convincing evidence that the different approaches to classification reviewed here all contribute to identifying psychopathology in early childhood (for reviews see[27,28]). Each of these approaches provides a particular window into understanding the phenomena of problematic behavioral and emotional dysregulation in young children. The clinician who provides mental health care to young children and their families should be familiar with each of these diagnostic, multiaxial mental health classifications.

COMPREHENSIVE, EVIDENCE-BASED PSYCHIATRIC ASSESSMENT OF YOUNG CHILDREN

In this next section, we provide an overview of the 6 essential components of a comprehensive mental health assessment of an infant, toddler or a young child: (1) multiple sessions (2) multiple informants (3) a multidisciplinary approach (4) a multicultural perspective (5) multiple modes of assessment and (6) a multiaxial diagnostic perspective. These components arise from the multidisciplinary, developmental, relationship-based, and family-centered orientations of the infant/early childhood mental health field's approach to understanding psychopathology in early childhood.[14] Although the principles of these components are applicable to the assessment of infants, there is much less empirical evidence about how to characterize, assess, and treat mental health problems in children younger than 2 years of age. We address the challenges of psychiatric assessment in infants and young toddlers at the end of this article.

Multiple Sessions

A first requirement is for *multiple sessions*. Despite the real reimbursement constraints that clinicians face, it is not possible to conduct an adequate psychiatric assessment of a young child in one session. Although it could be argued that this caveat is true for all of pediatric psychiatry, the rapid developmental changes that characterize the infant and preschool periods, as well as the young child's physical and emotional dependence on his/her primary caregivers, make it imperative that information be gathered about the child and his or her caregivers across sessions and across time. For example, a tired 3-year-old child seen after a long day at preschool may look quite different when seen in the morning after a good night's sleep. The child also has to be evaluated with and without his/her parent(s) or other primary caregiver to understand the relationship context of the problematic behaviors that brought the child to the evaluation in the first place. At some preschool clinics (see a description of the Duke Preschool Anxiety Clinic in[44]), the clinicians choose to see the parent(s) without the child for one of the sessions so as to obtain a detailed history of the child's, as well as the family history and current family functioning. It is essential to obtain information about current and past parental psychiatric and substance abuse problems and treatments, domestic violence in the home, and marital (or partner) difficulties, but it is not appropriate to discuss these issues in front of the child. Nor is it appropriate for the child to hear negative and demeaning comments about him or herself (eg, "he is a bad kid, just like my brother who is in jail."). Even if the child is seemingly absorbed in play in the corner of the office, one can be confident that the child is listening to the adult conversation. Clinicians who choose to have both the parent and the child present at the evaluation sessions must also allot time for "adult only" discussion either at one of the sessions (care will need to be available for the child) or a subsequent session. Evaluation sessions may also include additional daycare or preschool observations to see the child functioning with peers in an out-of-home setting and/or a home visit.

Multiple Informants

Multiple informants must contribute to the history and evaluation. Informants include parents (including mother and father, stepparents, and nonbiological parent figures), teachers/daycare providers, other important caregivers, such as a nanny, grandparent, and the child. However obvious it may seem, we must make this point emphatically and unequivocally: it is not possible to conduct a psychiatric assessment of a young child based solely on adult report. Every young child, whether an infant or a young 2-year-old with limited expressive language or a 5-year-old about to enter kindergarten, is a critical informant. Information can be obtained by speaking with and/or playing with the child (using structured or unstructured approaches) and observing the child interacting with parents, with another clinician, and with teachers/childcare providers or peers in school or daycare. Moreover, the clinician should make every effort to spend time alone with the child (severe separation anxiety is one example of a disorder that might make this very difficult, but that fact in itself is an important piece of clinical information).

Of course, an evaluation cannot be conducted without information from the child's biological parents or adults who are acting as parents, such as stepparents, grandmothers, or foster parents. An evaluation should include a three-generation genogram identifying the important parental figures and family members (and should include psychiatric and substance abuse history for each member). Ideally, if there are two parents in the home, both will attend the evaluation sessions and fill out all measures separately. Often each parent provides a somewhat different description of the child's symptoms. This does not undermine the validity of these reports but rather reflects the fact that the child shows different aspects of his/herself within different relationships. The divergence also reflects the reality that parents often have different interpretations and levels of concern about their child's behaviors. This information is diagnostically important and may be useful in guiding treatment planning. The parents will also provide information about themselves (eg, current psychiatric symptoms and treatment, parental and marital stress). Information must also be obtained from the child's nonparental caregivers, such as teachers/childcare providers, nannies, and babysitters, who spend a significant amount of time with the child. As described in more detail in the next section, other clinicians, such as the child's pediatrician or occupational therapists, are also critical informants.

Multidisciplinary Approach

Because a comprehensive mental health evaluation of a young child must include assessment of multiple domains, it is by necessity multidisciplinary and must include collaboration with other clinicians and care providers. The expertise of psychiatrists, developmental and clinical psychologists, school psychologists, pediatricians, neurologists, social workers, caseworkers, speech and language therapists, occupational therapists, early interventionists, child welfare providers, among others, will contribute to understanding the child's strengths and difficulties. Communication with psychiatrists, psychologists, other psychotherapists, substance abuse counselors, and/or marital or family therapists who are treating the child's parents/primary caregivers and/or siblings can also help to understand the child's family psychiatric history and treatment responses, as well as the child's family context.

The infant/early childhood mental health clinic, we believe, has an opportunity to integrate the data from these multiple sources to develop both a comprehensive diagnostic assessment and a meaningful treatment plan. For example, we know that many preschoolers with psychiatric disorders will also have speech and language delays and/or other developmental problems. A psychiatric treatment plan must include assessment of and a treatment plan for these delays, as well as for the primary psychiatric symptoms. Too often, families, already burdened by their child's symptoms (and by their own psychiatric and psychosocial problems), are asked to make multiple visits to multiple providers with no one taking the responsibility for putting all of this information together. The mental health provider assessing a young child should not only ensure that appropriate assessments across domains are completed but that the information from these assessments is integrated into a comprehensive treatment plan. Ideally, young-child assessments will be conducted within multidisciplinary mental health teams. The young-child mental health team will take responsibility for facilitating cross-domain assessment and treatment planning and coordinated interventions among providers. The aim is not to reify traditional hierarchical mental health clinical models with the physician at the apex of a pyramid but rather to create collaborative and integrative clinical models that clearly delineate the individual responsibilities within the team as well as an identified leader (from whatever discipline is most appropriate and effective in a particular clinical setting).

Multicultural Approach

It is important that the assessment include a *multicultural perspective*. The inclusion of a guide to cultural case formulation in the DSM-IV reflects the recognition in the psychiatric community that psychological functioning, assessment, and treatment occur within the context of specific cultural experiences, norms, and expectations of patients and of clinicians.[57] The impact of culture on infant/early childhood mental health assessment and treatment is now being addressed by clinicians and researchers. In a 2008 Zero to Three review of the impact of culture on early child development, culture is defined as "a shared system of meaning, which includes values, beliefs, and assumptions expressed in daily interactions of individuals within a group through a definite pattern of language, behavior, customs, attitudes, and practices."[58] For clinicians and scientists, inclusion of a multicultural perspective requires a genuine attempt to understand how culture shapes parents' understanding of their child's emotions, behaviors, and needs and affects the child's experiences within the home and within the wider community. Clinicians must also be aware of how their own cultural values, beliefs, and assumptions affect their understanding and interpretation of the child's experiences and needs. Christensen and colleagues' 2004 revisions to the DSM-IV cultural formulation text for use with infants and toddlers provide a framework for assessment of the clinical impact of culture. Areas of inquiry include cultural identity of child and caregivers; cultural explanation of the child's presenting problem; cultural factors related to the child's psychosocial and caregiving environment, including cultural beliefs about parenting and child development; cultural elements of the relationship between the child's caregiver(s) and the clinician; and how cultural considerations specifically influence comprehensive diagnosis and care of the child.[59]

Multiple Modes of Assessment

Because of the challenges of obtaining information about the emotions and experiences of young children, different modes of assessment, including structured screening and diagnostic measures, psychological/developmental testing, observational assessments, direct interviewing, laboratory tests, and structured and unstructured play, are necessary to obtain the multiple perspectives needed to understand the child and his/her symptoms within the context of his/her relationships and environment. As noted earlier, different informants will be able to provide various information and perspectives on the child's mental health and environment.

When possible, empirically tested measures with demonstrated reliability and validity should be used to assess child and family domains. Use of such measures not only provides a reliable baseline measure of the child's and the family's symptoms and functioning but also identifies valid targets for treatments. These measures can be then be administered during the course of treatment to evaluate the efficacy of the treatment. Documenting empirical data on the effectiveness of treatments is essential, particularly because there are few empirically validated treatments for psychiatric disorders in preschoolers at the present time.

Types of measures include symptom checklist measures, such as the CBCL 1.5–5,[35] the ITSEA for children 12 to 36 months old,[36,60] DSM-referenced rating scales, such as the Early Childhood Inventory-4 (ages 3–6 years),[61–64] or checklist measures of specific symptom clusters, such as the ADHD Rating Scale[65,66] or the Preschool Anxiety Scale.[67] Teacher/caregiver measures, such as the Caregiver-Teacher Report Form,[35] as well as measures assessing social skills and peer relationships, such as the Social Skills Rating System (SSRS),[68,69] are also useful.

In the future, structured diagnostic interviews for assessing young-child psychiatric symptoms and disorders will be the best way to obtain a comprehensive assessment of psychiatric symptoms in young children, but these measures are not yet "user-friendly" or feasible for use in clinical settings. The exception is the Autism Diagnostic Interview Schedule, which, when conducted in conjunction with the Autism Diagnostic Observational Assessment (ADOS), is considered the "gold standard" assessment for autism.[70,71] The Preschool Age Psychiatric Assessment (PAPA) is currently the only comprehensive parent psychiatric interview for assessing psychiatric symptoms and disorders in children aged 2 to 5 years, with demonstrated test-retest reliability and validity.[72] The entire interview takes 1 to 2 hours to administer and an additional hour to code. A version of the PAPA for assessing non-PDD symptoms in children with autism and other PDDs (PAPA-PDD) will be completed in 2009. The purpose of the PAPA-PDD will be to assess comorbid emotional and behavioral symptoms and disorders with children who have already been diagnosed with a PDD, usually with the Autism Diagnostic Interview and ADOS. The hope is that the PAPA-PDD will also be useful in assessing psychiatric symptoms in children with mental retardation, although additional modifications may have to be made to address the needs of these children. The ePAPA, a web-based version of the PAPA (and PAPA-PDD) that is administered on a tablet PC, has recently been developed and will be available for use in clinical settings in the future. The PAPA was not developed to assess symptoms in children younger than 24 months. As the infant/early childhood mental health field develops a clearer understanding of how psychiatric symptoms and disorders present in young toddlers and infants, it will be possible to develop empirically based measures to assess symptomatology in these very young children.

Direct "interviews" with the young child about his/her feelings and experiences are also be an essential component of a comprehensive assessment, particularly for the emotional disorders. Clearly, the child's developmental stage, particularly language level, will determine how the clinician approaches and conducts these interactions. In most clinical practice, unstructured play is used to learn about the child's emotions. Structured child interviews, such as the Berkeley Puppet Interview (BPI) and the MacArthur Story-Stem Battery (MSSB), show significant promise for older preschoolers. The BPI is an interactive interview for children 4 through 8 years old.[73,74] Children are interviewed with two identical puppets who present opposing statements about themselves (ie, "I am a sad kid" "I am not a sad kid") and then ask the child, "How about you?" The Symptomatology Scales of the BPI provide a child's report of emotional and behavioral symptoms. The MSSB,[75–83] which has been used with children as young as 3 years of age, consists of a systematic group of story beginnings, enacted in play with Lego figurines. The child is asked to complete the story by showing "what happens next," using the Lego toys. Warren's Narrative Emotional Coding[78] system can be used to assess the child's emotion regulation, anxiety, and depression. Available, as well, are story-stem measures that use dollhouses and family figure dolls (usually chosen by the child to represent his/her own family) as the props. Children are asked to complete stories that are specific to the symptomatology being assessed (eg, a loud sound in the middle of the night, stranger at the door). Some groups also use a schoolhouse and teacher dolls to address school/daycare anxiety (Jonathan Hill MRCPsych, Manchester, England, May 2005; Lynne Murray PhD, Reading, England, July, 2006; Helen Egger MD, Durham, NC; personal communications).

Observational assessments, particularly parent-child interactions and direct child observation, play an important role in assessments of young children. Excellent reviews of available measures can be found in the sources cited here.[15,17,59] Inspired by the success of the ADOS, a structured assessment for autism where the examiner "presses" for the symptoms with specific tasks, researchers have been developing similar diagnostic observational assessments for assessing disruptive behavior disorders in preschoolers (Disruptive Behavior-Diagnostic Observational Schedule [DB-DOS][50,84,85]). An observational measure of emotional disorders is under development (Lauren Wakschlag PhD, Chicago, IL, personal communication).

There are numerous standardized, developmentally specific measures for assessing the preschooler's status in cognitive, language, motor, and preacademic domains. Reviews of specific measures in this and the other areas mentioned in the section can be found in these sources.[15,17,46,59,86]

Multiaxial

A comprehensive psychiatric assessment of young children should be built on the foundation of a *multiaxial developmental framework* with coverage across multiple domains within the child and within the child's family and wider environment. Both the DSM/ICD and DC: 0-3 multiaxial approaches emerged from a "biopsychosocial" framework that seeks to understand the child's symptoms within the broad contexts of the child's internal and external environments. **Table 1** compares the DSM and DC: 0-3 axes. Clinicians who use the DC: 0-3 axes commonly make a "cross-walk" to the DSM axes since DSM/ICD codes are often needed for insurance reimbursement for services. **Box 1** provides a summary of the domains that should be assessed and recorded in the clinical history and then integrated into a multiaxial formulation.

Differences in the DC: 0-3 multiaxial structure from the DSM approach reflect the developmental and contextual perspectives that are critical components of the psychiatric assessment of a young child. First, information for each axis is gathered and integrated within a developmental context. A truly developmental assessment will arise from an understanding of the differences in the presentation of psychiatric symptoms from ages 2 through 5 years. Familiarity with the current consensus on developmentally appropriate psychiatric disorders and symptoms during the preschool period is essential. Valuable resources include those listed in the previous section on classification systems[21–23] as well as books including *The Handbook of Infant Mental Health*[17] (a revised version will be published in 2009), *The Handbook of Preschool Mental Health*,[46] and *Handbook of Infant, Toddler, and Preschool Mental Health Assessment*.[59]

The child's symptoms must also be understood within the child's current level of functioning across multiple developmental domains (eg, cognitive functioning,

	DSM-IV	DC: 0-3	DC: 0-3R
Table 1 **Comparison of axes in the DSM and DC: 0-3 systems**			
AXIS I	Clinical disorders	Primary diagnosis	Clinical disorders
AXIS II	Personality disorders Mental retardation	Relationship disorder classification	Relationship classification
AXIS III	General medical conditions	Medical and developmental disorders and conditions	Medical and developmental disorders and conditions
AXIS IV	Psychosocial and environmental problems	Psychosocial stressors	Psychosocial stressors
AXIS V	Global assessment of functioning	Functional, emotional developmental level	Emotional and social functioning

Bold indicates a difference between DSM-IV and DC: 0-3; Italics indicate a change from DC: 0-3 to DC: 0-3R.

expressive and receptive language, gross and fine motor skills, prekindergarten knowledge, social-emotional skills). These developmental assessments are important (1) for understanding the child's mental health symptoms within his/her developmental capacities (not simply the child's chronological age) and (2) for identifying developmental lags, deficits, and/or disorders that can be effectively addressed (eg, expressive language problems). Because children 3 years of age and younger (and in some states 5 years and younger) are eligible for early intervention services for developmental delays, it is critical that clinicians who are assessing young children identify these delays and provide appropriate treatment referrals.

The DC: 0-3 includes a separate axis (axis II) to record information about the nature and quality of the child's relationships with his/her primary caregivers and list relationship disorders. The Parent-Infant Relationship Global Assessment of Functioning scale and a relationship problems' checklist are included in the DC: 0-3R to guide the clinician in formulating an understanding of the child's relationships with his/her primary caregivers. The assessment of the context of the child's symptoms extends beyond this new axis. The qualities and characteristics of the child's relationships with the primary caregiver(s) are critical, but the nature of the child's relationships with others, including other adults and children (eg, siblings and peers), also informs the clinical formulation. The intensity and pervasiveness of the child's symptoms, across these relationships (as well as across different settings), will provide important information about the child's emotions and behaviors. For example, if a child has explosive tantrums that occur when the child is at home or at school and with the parent, as well as the child's daycare provider, the child may well be experiencing a symptom of a behavioral disorder. The child who has similar tantrums only when separating from her mother may be experiencing a symptom of an anxiety disorder. The child who has these tantrums only when being dropped off for a custody visitation with a divorced parent may be expressing distress that arises primarily from the difficulty of moving back and forth between two parental homes. The child who has tantrums only with his mother but shows good emotional and behavioral regulation with all other adults may be showing signs of a relationship disturbance with his mother. The infrequent tantrums that occur only when a child is exhausted (eg, after a long car trip traveling home from a vacation visit with Grandma) may very well be

Box 1
Domains to be assessed in the comprehensive psychiatric assessment of a young child

- Current and past history of emotional and behavioral symptoms, including frequency, duration, content, onset, relationship context, and triggers for positive symptoms

- Developmental history including history of pregnancy, maternal prenatal care (eg use of alcohol, tobacco, or drugs during pregnancy), neonatal history, and developmental milestones and delays (eg motor, language)

- Sleep, feeding and eating, and toileting history

- Child's play (eg content, enjoyment of, variety)

- Parent-child relationship (eg affect of parent and child during interaction, child's reactions to separation and reunion, level of conflict/coercion/intrusiveness)

- Current cognitive and developmental assessment of expressive/receptive language ability, gross and fine motor capacities, and adaptive functioning

- Medical history, including history of streptococcal infections, ear infections, hospitalizations, traumatic medical experiences, high lead levels, head injury, and central nervous system disorders, such as epilepsy

- Recent physical examination results, including height, weight, BMI, and blood pressure

- Medication history, including psychotropic medications and other medications, such as antibiotics and asthma medication (name, dosage, length of treatment, adverse side effects)

- Laboratory tests, including genetic testing, if indicated

- History of potentially stressful life events, including major traumas (eg death in the family, abuse, witness to violence), "minor" stressors (eg birth of sibling, changing daycare/school), and ongoing stressors (eg economic hardship, parental illness)

- Family structure and functioning, including discipline practices, such as use of corporal punishment

- Relationships with siblings, peers, and other-age children

- Child's and family's culture as well as appreciation of the impact of cultural differences/conflicts between this culture and the culture of the wider community

- Daycare/school experiences, including type of setting, teacher/child ratios, length of time in setting, relationship with teachers/childcare provider, and relationship with peers

- Three-generation family psychiatric/substance abuse/criminal history (ideally collected as a genogram) with a record of symptoms/diagnoses/events, age at onset, treatments, including in-patient and out-patient interventions, psychotherapy, and medications (name, dosage, any adverse side effects), including details about anxiety disorders and depression

- Current history of parental psychiatric symptoms, including symptoms of depression, anxiety, and substance use/abuse

- Current and past history of domestic violence between adults and between adult and child in the child's home

- Assessment of the child's impairment in activities and relationships from symptoms

- Assessment of the child's strengths and competencies

- Impact of the child's symptoms on the family's functioning (eg unable to leave the child with a babysitter due to the child's anxious distress)

- Degree of parental stress, both overall and in relationship to the child being evaluated

- Demographic and environmental information, including living conditions, parental employment, number of people living in the home, socioeconomic status and stress, neighborhood resources and violence, community participations, religious participation, and faith practices

developmentally normal. These examples highlight the importance of obtaining detailed examples of the child's behaviors with a focus on the characteristics and context of symptoms. Relevant questions include the following: What does the child do or say? How often does it happen? How long does it last? When did it start? What triggers the symptom? When, where, and with whom does the symptom occur? What helps? This descriptive information is not the same as asking the parent "why does your child do that?" Often, we do not know "why," but we can understand the symptom and how it clusters with other symptoms to move to an understanding of the nature of the disorder (eg, is it an anxiety disorder, behavioral disorder, or relationship disorder?).

Context also extends beyond relationships into the child's experiences within the family system and the wider community. In the DSM and DC: 0-3R systems, stressors and risk factors are listed on Axis IV. DC: 0-3R includes a broad (but not exclusive) checklist of known stressors, along with a place to indicate the age at onset, duration, severity, and context of these stressors, which is meant to serve as a guide to the assessment of this domain. Axis IV should reflect a careful review of the child's environments across multiple domains, including an understanding of (1) parental/family factors, such as a family history of psychiatric and substance abuse disorders, and treatment, including types and doses of psychotropic medications and types of psychosocial treatments (a history of postpartum depression should be obtained), family structure and functioning, including a careful assessment for physical or emotional abuse or neglect and sexual abuse, parent-partner relationship functioning, including an assessment of adult-adult domestic violence and emotional abuse, sibling relationships; (2) pregnancy and birth factors, including premature birth, low birth weight, maternal smoking or use of other substances during pregnancy, neonatal complications, maternal depression during or following the child's birth; (3) the child's school/daycare experiences, including teacher-child ratios, frequency of changes in child care settings and providers, amount of time child is away from parent(s), age when child started out of home care, peer relationships and relationships with nonparental child care providers; (4) neighborhood factors, including safety and proximity of relatives; (5) socioeconomic factors, including parental employment status, family's social economic status, and absence of health insurance to name a few. This list is not meant to be inclusive but rather a guide to the breadth and specificity of information that must be gathered. Chronic stressors or those that may seem "minor" (eg, change in daycare, moving to a new house) should also be recorded, since there is evidence from work with older children that the accumulation of multiple stressors with varying intensities may have as profound an impact on a child's mental health as a single traumatic event.[87–89] Both acute and cumulative stressors significantly raise the risk that the child will have 1 or more psychiatric disorders and be impaired.[1]

CLINICAL FORMATION AND TREATMENT PLANNING

Clinical formulation is an integrative process. The clinician pulls together a wide range of information from multiple sources and contexts and across many domains, to identify meaningful patterns that can be used to plan treatments or interventions that will address the child's and the family's needs. Clinical formulation emerges from the assessment of an individual child within the complexity of his or her specific family, community, and experiences. The clinical formulation section of the DC: 0-3R emphasizes that the diagnostic process occurs over time and that it must account for the developmental and contextual changes that characterize early childhood and the characteristics of this specific child.

When a comprehensive psychiatric evaluation has been conducted with a young child and his/her family and the DSM and/or DC: 0-3R axes have been completed, a treatment plan addressing each area of need should be developed. Clearly defined symptoms within the child must be identified, ideally using developmentally appropriate, reliable, and valid measures that are sensitive to change, so that the clinician will be able to assess the efficacy of the intervention and the outcome of treatment. Of course, a comprehensive assessment will also identify targets for treatment beyond the child's mental health symptomatology. For example, a treatment plan might include the following: referral of the child for speech or occupational therapy, recommendations that the parents seek an Individual Education Plan from the school system, referral of a parent for evaluation and treatment of his/her psychopathology, referral to marital therapy to address conflict in the parents' relationship, and/or recommendations for reducing parental stress, including respite care or regular exercise, or other opportunities for self-care for the primary caregiver.

It is quite clear that approximately 10% of children aged 2 to 5 years experience severe impairing psychiatric disorders, which cause suffering and put them at risk of ongoing emotional and developmental problems and impairment.[1] Reviews of types of current treatments for early childhood mental health disorders can be found in *The Handbook of Preschool Mental Health*, *The Handbook of Infant Mental Health*, and in this issue (see Tandon and colleagues, Lieberman and Horn, Shepard and Dickstein, Smyke and Zeanah, Gleason and Fanton). Unfortunately, the evidence base for psychiatric treatments for infants, toddlers, and preschoolers is very thin, with the exception of interventions for disruptive behavior disorders, ADHD, and some aspects of autism. The lack of treatment studies, as well as the potential risks of treatment, suggests that it is medically and ethically imperative that clinicians who treat young children for mental health disorders (1) acknowledge that there are limited data on evidence-based treatments and (2) develop thoughtful and empirically based strategies for providing mental health care to young children and their families. On one hand, children with mental health problems and their families deserve effective and safe treatment and cannot wait for the research base to catch up. On the other hand, clinicians and parents must weigh the risks of the disorder(s) with the risk of treatments and make cost-benefit decisions about how to best care for the child. Clinicians who treat preschoolers must know the current state of evidence on the assessment and treatment of early childhood psychopathology, know how to decide on and determine the efficacy of treatments that may not have been studied in young children, and be committed to keeping up with and incorporating new findings into their practice. Single-case experimental designs (eg, n-of-one trial) are the best way to manage these risks. A description of such an approach for treatment of preschool anxiety disorders can be found in Egger and Angold's work.[44] This treatment approach is particularly vital when use of psychotropic medication is being considered. The guidelines for psychopharmacological treatment of preschools (2007) recommend this empirically driven (and cautious) approach to treatment. Over the next decade, we can hope to see major advances in our understanding of the etiology and course of early onset mental health problems as well as development of effective treatments and preventive interventions.

CHALLENGES IN THE MENTAL HEALTH ASSESSMENT OF INFANTS

Classification of mental health symptoms and disorders in young toddlers and infants is still largely undeveloped. Measures such as the PAPA and clinical observational measures such as the DB-DOS are focused on the preschool child's emotions and behaviors, not the mental health needs of infants and toddlers. Few tools for assessing mental health symptoms in infancy exist. There are a number of excellent developmental assessments for infants and toddlers, which evaluate the child's functional capacities, development across domains including language and socialization, and the child's adaptive and coping capacities. However, a quantitative developmental evaluation is only one piece of a comprehensive clinical assessment of an infant. Mental health evaluations of all young children, but infants in particular, must include careful clinical observation of the child and of the all important caregiver-child relationship. There are a number of empirically valid observational and parent-report measures of the parent-child relationship, particularly attachment styles and disturbances of attachment for use in clinical practice. Behavioral observational paradigms, such as the Still-Face Paradigm[90] and the Strange Situation,[33,91] and the more recent Emotional Availability Scales,[92] have been valuable research tools for assessing the child's and the caregiver's social and emotional functioning, affect regulation, and interactions with and attachment to each other. Studies using these paradigms are advancing our understanding of normative infant development, individual differences in development, and the impact of clinically significant domains (eg, maternal depression, *in utero* drug exposure, autism) on the infant's and caregiver's capacities for emotion regulation and social interactions. although these methods have been used in some clinical settings, coding is time consuming.

These observational measures of the parent-child relationship assess domains that are shared by the symptoms and symptom patterns of clinically significant mental health problems (eg, infant affect, emotion regulation), but they do not encompass the full range of emotional and behavioral dysfunctions in infants and toddlers. The absence of mental health measures for very young children reflects the lack of consensus about how to characterize mental health problems in babies. We also do not know how to aggregate symptoms and classify syndromes in these young children. Measures for classifying and assessing emotional distress and behavioral dysregulation that go beyond familiar global constructs such as negative affectivity are urgently needed. We also need clinically focused, longitudinal studies of infants that use much more refined measures of emotional distress and behavioral dysregulation and other types of early emerging symptomatology. Most likely, infancy psychiatric syndromes will be defined by patterns of dysregulation across multiple domains. We need measures that will enable us to describe normative variation and patterns of dysregulation in crying, sleeping, eating, motor activity, sensory sensitivity, and disturbances in social relatedness (eg, not simply the presence of dysregulation but the intensity, frequency, duration, onset, and environmental and relational context of this dysregulation). These measures will help us to determine empirically the boundaries between normative and clinically significant presentations, just as we have done with mental health symptomatology in older toddlers and preschoolers. Measures such as Guedeney's and Fermanian' Infant Alarm Distress Scale, which assesses social withdrawal in infants,[93] or Wolke's assessment of regulatory disturbances in crying, sleep, and feeding in infancy[94,95] are promising examples of the types of measures and methods that will enable us to refine our current, rather crude, infancy criteria. In the absence of empirical evidence, the clinician should conduct assessments guided by the approaches outlined here for the assessment of toddlers and preschoolers. In particular, evaluation of family distress and dysfunction, severity of the infant's distress and impairment, and parental psychiatric symptoms and levels of impairment is critical, particularly because there is some evidence that interventions targeting parental disorders, rather than the child's symptoms, may be effective treatments for a child's distress.[96]

LIMITATIONS OF OUR CURRENT UNDERSTANDING OF EARLY CHILDHOOD PSYCHIATRIC DISORDERS

Many of the limitations facing the classification and assessment of psychiatric disorders in young children are simply mirrors of limitations facing all classification of psychopathology. Just as the DSM and ICD systems have undergone multiple iterations (DSM-V is slated for publication in 2011), the DC: 0-3 will continue to be revised. One can hope that eventually the best aspects of the developmental, relationship-based, and context-specific DC: 0-3 approach will be represented in the DSM/ICD systems. We can also anticipate that classification of psychopathology based on clinical observations of clusters of specific behaviors and emotional states will evolve as we understand more about the relationship between multiple biological systems and behaviors. In the future, we should be able to develop a clinically and biologically meaningful classification system of mental health disorders that enables us to find better ways to identify and alleviate the suffering of young children. Until then, there is reason to believe that we currently have "good enough" classifications and measurement tools and assessment approaches to push the infant/early childhood mental health field forward and enable us to better care for young children with impairing emotional and behavioral problems.

REFERENCES

1. Egger HL, Angold A. Common emotional and behavioral disorders in preschool children: presentation, nosology, and epidemiology. J Child Psychol Psychiatry 2006;47(3/4):313–37.
2. US Government. Fed Regist 1993;58:29425.
3. Lavigne JV, Gibbons RD, Christoffel KK, et al. Prevalence rates and correlates of psychiatric disorders among preschool children. J Am Acad Child Adolesc Psychiatry 1996;35(2):204–14.
4. Costello EJ, Egger HL, Angold A. 10-Year research update review: the epidemiology of child and adolescent psychiatric disorders: I. Methods and public health burden. J Am Acad Child Adolesc Psychiatry 2005;44(10):972–86.
5. Kessler RC, Wai Tat Chiu AM. Prevalence, severity, and comorbidity of 12-month DSM-IV disorders in the national comorbidity survey replication. Arch Gen Psychiatry 2005;62:617–27.
6. Briggs-Gowan MJ, Carter AS, Skuban EM, et al. Prevalence of social-emotional and behavioral problems in a community sample of 1- and 2-year old children. J Am Acad Child Adolesc Psychiatry 2001;40:811–9.
7. Lavigne JV, Arend R, Rosenbaum D, et al. Psychiatric disorders with onset in the preschool years: I. Stability of diagnoses. J Am Acad Child Adolesc Psychiatry 1998;37:1246–54.
8. Lavigne JV, Arend R, Rosenbaum D, et al. Psychiatric disorders with onset in the preschool years: II. Correlates and predictors of stable case status. J Am Acad Child Adolesc Psychiatry 1998;37:1255–61.
9. Lavigne JV, Cicchetti C, Gibbons RD, et al. Oppositional defiant disorder with onset in preschool years: longitudinal stability and pathways to other disorders. J Am Acad Child Adolesc Psychiatry 2001;40:1393–400.
10. Fombonne E. The epidemiology of autism: a review. Psychol Med 1999;29(4): 769–86.
11. Dawson G. On the origins of a vulnerability to depression: the influence of the early social environment on the development of psychobiological systems related to risk

for affective disorder. In: Nelson CA, editor. The Effect of early adversity on neurobehavioral development. Mahwah (NJ): L. Erlbaum Associates; 2000. p. 245–79.

12. Carter AS, Garrity-Rokous FE, Chazan-Cohen R, et al. Maternal depression and comorbidity: predicting early parenting, attachment security, and toddler social-emotional problems and competencies. J Am Acad Child Adolesc Psychiatry 2001;40:18–26.

13. Horwitz SM, Gary LC, Briggs-Gowan MJ, et al. Do needs drive services use in young children? Pediatrics 2003;112(6 Pt 1):1373–8.

14. Emde RN, Bingham RD, Harmon RJ. Classification and the diagnostic process in infancy. In: Zeanah CH Jr, editor. Handbook of infant mental health. 1st editon. New York: Guilford Press; 1993. p. 225–35.

15. Carter AS, Briggs-Gowan MJ, Davis NO. Assessment of young children's social-emotional development and psychopathology: recent advances and recommendations for practice. J Child Psychol Psychiatry 2004;45:109–34.

16. Angold A, Egger HL. Psychiatric diagnosis in preschool children. In: DelCarmen-Wiggins R, Carter A, editors. Handbook of infant, toddler, and preschool mental health assessment. New York: Oxford University Press; 2004. p. 123–39.

17. Zeanah CH Jr, editor. Handbook of infant mental health. Second edition. New York: Guilford Press; 2000.

18. Sameroff AJ, Chandler M. Reproductive risk and the continuum of caretaking casualty. In: Horowitz FD, editor, Review of the child development research, vol. 4. Chicago: University of Chicago Press; 1976. p. 87–244.

19. American Psychiatric Association. Diagnostic and Statistical Manual of Mental Disorders. Text Revision. 4th edition. Washington, DC: American Psychiatric Press; 2000.

20. World Health Organization. ICD-10: the ICD-10 classification of mental and behavioral disorders: clinical descriptions and diagnostic guidelines. Geneva, Switzerland: World Health Organization; 1992.

21. Zero to Three. Diagnostic classification: 0-3: diagnostic classification of mental health and developmental disorders of infancy and early childhood. Arlington (VA): National Center for Clinical Infant Programs; 1994.

22. Zero to Three. Diagnostic classification: 0-3r: diagnostic classification of mental health and developmental disorders of infancy and early childhood: revised edition. revised edition. Washington, DC: Zero To Three Press; 2005.

23. Task Force on Research Diagnostic Criteria: Infancy and Preschool. Research diagnostic criteria for infants and preschool children: the process and empirical support. J Am Acad Child Adolesc Psychiatry 2003;42:1504–12.

24. McClellan JM, Speltz ML. Psychiatric diagnosis in preschool children. J Am Acad Child Adolesc Psychiatry 2003;42:127–8.

25. Burke MG. Depression in preschool children. J Am Acad Child Adolesc Psychiatry 2003;42:263–4.

26. Rutter M, Gould M. Classification. In: Rutter M, Hersov L, editors. Child and adolescent psychiatry: modern approaches, 2nd Edition. Oxford: Blackwell Scientific Publications; 1985. p. 304–21.

27. Angold A, Egger HL. Preschool psychopathology: lessons for the lifespan. J Child Psychol Psychiatry 2007;48(10):961–6.

28. Egger HL, Angold A. Classification of psychopathology in early childhood In: Zeanah C, editor. Handbook of mental health (3rd Edition). New York: Guilford; in press.

29. Spitz R. Anaclitic depression. Psychoanal Study Child 1946;2:313–42.

30. Zeanah CH, Fox NA. Temperament and attachment disorders. J Clin Child Adolesc Psychol 2004;33(1):32–41.

31. Boris N, Wheeler E, Heller S, et al. Attachment and developmental psychopathology. Psychiatry 2000;63:75–84.
32. Bates J, Bayles K. Attachment and the development of behavior problems. In: Belsky J, Nezworski T, editors. Clinical implications of attachment. Hillsdale (NJ): Lawrence Erlbaum Associates; 1988. p. 253–99.
33. Ainsworth MD, Blehar MC, Waters E, et al. Patterns of attachment: a psychological study of the strange situation. Hillside (NJ): Lawrence Erlbaum Associates; 1978.
34. Bowlby J. Attachment and loss: vol. 2. separation. New York: Basic Books; 1973.
35. Achenbach TM, Rescorla LA. Manual for the ASEBA preschool forms and profiles: an integrated system of multi-informant assessment. Burlington (VT): University of Vermont Department of Psychiatry; 2000.
36. Carter AS, Briggs-Gowan, Margaret J, et al. The Infant-Toddler Social and Emotional Assessment (ITSEA): factor structure, reliability, and validity. J Abnorm Child Psychol 2003;31(5):495–514.
37. Rothbart MK. Longitudinal observation of infant temperament. Dev Psychol 1986; 22(3):356–65.
38. Kraemer HC, Noda A, O'Hara R. Categorical versus dimensional approaches to diagnosis: methodological challenges. J Psychiatr Res 2004;38(1):17–25.
39. Pickles A, Angold A. Natural categories or fundamental dimensions: on carving nature at the joints and the rearticulation of psychopathology. Dev Psychopathol 2003;15:529–51.
40. Rutter M. Genetic studies of autism: from the 1970s into the Millennium. J Abnorm Child Psychol 2000;28:3–14.
41. Volkmar FR, Lord C, Bailey A, et al. Autism and pervasive developmental disorders. J Child Psychol Psychiatry 2004;45(1):135–70.
42. Fombonne E. Epidemiological surveys of autism and other pervasive developmental disorders: an update. J Autism Dev Disord 2003;33(4):365–82.
43. Fombonne E, Simmons H, Ford T, et al. Prevalence of pervasive developmental disorders in the British nationwide survey of child mental health. Int Rev Psychiatry 2003;15(1–2):158–65.
44. Egger HL, Angold A. Anxiety Disorders. In: Luby J, editor. Handbook of preschool mental health: development, disorders, and treatment. New York: Guilford Press; 2006. p. 137–64.
45. Luby J, Mrakotsky C, Heffelfinger A, et al. Modification of DSM-IV criteria for depressed preschool children. Am J Psychiatry 2003;160:1169–72.
46. Luby J, editor. Handbook of preschool mental health: development, disorders, and treatment. New York: Guilford Press; 2006.
47. Scheeringa MS, Peebles CD, Cook CA, et al. Toward establishing procedural, criterion, and discriminant validity for PTSD in early childhood. J Am Acad Child Adolesc Psychiatry 2001;40:52–60.
48. Scheeringa MS, Zeanah C, Myers L, et al. New findings on alternative criteria for PTSD in preschool children. J Am Acad Child Adolesc Psychiatry 2003;42:561–71.
49. Scheeringa MS, Zeanah CH, Myers L, et al. Predictive validity in a prospective follow-up of PTSD in preschool children. J Am Acad Child Adolesc Psychiatry 2005;44(9):899–906.
50. Wakschlag LS, Leventhal B, Briggs-Gowan, et al. Defining the "disruptive" in preschool behavior: what diagnostic observation can teach us. Clin Child Fam Psychol Rev 2005;8(3):183–201.
51. Keenan K, Wakschlag LS. Are oppositional defiant and conduct disorder symptoms normative behaviors in preschoolers? A comparison of referred and nonreferred children. Am J Psychiatry 2004;161:356–8.

52. Keenan K, Wakschlag LS. Can a valid diagnosis of disruptive behavior disorder be made in preschool children? Am J Psychiatry 2002;159:351–8.
53. Lahey BB, Pelham WE, Loney J, et al. Instability of the DSM-IV subtypes of ADHD from preschool through elementary school. Arch Gen Psychiatry 2005;62(8): 896–902.
54. Eley TC, Bolton D, O'Connor TG, et al. A twin study of anxiety-related behaviours in pre-school children. J Child Psychol Psychiatry 2003;44:945–60.
55. Spitzer RL, Endicott J, Robins E. Research diagnostic criteria: rationale and reliability. Arch Gen Psychiatry 1978;35:773–82.
56. Emde RN. RDC-PA: a major step forward and some issues. J Am Acad Child Adolesc Psychiatry 2003;42:1513–6.
57. American Psychiatric Association. Diagnostic and statistical manual of mental disorders fourth edition (DSM-IV). Washington, DC: American Psychiatric Press, Inc.; 1994.
58. Maschinot B. The changing face of the United States: the influence of culture on early child development. Washington, DC: Zero to Three; 2008.
59. DelCarmen-Wiggins R, Carter A, editors. Handbook of infant, toddler, and preschool mental health assessment. New York: Oxford University Press; 2004.
60. Briggs-Gowan MJ. Preliminary acceptability and psychometrics of the Infant-Toddler Social and Emotional Assessment (ITSEA): a new adult-report questionnaire. Inf Mental Hlth J 1998;19(4):422–45.
61. Gadow KD, Sprafkin J, Nolan EE. DSM-IV symptoms in community and clinic preschool children. J Am Acad Child Adolesc Psychiatry 2001;40:1383–92.
62. Gadow KD, Sprafkin J. Early childhood symptom inventory-4 norms manual. Stony Brook (NY): Checkmate Plus; 1997.
63. Gadow KD, Sprafkin J. Early childhood symptom inventory-4 screening manual. Stony Brook (NY): Checkmate Plus; 2000.
64. Sprafkin J, Gadow KD. Early childhood inventories manual. Stony Brook (NY): Checkmate Plus; 1996.
65. DuPaul GJ, Power TJ, Anastopoulos AD, et al. Manual for the AD/HD rating scale-IV. New York: Guilford Press; 1998.
66. Gimpel G, Kuhn B. Maternal report of attention deficit hyperactivity disorder symptoms in preschool children. Child Care Health Dev 2000;26:163–79.
67. Spence SH, Rapee R, McDonald C, et al. The structure of anxiety symptoms among preschoolers. Behav Res Ther 2001;39:1293–316.
68. Gresham F, Elliott S. Social skills rating system manual. Circle Pines (MN): American Guidance Service; 1990.
69. Fantuzzo J, Manz P, McDermott P. Preschool version of the social skills rating system: an empirical analysis of its use with low-income children. J Sch Psychol 1998;36(2):199–224.
70. Lord C, Rutter M, DiLavore PC, et al. Autism Diagnostic Observation Schedule (ADOS). Los Angeles (CA): Western Psychological Services; 2003.
71. Le Coureur A, Lord C, Rutter M. Autism Diagnostic Interview, Revised (ADI-R). Los Angeles (CA): Western Psychological Services; 2003.
72. Egger HL, Erkanli A, Keeler G, et al. The test-retest reliability of the Preschool Age Psychiatric Assessment (PAPA). J Am Acad Child Adolesc Psychiatry 2006;45(5): 538–49.
73. Measelle JR, Ablow JC, Cowan PA, et al. Assessing young children's views of their academic, social, and emotional lives: an evaluation of the self-perception scales of the Berkeley Puppet Interview. Child Dev 1998;69:1556–76.

74. Ablow JC, Measelle JR, Kraemer HC, et al. The MacArthur Three-City Outcome Study: evaluating multi-informant measures of young children's symptomatology. J Am Acad Child Adolesc Psychiatry 1999;38:1580–90.
75. Warren SL, Oppenheim D, Emde RN. Can emotions and themes in children's play predict behavior problems? J Am Acad Child Adolesc Psychiatry 1996;35:1331–7.
76. Oppenheim D, Emde RN, Warren S. Children's narrative representations of mothers: their development and associations with child and mother adaptation. Child Dev 1997;68:127–38.
77. Oppenheim D, Nir A, Warren S, et al. Emotion regulation in mother-child narrative co-construction: associations with children's narratives and adaptation. Dev Psychol 1997;33:284–94.
78. Warren SL, Emde RN, Sroufe A. Internal representations: predicting anxiety from children's play narratives. J Am Acad Child Adolesc Psychiatry 2000;39:100–7.
79. Oppenheim D, Emde RN, Wamboldt FS. Associations between 3-year-olds' narrative co-constructions with mothers and fathers and their story completions about affective themes. Early Development and Parenting 1996;5:149–60.
80. Toth SL, Cicchetti D, Macfie J, et al. Representations of self and other in the narratives of neglected, physically abused, and sexually abused preschoolers. Dev Psychopathol 1997;9:781–96.
81. Warren SL, Schmitz S, Emde RN. Behavioral genetic analyses of self-reported anxiety at 7 years of age. J Am Acad Child Adolesc Psychiatry 1999;38:1403–8.
82. Petrill SA, Saudino K, Cherny SS, et al. Exploring the genetic and environmental etiology of high general cognitive ability in fourteen- to thirty-six-month-old twins. Child Dev 1998;69:68–74.
83. Macfie J, Toth SL, Rogosch FA, et al. Effect of maltreatment on preschoolers' narrative representations of responses to relieve distress and of role reversal. Dev Psychol 1999;35:460–5.
84. Wakschlag L, Hill C, Carter A, et al. Observational assessment of preschool disruptive behavior Part II: validity of the Disruptive Behavior Diagnostic Observation Schedule (DB-DOS). J Am Acad Child Adolesc Psychiatry 2008;47(6): 632–41.
85. Wakschlag L, Hill C, Carter A, et al. Observational assessment of preschool disruptive behavior Part 1: reliability of the Disruptive Behavior Diagnostic Observation Schedule (DB-DOS). J Am Acad Child Adolesc Psychiatry 2008;47(6): 622–31.
86. Bracken B, editor. The Psychoeducational assessment of preschool children Mahaw (NJ): Lawrence Eribaum Associates; 2004.
87. Copeland W, Keeler G, Angold A, et al. Traumatic events and posttraumatic stress in childhood. Arch Gen Psychiatry 2007;64:577–84.
88. Costello EJ, Erkanli A, Keeler G, et al. Distant trauma: a prospective study of the effects of 9/11 on rural youth. Appl Dev Sci 2004;8(4):211–20.
89. Scheeringa MS, Zeanah CH. Symptom expression and trauma variables in children under 48 months of age. Inf Mental Hlth J 1995;16:259–70.
90. Tronick ER, Cohn JF. Infant-mother face-to-face interactions: age and gender differences in coordination and the occurrences of miscoordination. Child Dev 1989;60:85–91.
91. Ainsworth MDS, Wittig BA. Attachment and exploratory behavior of one-year olds in a strange situation. Determinants of infant behavior IV. London: Methuen & Co.; 1992. p.111–36.
92. Biringen Z. Training and reliability issues with the Emotional Availability Scales. Inf Mental Hlth J 2005;26(4):404–5.

93. Guedeney A, Fermanian J. A validity and reliability study of assessment and screening for sustained withdrawal reaction in infancy: the Alarm Distress Baby scale. Inf Mental Hlth J 2001;22(5):559–75.
94. Wolke D. [Classification of regulatory disturbance in infancy]. Deutsche Gesellschaft fur Kinder-und Jugendpsychiatrie und Psychotherapie 2007 [German].
95. Wolke D, Meyer R, Gray P. Validity of the Crying Pattern Questionnaire in a sample of excessively crying babies. J Reprod Infant Psychol 1994;12(2):105–14.
96. Weissman MM, Pilowsky DJ, Wickramaratne PJ, et al. Remissions in maternal depression and child psychopathology: a STAR*D-child report. JAMA 2006; 295(12):1389–98.

Relationship Assessment in Clinical Practice

Mary Margaret Gleason, MD[a,b],*

KEYWORDS

• Early childhood • Infant • Mental health
• Parent-child relationship • Assessment

Parent-child relationship assessment is a critical part of a comprehensive assessment in an infant or early childhood mental health assessment. In early childhood, the parent-child relationship is arguably among the most powerful contexts of a child's experience. For infants, toddlers, and preschoolers, this relationship is the buffer through which they experience the world and can selectively transmit or block positive and negative environmental factors.

The relationship assessment serves a number of functions in clinical practice. First, a robust literature demonstrates the association between parent-child relationship characteristics and the very young child's current and future clinical status.[1–4] Thus, understanding the parent-child relationship patterns provides an important level of understanding of the child's clinical presentation and allows a clinician to make a more sophisticated formulation about the clinical presentation.[5] Second, the traditional child psychiatric assessment strategies rely heavily on parent report. Although use of multiple reporters and observational measures help to reduce the influence of any single reporter's perspective (see the article by Egger, elsewhere in this issue), clinicians who assess a parent's internal representation of the child (ie, the lens through which the parent sees the child and provides the history) can understand the parent reports in the context of the internal representation. This allows the clinician to integrate all available information into a comprehensive case formulation. For example, domestic violence perpetrated by the father of the infant may distort the lens through which the mother sees her infant, and she may attribute aggressive intent to developmentally appropriate behaviors such as kicking legs during a diaper change. Attention to this distortion allows the clinician to understand the mother's description of the infant's behaviors into this more complex clinical setting that

a Department of Pediatrics, Tulane University School of Medicine, 1440 Canal Street, TB 52, New Orleans, LA 70112, USA
b Department of Psychiatry & Neurology, Tulane University School of Medicine, 1440 Canal Street, TB 52, New Orleans, LA 70112, USA
* Corresponding author. Department of Pediatrics, Tulane University School of Medicine, 1440 Canal Street, TB 52, New Orleans, LA 70112.
E-mail address: mgleason@tulane.edu

Child Adolesc Psychiatric Clin N Am 18 (2009) 581–591
doi:10.1016/j.chc.2009.02.006   childpsych.theclinics.com
1056-4993/09/$ – see front matter © 2009 Elsevier Inc. All rights reserved.

includes her own internal representational world. Third, the assessment of the relationship guides treatment planning. Most effective interventions in early childhood mental health use the interventions focused on the parent and parent-child relationship to affect the child's emotional well-being.[6-10] A sophisticated understanding of the parent-child relationship allows treatment to focus on the areas of strength within the relationship and to build those strengths. In the example above, effective treatment for that dyad would recognize the parent's distorted internal representation of her child as an aggressor and her own experiences of the world as unsafe and build on her positive and developmentally appropriate attributions rather than focusing specifically on child behaviors.

COMPONENTS OF THE RELATIONSHIP ASSESSMENT

Bruschweiler-Stern and Stern presented a model that facilitates a systematic approach to relationship assessment.[11] This model conceptualizes parent-child relationships as the result of four components: the parent's internal representations, the parent's behaviors, the child's behaviors, and the child's internal representations (**Fig. 1**). Importantly, this model reminds clinicians to include internal representational experiences as part of the definition of parent-child relationships. This simple structure can guide clinical assessment, as clinicians can develop an assessment strategy that focuses on most of the components. Parental representations and behaviors can be measured in a systematic way, as can infant behaviors. Infant internal representations must be inferred from the child's behaviors.

The attachment relationship provides an excellent example of a relationship's component that can be described using these four components. Attachment theory, developed by Bowlby, Main, and elaborated by many other investigators, posits that humans have a biologically driven attachment drive, which promotes proximity seeking to a primary caregiver in times of stress or distress.[12] This drive is counterbalanced by the exploratory system, which promotes exploration of the child's environment. The caregiver's patterns of behavior as a source of support and comfort influence the child's developing patterns of attachment behaviors. A child's attachment behaviors reflect past experiences with this caregiver. Parent's patterns of behaviors in response to a child's distress are thought to allow the child to develop expectations of those responses in new episodes of distress. For example, consistent, nurturing parental responses to child distress allow the child to act with the expectation of being comforted in new episodes of distress. Although we cannot reliably measure the child's internal representations below the age of 3 to 4 years, it is thought that the child's confident approach behavior and easy soothability reflect a belief that the parent will comfort him or her this time as they have so many other times. Parental internal representations of themselves in caregiving relationships and of the child guide the parent's interactions with the child.[13,14] Newer research investigating

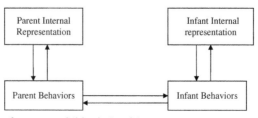

Fig. 1. Components of a parent-child relationship.

attachment has highlighted the importance of parental insight about the child's internal motivations and observable sensitivity to the child's needs as key parental cognitive and behavioral contributions to a healthy attachment relationship in infants and young children.[15,16] The quality of an attachment relationship predicts child relationship skills, emotional and behavioral regulation, psychophysiological markers, and mental health in early childhood, school age, adolescence, and adulthood (e.g.[17–25]). Although most research focused on attachment focuses on a dyadic relationship, it is also clear that family functioning and the parent-parent-child triad are important factors in child well-being as well.[26]

Other components of the parent-child relationship warrant clinical attention as well, including the quality of interactions of child and parent in play, teaching/learning, emotional regulation, and limit setting.[27] Clinical assessment strategies should pay attention to all of these domains.

INFORMAL ASSESSMENTS

Often in clinical practice, the traditional psychiatric interview precedes formal relationship procedures in early childhood mental health practice. This interview and mental status examination provide background information and may alert the clinician to areas of risk or strength within the relationship.

When obtaining a history, a clinician can attend to the quality of the parent's description of the child. What is the parent's tone when talking about the child? Is there flexibility in identifying strengths as well as concerns? To what or whom does the parent attribute the current clinical concern? How does he or she interpret the symptoms? Can the parent focus on the child's experiences or is it difficult to redirect the parent away from talking only about his or her own distress in relationship to the child's symptoms? These questions allow a clinician to begin to focus on the parent's internal representation of the child. It is useful to remember that asking a parent about the quality of a relationship may be less fruitful than observing the manner in which the parent talks about the child. At the end of the interview, it can be useful for the clinician to assess whether the history provided a relatively vivid and complex "picture" of the child and the degree to which that picture is multidimensional, balanced, flexible, and distinguishable from the parent's picture of herself. Although empirical data are lacking in the predictive value of these qualities as assessed informally, anecdotal experience suggests that parents who hold fixed, distorted, and overly negative internal representations of their children require clinical intervention that addresses these representations.

Traditional assessments also provide opportunities for observations of parent-child interactions. The waiting room provides the first opportunity for informal observation and sometimes can provide the richest data, because the interactions tend not to be affected by the act of the observation itself. Domains of parent-child interactions that can be observed informally in the waiting room and assessment room include the child's use of the parent for the sharing of joy and discovery, assistance, comfort seeking, and as a partner in play and authority figure as well as the parent's attention to the child's needs, responsiveness to the child's bids for attention, and ability to help the child organize overwhelming feelings or activities, to set limits, and enjoy the interactions. Similar patterns of parent behaviors can be observed in infant-parent interactions, in which infant regulatory patterns, such as ability to be soothed when crying, feeding patterns, and social engagement with the parent, are important patterns. Training the nonclinical staff (eg, receptionists, administrators) to report extreme interactions to the clinician can be quite useful.

Another unique opportunity for assessment of relational factors is when the clinician introduces himself or herself to the family, because at that moment, the clinician is a complete stranger to a child at least 7 to 9 months old, who would be expected to have developed a focused attachment relationship, and the associated stranger distress.[28] Clinicians can observe the child's response to meeting a stranger, with attention to whether the child references the parent before engaging with the clinician, the degree of inhibition in response to meeting a stranger, or if the child is overly friendly toward the new stranger. Normative development plays some role in these patterns, as children who attend out-of-home childcare settings are more accustomed to meeting new adults. However, it is not unusual in clinical settings to see children demonstrate extreme responses to the "stranger," either by shutting down and hiding or running to the clinician and trying to give a hug. Both extremes suggest that the child is not able to use the parent effectively for support during this new experience and prime the clinician to continue to observe patterns of effective or ineffective strategies for receiving comfort from the parent. Parent and child factors, including parental availability and sensitivity as well as the clarity or appropriateness of the child's signals for comfort, can influence the development of these patterns. With children of at least age 7 to 9 months, it can be informative to create an opportunity to observe a separation and reunion during the evaluation to provide an indicator of how the dyad copes with the stress of a brief separation upon reunion. Parents can demonstrate sensitivity by preparing a child for the separation and clinicians can learn about child temperament by the distress response to the separation.[29] However, the information most reflective of the quality of the attachment is the dyad's ability to resolve separation distress together during the reunion.[30,31]

Observations of child-parent interaction and attention to the manner in which the parent talks about the child allow a clinician to develop clinical hypotheses as part of the clinical formulation. In most cases, however, a formal assessment helps to guide treatment, especially with infants, toddlers, and younger preschoolers.

FORMAL ASSESSMENT

A number of formal, clinically useful relationship assessment strategies can inform early childhood mental health assessment and treatments. Formal assessment strategies, like systematic approaches to other parts of the clinical assessment, offer a number of advantages. Standardized approaches allow comparison across children and across time without the variability associated with informal observations.[32] Clinicians can also have meaningful discussions with other providers, allowing a shared understanding of the parent-child relationship. When programs use formal assessment strategies in a systematic way, parents can be reassured that these potentially sensitive areas are topics of attention for all patients in the program. Formal assessments do not resolve the challenge of identifying relationship-specific patterns. A child's interaction pattern with one caregiver does not reflect the interactions with another caregiver, and relationship observations cannot be generalized. A second limitation is that formal assessments are often time consuming and require trained staff. Some formal assessments, such as the well known Strange Situation Procedure,[33] were developed as research tools and are difficult to translate effectively into the clinical arena. The assessments described here have been chosen, because they can be performed in clinical settings and provide valuable clinical information.

Parent-Child Interactions

One effective way to assess patterns of attachment systematically is the *Disturbances in Attachment Interview*[23] (Smyke AT, Zeanah CH, unpublished data, 1999). This semistructured interview allows the clinician to explore a child's patterns of attachment behavior with the caregiver. The 12-item interview includes one question intended to identify whether or not the child has a focused attachment relationship with one or a small number of important caregivers. There are four items focused on symptoms associated with inhibited reactive attachment disorder, including not seeking comfort when distressed, not being able to be comforted, limited positive reciprocal interactions, inhibited, or limited, positive affect, and poor mood regulation. The next three items focus on patterns of indiscriminant attachment behaviors, including not checking back with a parent in a new setting, indiscriminant approach toward new adults, and willingness to go off with a stranger. The last four items focus on the proposed symptoms of disturbed attachment not represented in the Diagnostic and Statistical Manual of Mental Disorders, fourth edition (DSM)-IV, including provocative risk taking, excessive clinginess in new situations, hypervigilance, and role reversal. After sufficient probing, items are scored on a 0, 1, 2 non-Likert scale, with "0" representing healthy behaviors, "2" representing clear evidence of a symptom of an attachment disorder, and "1" being used when the symptom is sometimes or somewhat present. The interview takes approximately 20 minutes to complete. Internal consistency for the two first subscales is adequate (Crohnbach's alpha 0.8 and 0.83, respectively), and interrater reliability is also strong.[34] The measure differentiates a group of children who resided in a typical Romanian institutional unit from a comparison group that had been placed on a pilot unit. This pilot unit was characterized by a staffing schedule that provided more consistent time spent with the children and which provided an opportunity for the children to develop focused attachment relationships.[34] Although attachment disorder symptoms are rare in healthy populations, it is not uncommon to identify symptoms of attachment disturbance in high-risk populations, including children exposed to homelessness or maltreatment,[35] and in clinical samples.

Parent-child interaction can also be assessed by observation as well. In the Crowell procedure,[36] the parent and child (of at least 6 months developmental age) are observed in a series of nine episodes (access at: www.infantinstitute.org). Throughout the procedure, the clinician assesses a number of domains of the parent-child relationship including reciprocal emotions, protection and safety, comforting and comfort seeking, teaching and learning, play, discipline and response to limits, and parental structure and child's self-regulation. The assessment can provide more depth of understanding of the dyad's interactions, capacity for joy, and ability to negotiate stressful situations. The procedure begins with a free-play period that allows the clinician to observe the dyad in a low-stress situation and to attend to the level of mutual enjoyment, familiarity with play, parent's ability to engage in the child's play, and the child to include the parent in the play. For most dyads, this session allows the parent to become more comfortable with the procedure.[37] The next episode is a cleanup period, which places mild stress on the child when stopping an enjoyable activity and provides an opportunity to observe the dyad's ability to negotiate the situation and collaborate. A bubble sequence follows cleanup, with the goal of eliciting the sharing of joy and other positive affects. The sequence that follows includes puzzle tasks that are arranged by the clinician in order of increasing difficulty. By starting with a task that is easy for the child, the parent ideally can be expected to encourage and praise the child. By progressively moving to tasks that are beyond the child's developmental level, the parent needs to be able to scaffold the tasks so that the child can complete them. The procedure ends with a separation that allows observation of the child's and the parent's ability to tolerate the separation. This is followed by a reunion, which allows the clinician to observe how the child uses the parent for comfort after the mild stressor of the separation. Children who approach the parent and effectively seek comfort show evidence of a healthy attachment relationship. This procedure does not allow formal classification of attachment status but does allow the clinician to identify some patterns of reunions that may be concerning. Examples of such patterns include when a distressed child actively avoids a parent, when a child shows alternating approach-avoidant patterns or resists the parent's comfort, or when a child seems to have no consistent strategy for resolving the distress. The reunion behaviors provide valuable information about how the child does or does not experience the parent as someone from whom he can elicit comfort.

The Insightfulness Assessment (IA) uses parent-child interactions to explore a parent's insightfulness about his or her child. Oppenheim and Koren-Karie[16] define insightfulness as the capacity "to see things from the child's point of view, and is based on insight into the child's motives, a complex view of the child, and openness to new information about the child." This capacity is associated with a parent's ability to respond sensitively to a child's needs, to use positive parenting practices, and the development of a secure attachment relationship. The IA includes a play episode with the child and parent, which is videotaped for review. In the assessment portion of the procedure, the parent views brief videotaped clips of the play interaction and is asked to comment on the child's thoughts, feelings, and motivations during the clips. In research settings, the transcripts are transcribed and coded into "Positively Insightful," "One Sided," "Disengaged," or "Mixed." Parents who are coded as positively insightful are able to recognize their child's motives for behaviors, are open to the idea that the child may change with development or experiences, are able to maintain their focus on the child during the interview, describe the child as a complex person, and provide a coherent story about the child. Parents coded as one-sided seem to have a preset representation of the child that is not affected by the behaviors in the video clips. Those classified as disengaged show limited emotional connection to the child during the interview and do not value understanding the child's internal experiences. Insightfulness is associated with secure attachment classification, observed maternal sensitivity, and with clinician-rated improvement of clinical symptoms with treatment (as reviewed in[16]).

Parent Internal Representations

The Working Model of the Child Interview (WMCI)[38] is a 1-hour interview that invites a parent to tell the story of his or her child and of the relationship they share (available through http://www.infantinstitute.com/training.htm). The interview begins with questions about the child's prenatal history and birth story, with an emphasis on the relational and emotional factors rather than the traditional information of "facts and figures." The interview continues by asking the parent about the child's personality, first generally, and then asking the parent to choose five words to describe the child and to provide specific examples of events that demonstrate this pattern. Parents are invited to talk about challenging behaviors, how they handle those, and their emotional responses to the difficult interactions. The interviewer asks the parent to talk about how the child is similar to each parent as well. The same sequence occurs when asking about the parent's view of her relationship with the child as related to the child's personality. During the interview, the interviewer also asks the parent to talk about what is special, unique, or different about the child, hopes for the child, and challenges the parent anticipates.

Parents' responses can provide useful information about the parent's experience of the infant or young child. However, this interview follows in a tradition of using the quality of narrative in response to interview questions to understand the interviewee's internal representations.[39] This interview is intended to provide information about the parent's internal representation of the child, as demonstrated by narrative character- istics. These characteristics include the following:

- Richness of perception: level of details provided that allows the clinician to "see" the internal representation of the child that the parent holds in her mind.
- Affective tone: Joy and pride about the child should be evident.
- Openness to change/flexibility: the degree to which the parent can imagine the child developing and changing over time and with new experience, particularly with respect to the clinical presenting problem.
- Coherence: clarity, consistency, and plausibility all contribute to the assessment of coherence. Coherence is achieved when an interview provides a picture of a child that "makes sense."
- Acceptance: the ability of the parent to accept the balance of the caring for the child and appreciating the developing independence in young children.
- Caregiving sensitivity: recognition of the child's current developmental needs and internal experiences.
- Child difficulty: Ability to recognize the child's clinical problems (if present) without a sense of being burdened by the child. This is a particularly important factor in clinical settings where children are perceived to have notable difficult patterns and parents may be at higher risk for negative attributions.
- Irrational fear of loss: fears of the child's death or excessive fears about the child's safety.
- Finally, affective tone and the balance of positive or negative tones and modula- tion of tone are important prognostic signs.[40]

In clinical practice, videotaping these interviews can be useful both for further review by the clinician across different domains (ie, content, narrative coherence, affective expression, nonverbal communication, and gestures, etc) as well as to play back and review with the parent.

This interview has been used in research and produces three classifications: balanced, disengaged, and distorted based on the narrative coherence and affective tone. The stability of the WMCI classifications is also notable and highlights the non- child influences on the parent's internal representation of the child. In one study, WMCI done prenatally predicted the WMCI classification at 11 months in 80% of chil- dren.[41] In the same study, prenatal WMCI accurately predicted attachment classifica- tion in nearly three-quarters of children at 12 months. Using the research classifications, the interview can differentiate between clinically referred and nonclini- cally referred infants.[41] In addition, a balanced WMCI classification is associated with attachment classification in the Strange Situation Procedure.[38]

Child Internal Representations

In infants, we must depend on behaviors to make inferences about the child's internal representations. However, innovative research procedures provide useful information about the child's internal representations. A young child's view of self is thought to be associated with the experiences that he has had with caregivers. Safe, nurturing inter- actions with a caregiver convey to a child that he is protected and loved and such experiences contribute to a positive view of self.[42] With young children, semistruc- tured interactions with puppets or dolls can be used as aids to elicit a child's view of himself or of his caregiving relationship.

In the Puppet Interview,[42] children are asked to "speak" for the puppet and answer questions such as, "do you like [the child]?" Child responses are thought to represent the child's perception of how other people ("the unspecific other") view him or her. The interview can be rated on two major dimensions—affective positiveness and openness to recognizing imperfections in self. Both dimensions are associated with teacher reports and parent reports of behavioral and social competence.[43] Concurrent positive sense of self-competence and openness or flexible view of self are associated with attachment observed behaviors.[44] A second approach to using dolls to understand children's internal representations examines the child's perception of the parent, as in the MacArthur Story Stem Battery[11] (Bretherton I, Oppenheim D, Buchsbaum H, and colleagues, unpublished data, 1990). These procedures use dolls or puppets to start a story and ask the child to complete the story. Story stems can involve mild stressors, such as the child being awakened in the middle of the night by a noise. The way the child completes the story is thought to reflect the way the child sees himself in the relationship with the caregiver, specifically, whether the child feels accepted and valued and that the child feels safe within the relationship.[42] In the MacArthur Story Stem Battery, responses are categorized into positive, negative, and disciplinary representations.[45,46] Story completion measures have also been coded according to global attachment classification (secure, avoidant, bizarre/ambivalent) and an overall security score. This score is moderately correlated with the child's view of self and with observed attachment behaviors.[42,43] Like other measures of attachment status, positive representations about parents are moderately associated with parent and teacher reports of child prosocial behaviors, and negative representations are inversely associated with prosocial behaviors.[47]

Both self-representations and representations of the relationship are associated with security of attachment, with securely attached preschoolers demonstrating higher levels of positive affect toward themselves, assigning positive attributes to the relationship with the mother.[42]

In research settings, coding of both these measures is done by trained reviewers who are blind to the child's clinical status or other assessments. Although these measures have not been adapted for routine clinical use, they provide promising strategies to expanding our clinical understanding of the internal worlds of very young children. Clinicians can use three factors in the child's responses to either procedure: coherence of the response, dominant themes, and child's behavior during the response to help inform a clinical assessment.[45]

SUMMARY

In infants and very young children, traditional psychiatric assessments must be considered in the context of the early caregiving relationships. A strong literature supports the importance of the caregiving relationship as a predictor of child social emotional well-being into adulthood. Informal and formal measures of parent and child interactions within their relationship and of representational processes involved in the relationship can be used in clinical settings to guide the clinical formulation and treatment planning. These assessments do not replace other components of the psychiatric assessment; a clinical formulation includes the child's psychiatric symptoms, developmental path and current functioning, medical conditions, possible genetic loading for psychiatric conditions, exposure to family psychopathology, and the influence of family and community stressors or protective factors. However, careful assessment of the strengths and qualities of the parent-child relationship informs how a clinician interprets parent report, how the parent experiences the child, and provides rich information about the messages and feelings a child receives from the important caregivers in his or her life. For example, in a child who has a history of prematurity and extreme separation symptoms, an assessment of the parent-child relationship may help shift a clinical assessment of aggressive behaviors from "anxiety disorder not otherwise specified" to "anxiety disorder in the context of persistent and distorted paternal attributions of child vulnerability, extreme parental protective behaviors, and child's negative self attributions." The latter assessment identifies underlying dynamics that become targets for treatment that may prove more meaningful than a nondyadic approach to anxiety disorders. Child psychiatrists in the twenty-first century have the opportunity to integrate the tools of the medical model with the relationship-focused evidence base of infant mental health to develop truly biopsychosocial formulations of each child and family we see, in order to provide individualized treatment plans for our patients.

REFERENCES

1. Deklyen M. Disruptive behavior disorder and intergenerational attachment patterns: A comparison of clinic-referred and normally functioning preschoolers and their mothers. J Consult Clin Psychol 1996;64:357.
2. Lyons-Ruth K. Attachment relationships among children with aggressive behavior problems: the role of disorganized early attachment patterns. J Consult Clin Psychol 1996;64:64.
3. Oppenheim D, Goldsmith D, Koren-Karie N. Maternal insightfulness and preschoolers' emotion and behavior problems: reciprocal influences in a therapeutic preschool program. Infant Ment Health J 2004;25:352.
4. Shonkoff JP, Phillips D. From neurons to neighborhoods: The science of early childhood development. Washington, DC: National Academy Press; 2000.
5. Jellinek MS, McDermott JF. Formulation: putting the diagnosis into a therapeutic context and treatment plan. J Am Acad Child Adolesc Psychiatry 2004;43:913.
6. Dozier M. Attachment and biobehavioral catch-up: an intervention for caregivers of babies who have experienced early adversity, in Boston Institute for the Development of Infants and Parents. Lexington (MA); 2006.
7. Hood KK, Eyberg SM. Outcomes of parent-child interaction therapy: mothers' reports of maintenance three to six years after treatment. J Clin Child Adolesc Psychol 2003;32:419.
8. Lieberman AF, Ippen CG, Van Horn PJ. Child-parent psychotherapy: 6 month follow-up of a randomized controlled trial. J Am Acad Child Adolesc Psychiatry 2006;45:913.
9. Toth SL, Maughan A, Manly JT, et al. The relative efficacy of two interventions in altering maltreated preschool children's representational models: implications for attachment theory. Dev Psychopathol 2002;14:877.
10. Webster-Stratton C, Reid MJ, Hammond M. Treating children with early-onset conduct problems: intervention outcomes for parent, child, and teacher training. J Clin Child Adolesc Psychol 2004;33:105.
11. Bruschweiler-Stern N, Stern D. A model for conceptualizing the role of the mother's representational world in various mother–infant therapies. Infant Ment Health J 1989;10:142.
12. Bowlby J. A secure base: parent-child attachment and healthy human development. New York: Basic Books; 1988.
13. Goldberg S, Benoit D, Blokland K, et al. Atypical maternal behavior, maternal representations, and infant disorganized attachment. Dev Psychopathol 2003; 15:239.

14. Lieberman AF, Padron E, Van Horn P, et al. Angels in the nursery: the intergenerational transmission of benevolent parental influences. Infant Ment Health J 2005; 26:504.
15. Koren-Karie N, Oppenheim d, Dolev S, et al. Mother's insightfulness regarding their infants' internal experience: relations with maternal sensitivity and infant attachment. Dev Psychol 2002;38:534.
16. Oppenheim D, Koren-Karie N. Mothers' insightfulness regarding their children's internal worlds: The capacity underlying secure child-mother relationships. Infant Ment Health J 2002;23:593.
17. Carlson E. A prospective longitudinal study of attachment disorganization/disorientation. Child Dev 1998;69:1107.
18. Cassidy J. Emotion regulation: Influences of attachment relationships. Child Dev 1994;59:228.
19. Easterbrooks MA, Robyn A. Windows to the self in 8-year-olds: bridges to attachment representation and behavioral adjustment. Attach Hum Dev 2000;2:85.
20. Erickson MF, Sroufe LA, Egeland B. The relationship between quality of attachment and behavior problems in preschool in a high-risk sample. Monogr Soc Res Child Dev 1985;50:147.
21. Greenberg MT, Speltz ML, Deklyen M, et al. Attachment security in preschooler with and without externalizing behavior problems: a replication. Dev Psychopathol 1991;3:413.
22. Nachmias M, Gunnar M, Mangelsdorf S, et al. Behavioral inhibition and stress reactivity: the moderating role of attachment security. Child Dev 1996;67:508.
23. Sroufe L. Attachment and development: a prospective, longitudinal study from birth to adulthood. Attach Hum Dev 2005;7:349.
24. Warren SL, Huston LMA, Egeland B, et al. Child and adolescent anxiety disorders and early attachment. J Am Acad Child Adolesc Psychiatry 1997;36:637.
25. Weinfield N, Whaley G, Egeland B. Continuity, discontinuity, and coherence in attachment from infancy to late adolescence: sequelae of organization and disorganization. Attach Hum Dev 2004;6:73.
26. Hayden LC, Schiller M, Dickstein S, et al. Levels of family assessment: Family, marital, and parent-child interaction. J Fam Psychol 1998;12:7.
27. Crowell JA. Assessment of attachment security in a clinical setting: Observations of parents and children. J Dev Behav Pediatr 2003;24:199.
28. Gleason MM, Zeanah CH. Assessing infants and toddlers. In: Weiner JM, Dulcan MK, editors. Textbook of child and adolescent psychiatry. New York: American Psychiatric Publishing; 2008.
29. Gunnar MR, Larson MC, Hertsgaard L, et al. The stressfulness of separation among nine-month-old infants: effects of social context variables and infant temperament. Child Dev 1992;63:290.
30. Boris NW, Fueyo M, Zeanah CH. The clinical assessment of attachment in children under five. J Am Acad Child Adolesc Psychiatry 1997;36:291.
31. Zeanah CH, Larrieu JA, Valliere J, et al. Infant-parent relationship assessment. In: Zeanah CH, editor. Handbook of infant mental health. New York: Guilford Press; 2000. p. 222.
32. Carter A, Briggs-Gowan MJ, Davis NO. Assessment of young children's social-emotional development and psychopathology: recent advances and recommendations for practice. J Child Psychol Psychiatry 2004;45:109.
33. Ainsworth MDS, Blehar M, Waters E, et al. Patterns of attachment. Hillsdale (NJ): Erlbaum; 1978.

34. Smyke AT, Dumitrescu A, Zeanah CH. Attachment disturbances in young children: The caretaking casualty continuum. J Am Acad Child Adolesc Psychiatry 2002;41:972.
35. Boris NW, Hinshaw-Fuselier SS, Smyke AT, et al. Comparing criteria for attachment disorders: establishing reliability and validity in high-risk samples. J Am Acad Child Adolesc Psychiatry 2004;43:568.
36. Crowell JA, Feldman SS. Mothers' internal models of relationships and children's behavioral and developmental status: a study of mother-child interaction. Child Dev 1988;59:1273.
37. Zeanah CH, Boris NW, Heller SS, et al. Relationship assessment in infant mental health. Infant Ment Health J 1997;18:182.
38. Zeanah CH, Benoit D, Hirschberg L, et al. Mothers' representations of their infants are concordant with infant attachment classifications. Developmental Issues in Psychiatry and Psychology 1994;1:9.
39. George C, Kaplan N, Main M. Adult attachment interview, unpublished protocol. Berkeley: Department of Psychology, University of California; 1996.
40. Zeanah CH, Benoit D. Clinical applications of a parent perception interview in infant mental health. Child Adolesc Psychiatr Clin N Am 1995;4:539.
41. Benoit D, Parker KCH, Zeanah CH. Mothers' representations of their infants assessed prenatally: stability and association with infants' attachment classifications. J Child Psychol Psychiatry 1997;38:307.
42. Cassidy J. Child-mother attachment and the self in six-year-olds. Child Dev 1988; 59:121.
43. Verschueren K, Marcoen A, Schoefs V. The internal working model of the self, attachment, and competence in five-year-olds. Child Dev 1996;67:2493.
44. Clark SE, Symons DK. A longitudinal study of Q-sort attachment security and self-processes at age 5. Infant Child Dev 2000;9:91.
45. Oppenheim D. Child, parent, and parent–child emotion narratives: Implications for developmental psychopathology. Dev Psychopathol 2006;18:771.
46. Oppenheim D, Emde RN, Warren S. Children's narrative representations of mothers: their development and associations with child and mother adaptation. Child Dev 1997;68:127.
47. Stadelmann S, Perren S, von Wyl A, et al. Associations between family relationships and symptoms/strengths at kindergarten age: what is the role of children's parental representations? J Child Psychol Psychiatry 2007;48:996.

Internalizing Disorders in Early Childhood: A Review of Depressive and Anxiety Disorders

Mini Tandon, DO*, Emma Cardeli, AB, Joan Luby, MD

KEYWORDS

- Preschool • Early childhood • Depression
- Anxiety • Internalizing

The understanding of internalizing disorders in young children has lagged behind advances in our understanding of other areas of psychopathology in this age group. One factor contributing to the relatively slower progress in this domain might be that, as a group, internalizing disorders tend to be viewed as less problematic by parents, teachers, and other caregivers. This may be related to the fact that such disorders are most often characterized by quiet, internal distress sometimes referred to as "intropunitive," rather than overtly, socially negative, or disruptive behavior. Such features may also make these disorders more difficult to detect in the very young who have less well-developed verbal skills in general and specifically an even more limited capacity to describe internal feeling states.

Despite these impediments, a major shift, and advance in this area, has been the study of more discrete differentiated disorders instead of lumping of all internalizing symptoms into one broad category of the two-dimensional internalizing versus externalizing taxonomy of childhood psychopathology. This shift in the conceptualization and categorization of psychopathology, although still an area of considerable debate, has allowed systematic investigation of diagnostic nosologic classifications used in older children and adults and has contributed to our understanding of the differentiation between mood and anxiety disorders in early childhood and differences between preschoolers and school-age children. In older children, some investigations have provided data that dispute this distinction, suggesting that some anxiety disorders (eg, generalized anxiety disorder) should be categorized with major depressive disorder (MDD).[1,2] However, several investigations in young children have supported

Funding for the preparation of this manuscript was provided by the NIMH grant R01 MH 64769-01 to Joan Luby, M.D.
Department of Psychiatry, Washington University School of Medicine, Campus Box 8134, 660 South Euclid, St. Louis, MO 63110, USA
* Corresponding author.
E-mail address: tandonm@psychiatry.wustl.edu (M. Tandon).

Child Adolesc Psychiatric Clin N Am 18 (2009) 593–610
doi:10.1016/j.chc.2009.03.004
1056-4993/09/$ – see front matter © 2009 Elsevier Inc. All rights reserved.

childpsych.theclinics.com

a meaningful distinction between mood and anxiety disorders in general.[3,4] The question of whether to lump or split mood and anxiety disorders, and how to split them in early childhood, remains a relatively empirically unexplored area in need of further study.

The shift to a categorical and more differentiated view of mood and anxiety disorders in early childhood has also created a gap in our ability to link this newer literature to the large and rich older body of literature on young children that used these broader dimensional measures of psychopathology.[5–7] As in other areas of young child psychopathology, the recent development of age-appropriate measures of psychopathology has catalyzed this area of research, with findings moving beyond the traditional two-dimensional taxonomy as offered by the widely used Child Behavior Checklist (CBCL). In addition to the development of new diagnostic measures (in the article by Egger and colleagues, elsewhere this issue), another important advance has been the application of methodologies integral to the assessment of developmental and clinical psychopathology research in young children. This includes the use of observational measures as well as semiprojective or narrative measures and age-adapted (eg, puppet based) interview approaches. Such methods, although potentially elucidating to all forms of early psychopathology, are particularly important for internalizing disorders, where understanding the young child's internal emotional experience is critical to recognizing symptoms.

The Diagnostic and Statistical Manual of Mental Disorders (DSM) taxonomy has included a distinction between mood and anxiety disorders in all of its iterations to date. Since a new iteration of the DSM system is in development, some have argued that mood and anxiety disorders should be lumped across the age span.[8] However, given the well-established need for developmentally sensitive distinctions in this domain,[9] how this applies, or fails to apply, to young children remains unclear and understudied. This issue is an important step toward advancing the treatment of these disorders in early childhood, because it is necessary to have a clear and well-validated nosology before age-appropriate treatments can be designed and tested. A challenge common to diagnosis of any disorder in preschoolers, and highly pertinent to anxiety disorders, remains the limited ability of the child to articulate his or her own internal emotional states reliably. The American Academy of Child And Adolescent Psychiatry Work Group on Research has developed Research Diagnostic Criteria-Preschool Age (RDC-PA)[10] to address such quandaries in diagnosis in this age group. Pertinent to anxiety disorders, the group suggested, for example, modification of criteria so that emphasis would be placed on behavioral *observation* of withdrawal in social situations rather than expressed anxieties. Research examining the validity of these modified criteria for use in the preschool period is inconclusive and ongoing.[11]

Another diagnostic dilemma is the appropriateness of the duration criteria as currently required in DSM-IV for preschoolers. For example, the requirement that social phobia (SP) must persist for at least 6 months may exclude a young child with these symptoms who is significantly impaired.[12,13] For preschoolers, 6 months is an extremely long period of time, representing a high proportion of their lifespan, and, thus, perhaps a developmentally inappropriate criterion. More longitudinal research examining samples of preschoolers with anxiety symptoms is warranted to clarify such diagnostic ambiguities.

Toward this end, this article reviews the current empiric and descriptive database on the nosology and treatment of mood and anxiety disorders in young children, identifying advances and areas in which future studies are needed.

THE BROAD DIMENSION OF INTERNALIZING PSYCHOPATHOLOGY

Although externalizing disorders have received considerably more attention in preschool research in the past, the literature examining internalizing disorders and the pathways that connect the two is a recent development.[9,14–17] Empiric research supports the distinction between these 2 broad categories even as early as infancy.[18] Longitudinal investigations have described the stability of internalizing symptoms even when identified as early as infancy. For example, Briggs-Gowan and colleagues[19] found 1-year internalizing symptom persistence rates of 37.8% in a general population-based birth cohort of toddlers aged 1 to 3 years, and no significant gender differences were found. Preschoolers with internalizing disorders assessed in a general population cohort at ages 2 and 3 years have 3 times the risk for similar internalizing psychopathology 8 years later based on parent interview.[16] Toddler twin studies suggest that genetic factors account for 50% of the variance and shared environment for about 30% of the variance in the internalizing scales of the Infant Toddler Social and Emotional Assessment.[20,21] More recent literature has shown that internalizing children were more prone to sadness and less impulsive compared with those with externalizing disorders in a study of emotionality and "effortful control" as a form of regulation in 4- to 8-year-old children.[14] High levels of effortful control (the ability to suppress a dominant response in favor of exhibiting a less dominant response) appear to be associated with *internalizing* symptoms, or apparent overcontrol, whereas low levels of effortful control are associated with *externalizing* symptoms. Moderate levels of effortful control are associated with more adaptive regulation.[22,23] Consistent with less impulsivity, these children appear behaviorally inhibited, constrained, and prone to internalizing symptoms such as anxiety.[14,24]

Because of the self-directed nature of internalizing symptoms, patterns of reported internalizing symptoms vary by reporter. Longitudinal studies using multiple informants have suggested that fathers' reporting of internalizing symptoms in a child at age 3 years significantly predicted similar symptoms at age 5 years.[25] Other studies have suggested that parents' report, as opposed to teacher report, of internalizing symptoms may better predict observed, internalizing play behavior among preschoolers.[6]

Diagnostic outcomes in internalizing disorders have also been shown to be heterogeneous, and this may be related to the complex comorbidities that can go undetected in the assessment of young children. Along this line, internalizing disorders co-occur with themselves and with externalizing disorders more often than chance would predict.[26,27]

DEPRESSIVE DISORDERS
Major Depressive Disorder

Throughout history, the application of psychiatric diagnoses to preschool-aged children (aged 3–6 years) has been met with a great deal of skepticism and, in some cases, opposition. Diagnoses of clinical depression, in particular, have caused considerable unease. In the 1940s, Spitz provided compelling case reports of depressed affect in infants between the ages of 12 and 18 months.[28] Surprisingly however, there was little investigation of mood disorders in young children for decades after these observations were published. Theoretical literature subsequently refuted the idea that young children were capable of demonstrating depressed affect, believing that preschoolers were too immature to experience complex emotions, such as grief and melancholy.[29] Recent empiric data have disproved this claim, demonstrating that infants and toddlers exhibit a higher level of emotional sophistication than previously recognized.[30,31] Nonetheless, the study of preschool depression remained latent until the 1980s when Kashani and colleagues[32–37] provided evidentiary support for depression in the preschool period. Looking at a sample of schoolchildren in both clinical and community settings, Kashani and colleagues were able to identify a subgroup of preschoolers who met standard DSM-III criteria for MDD. Yet due to the fact that a portion of the sample failed to meet diagnostic criteria although they displayed clinically relevant symptoms,[34] this study raised questions about the use of standard diagnostic criteria, identifying the need for specific, developmentally appropriate diagnostic criteria for application to preschool-aged children.

The recently published "Diagnostic Classification of Mental Health and Development Disorders in Infancy and Early Childhood-Revised" aimed to provide symptom descriptions of depression as they manifest in early childhood.[38] In 2003, the American Academy of Child and Adolescent Psychiatry task force also proposed revisions of DSM criteria for use in future research on preschool psychopathology.[10] Where possible, the task force used empiric evidence to inform the modifications. Preliminary research by Luby and colleagues[39] guided the amendments concerning MDD, which included the addition of a new symptom, "persistent engagement in activities or play themes with death or suicide." Luby's work additionally provided evidence that a stable and specific depressive symptom constellation may develop in preschool children aged 3 years to 5 years and 6 months.[39]

In a controlled study of preschool depression, Luby and colleagues[39] assessed the validity of developmentally translated standard DSM-IV symptoms using a modified version of the Diagnostic Interview Schedule for Children, IV-Young Child (DISC-IV-YC).[40] These modifications included queries on "activities and play" rather than schoolwork, as preschoolers have limited exposure to conventional academic settings; the use of terms such as "sad and unhappy" in the place of "sad and depressed" to better reflect parents' perceptions of their child's mood states; and the framing of questions regarding "preoccupation with death themes and suicidality" around themes of play to account for young children's limited direct verbal capacities and tendency to express such thoughts in the context of play.

The duration criterion was an additional item in need of modification for young children, as research has demonstrated that younger children tended to experience greater variability in mood than older children and adults.[41] Nearly 80% of the preschoolers identified as depressed did not meet the traditional, DSM-IV 2-week duration criterion (as described in the DISC-IV-YC) despite demonstrating multiple markers of depression.[42] As a result, Luby and colleagues proposed a softening (or setting aside) of the DSM duration criteria, requiring only that symptoms be present over a 2-week period, though not necessarily with persistence.

Using these modifications of symptom descriptions and duration criteria, Luby and colleagues were able to identify a subsample of depressed preschoolers in accordance with markers of a valid psychiatric syndrome, as proposed by Robins and Guze.[43] These markers include family history of related disorders, evidence of impairment, biologic markers, and a stable symptom constellation.[39] Despite historical beliefs that younger children are more likely to exhibit masked symptoms (such as "somatization") instead of typical symptoms,[44] Luby and colleagues[45] discovered that typical symptoms occurred at higher rates, and therefore, function as more useful clinical markers of the disorder. Each of the depressive symptoms, with the sole exception of irritability, were found to occur more frequently in depressed preschoolers than in both healthy (no disorder) and psychiatric (meeting criteria for DSM-IV attention-deficit/hyperactivity disorder (ADHD) and/or disruptive disorders) comparison groups. Irritability/sadness (assessed jointly) was found to be the most sensitive symptom, as it was identified in 98% of depressed preschoolers, whereas anhedonia was found to be the most specific, because it was evidenced in solely the depressed group. As would be expected of a valid clinical syndrome, this study reported high internal consistency of depressive symptoms.[45]

Due to its evident specificity, Luby and colleagues[46] later compared the group of depressed preschoolers displaying anhedonia (54% of the depressed sample) to depressed preschoolers without this symptom, as well as to healthy and psychiatric controls, finding that anhedonically depressed preschoolers had the highest depression severity scores of the four subgroups. Furthermore, anhedonically depressed preschoolers evidenced features of depression similar to those exhibited by depressed adults, such as neurovegetative signs, lack of brightening, and alterations in stress cortisol reactivity. These results suggest that anhedonia may be a marker of a more severe, depressive subtype in preschoolers, as has been demonstrated in studies of older children and adults.[47]

Evidence of impairment is also key to the validation of a clinically significant symptom constellation, alhough capturing impairment in preschoolers requires the use of more developmentally sensitive measures due to their reliance on caretakers for daily functioning.[48] As such, Luby and colleagues were able to identify evidence of impairment by focusing on measures of social development, which was determined to best represent a preschooler's overall competence and adaptive functioning. Notably, impairment in social development was found in this sample of depressed preschoolers, as demonstrated by significantly lower scores on the Vineland socialization subscale in comparison with that of healthy controls.[39] Similar to findings of specific cognitive deficits in older children and adults suffering from depression,[49–51] this subsample also showed impairments in cognitive functioning—specifically visual spatial skills. In comparison with healthy controls, preschoolers identified as depressed performed more poorly on a block construction task than healthy controls.[52]

In a larger and more comprehensive second-stage investigation, impairment was assessed using the full Vineland[53] as well as other scales, such as the Preschool and Early Childhood Functional Assessment Scale (PECFAS).[54] This study further replicated and expanded upon previous findings of impairment, evidencing impairment in a sample of depressed preschoolers across multiple domains (all seven PECFAS domains) and according to multiple informants.[4] Notably, in this larger study, there were no significant delays in development overall, as measured by the Vineland.

Although markers such as family history of depression and evidence of impairment are important in establishing the validity of a psychiatric disorder, biologic markers are crucial to understanding the pathophysiology of a disorder, and therefore, to achieving the next level of scientific validity. Toward this end, Luby and colleagues used biologic measures in their study of preschool depression as well. According to research on depression in adulthood conducted by Nemeroff and others, a fundamental element of the pathophysiology, and perhaps to the etiology of depression, is a dysfunctional stress response.[55,56] This finding has been supported by additional research on depressed adults focusing on alterations of the stress response.[57–61] To begin to investigate this issue in preschool children, Luby and colleagues[62] measured salivary cortisol during and subsequent to mildly stressful laboratory tasks. Results showed that depressed preschoolers displayed unique patterns of stress cortisol reactivity when compared with those of healthy controls. Specifically, although healthy controls exhibited a decrease in cortisol levels over the course of the assessment compatible with steady adaptation to the laboratory environment, cortisol levels of depressed preschoolers showed persistent elevations. These findings are the first reported evidence of biologic correlates of preschool depression.

Dysthymic Disorder

Though very little research has been conducted on preschool dysthymic disorder, Kashani and colleagues[63] were able to identify a subsample of clinically referred preschool children using traditional, DSM-IV diagnostic criteria as well as proposed alternative research criteria, supporting the existence of dysthymic disorder in the preschool period. Because it was necessary for preschoolers to meet both traditional and alternative DSM-IV criteria, a conservative approach to diagnosis was used. Furthermore, preschoolers were required to verbally endorse symptoms of irritability and sadness, which, given the limited verbal capacities of preschool-aged children, further restricted criteria for diagnosis. Nevertheless, in a sample of 300 clinically referred preschoolers, 2.7% (n = 8) met criteria for dysthymic disorder. All of these children had a family history of psychiatric disorders. In addition, aggressive behavior and somatic complaints were endorsed by 100% of this subsample. Since dysthymia is generally considered to be a diagnosis associated with less acute morbidity than MDD, it is not surprising that none of the identified, dysthymic preschoolers demonstrated hopelessness, persistent loss of interest, and brooding, all of which are symptoms suggestive of a more depressive subtype. However, if left untreated, it is possible that a more severe syndrome could manifest. As a result, more research in this area is necessary to better understand dysthymic disorder in preschool-aged children.

FAMILY HISTORY AND RISK FACTORS

Depressive disorders are known to be transmitted through both genetic and psychosocial mechanisms—a finding that is evidenced in studies of older children and adults.[64–68] Consistent with this finding, Luby's sample of depressed preschoolers had a greater family history of depression compared with controls, as indicated by data on first- and second-degree relatives obtained from the parent informant.[39] In addition, a recent study that examined the associations between psychopathology in first- and second-generation relatives with behavior problems in the grandchild identified a significant interaction between both grandparental and parental MDD and internalizing symptoms in children aged 24 months, as measured by the CBCL.[69] Furthermore, even in the absence of parental MDD, an association between MDD in the second-generation relative (grandparent) and internalizing problems in the grandchild was still evident. Nonetheless, the presence of MDD in both the grandparental and parental generation did not convey a higher risk for the grandchildren than either risk factor independently.

Interestingly, having a family history of depression has also been shown to be associated with alterations in brain activity known in depression, as evidenced by frontal EEG asymmetries detected in depressed mothers and their newborns.[70] In previous studies examining EEG asymmetry in depressed adults, depressed subjects demonstrated decreased left-sided frontal activation in comparison with healthy controls.[71,72] Additional research has shown that frontal EEG asymmetry is related to affect processing in both infants and adults,[73,74] such that right-frontal EEG activation is associated with negative affect, and left-frontal EEG activation is associated with positive affect. Consistent with this idea, numerous studies have shown greater right-frontal EEG asymmetry in infants of depressed mothers, suggesting a relationship between asymmetries in frontal lobe activation and infants' display of negative emotions.[75–77] Behavioral differences observed in naturalistic, dyadic interactions between depressed mothers and their newborns have also been linked to decreased left-frontal EEG activation in infants;[76] an interesting finding as infants characteristically display greater activation in the left-frontal area during pleasurable interactions.[78]

These atypical patterns of brain activity generalized to positive interactions with nondepressed strangers as well,[76] although it remains unknown whether similar patterns of brain activity would be noted in interactions between infants of depressed mothers and other caregivers. Nevertheless, due to the fact that the frontal region plays such a crucial role in mediating emotional behavior in infants,[79] these findings have interesting implications for frontal EEG asymmetry as a possible risk marker for high negative affect later in life.

PROGNOSIS

Since the investigation of preschool-onset mood disorders is relatively new, there is little information regarding the stability and course of preschool depression into later childhood and adolescence. The population prevalence of preschool depression also remains somewhat ambiguous due to lack of clinical variability in diagnosing the disorder.[80] However, a recent epidemiologic study conducted by Egger and colleagues[81] reported a prevalence rate of 1.4% for MDD, 0.7% for depression not otherwise specified, and 0.6% for dysthymia, based on parent report of symptoms. Earlier studies have shown stability of general, preschool-onset psychopathology over a 4-year period.[82] Luby and colleagues[39] have reported that preschool depression was stable over a 6-month follow-up period. This is especially noteworthy because difficulties exhibited during the preschool period are commonly regarded as transient despite growing evidence to the contrary.[83,84] New findings demonstrating the 2-year stability and homotypic continuity of preschool-onset depression in the context of a remitting and relapsing course have recently become available as well, indicating that preschool depression is neither a transient, nor a nonspecific, early condition (J. Luby and colleagues, unpublished data, in press). Notably, 57% of depressed preschoolers had at least one recurrence of depression in the 2-year follow-up period, whereas 18% evidenced a persistent course over the 2 years.

Due to societal expectations of the preschool period as one in which positive emotion is high and emotional suffering is not experienced under normal conditions, it is difficult for many to accept the idea that depression could arise during this "carefree" time. Furthermore, at an age in which wide variations in behavior and emotional expression frequently arise and are often ephemeral, some express concern that applying psychiatric diagnoses to preschoolers may pathologize normative behavioral extremes. In spite of these misconceptions and ambiguities, empiric research has shown that preschoolers can meet criteria for clinical depression and show significant impairment in functioning related to the depressive symptoms. Although slight modifications to the diagnostic criteria were necessary, Luby and colleagues[39] were able to identify a sample of depressed preschoolers who displayed several markers of a valid psychiatric syndrome. The modifications include the incorporation of play themes in questions regarding preoccupation with death and suicidality and alterations of standard duration criterion. Additionally, data from two independent samples have now shown that depressed preschoolers exhibited typical symptoms of depression more frequently than masked symptoms;[45] this is an important finding given traditional beliefs that younger children are incapable of displaying the typical symptoms evidenced in adults.[44] This was noted in anhedonically depressed preschoolers in particular, who exhibited more acute features of depression comparable to those known in anhedonically depressed adults.[46] As a result, it is possible that anhedonia may be an indicator of a more severe, depressive subtype in preschool-aged children as well. Given these findings, it is clear that preschoolers may experience clinically significant depression that warrants clinical attention. Yet to better identify, diagnose, and treat preschool depression, more research in this area is needed with the aim of applying earlier and potentially more efficacious treatment interventions.

ANXIETY DISORDERS
Distinguishing Between Normative and Pathologic Fears

Anxiety symptoms have long been recognized in preschool-age children. Multiple early longitudinal epidemiologic studies have demonstrated that it is not uncommon for preschoolers to have fears in general, but most notably, fears of the dark and fears of animals.[85–88] In decreasing order of prevalence, common fears include fear of noises, strange situations, pain or sensory novelties, heights, animals, and sudden changes. Fears of physical injury are also prominent among preschool children.[89] Although some fears are normative and transient in development, it is now known that other anxiety patterns can be distressing and impairing to preschoolers and their families, persist, worsen in severity, and are associated with additional comorbidities in later childhood.[90] The degree of impairment, distress, uncontrollability, pervasiveness, and persistence all may help to distinguish between normative development and psychopathology.[12]

Diagnosing Discrete DSM-IV Anxiety Disorders

The DSM-IV categorizes anxiety disorders into multiple discrete categories, including separation anxiety disorder (SAD), SP, obsessive-compulsive disorder (OCD), and generalized anxiety disorder (GAD). Panic disorder is thought to occur more commonly in older children and adults with onset at puberty, and, therefore, is rarely observed in early childhood.[91–93] Posttraumatic stress disorder (PTSD) is also an anxiety disorder well known during the preschool period and more extensively studied to date. Consequently, it is covered separately in this special issue (see the article by Coates and Gaensbauer, elsewhere this issue). The question of whether GAD and SAD represent truly discrete and separable disorders in the preschool period remains largely uninvestigated. Both disorders have been suggested as loading onto one broader *anxiety* factor in the preschool period.[89] Other emerging research suggests that anxiety should continue to be studied as separate, distinct disorders, as specificity has been observed in very young children, and each disorder may necessitate a distinct treatment.[90,94]

A confirmatory factor analysis using current DSM-IV nosology suggested that preschool anxiety symptoms could be differentiated into five dimensions: GAD, SAD, social anxiety, obsessive compulsive symptoms, and fears, supporting the notion that anxiety disorders are distinct even as early as the preschool period.[89,94] This notion was further supported in a larger study (n = 1073) of preschoolers from a pediatric clinic, which found "emotional syndromes" differentiated into three factors: MDD/GAD, SAD, and SP.[3] OCD and PTSD were excluded from the analyses due to limited numbers of subjects with these disorders within the larger sample.[3] Sterba and colleagues[3] concluded that anxiety disorders are not undifferentiated despite this young age and that the use of DSM-IV in preschoolers is as applicable and valid as its use in older children. These findings from a confirmatory factor analysis provide support for the idea that anxiety disorders be studied as discrete disorders rather than as a broader group in the preschool period.[3] Despite such diagnostic challenges, one epidemiologic study of preschoolers estimated the prevalence of anxiety disorders defined by the RDC criteria as 9.4% in a primary care setting.[95] This need for specificity in diagnosis, even if for purposes of treatment, is well illustrated by the example of selective mutism. Although not incorporated in anxiety disorders according to

DSM-IV, the diagnosis of selective mutism (listed under the category of "disorders usually first diagnosed in early childhood") has been associated with familial anxiety disorders, has a unique and highly specific symptom constellation, and may warrant unique treatment,[96–98] as in OCD. Studies and clinical reports of OCD are rare overall in the extant preschool literature; however, the level of impairment in functioning and internal distress associated with these symptoms cannot be underestimated.

Diagnostic Continuity

Although many fears arising in early childhood may indeed be developmentally normative, children exhibiting impairing clinically significant anxiety disorders have been shown to have persisting disorders and are at risk for the development of comorbid conditions.[99,100] Many longitudinal studies of anxiety have included some preschoolers as part of older samples. Although these data are of interest, studies focusing on preschool-age samples may better inform the longitudinal course of preschool-onset anxiety disorders.[82]

Comorbidity

Anxiety is often accompanied by comorbid disorders in the preschool period. Most often, anxiety disorders co-occur with other anxiety disorders, followed by depression, ADHD, oppositional defiant disorder, and conduct disorder.[12] Comorbidity rates in an epidemiologic study in primary care centers were reported highest for specific phobia (100%), SAD (79%), selective mutism (59%), SP (55%) and GAD (53%).[12]

FAMILY HISTORY AND RISK FACTORS / EARLY PRECURSORS OF ANXIETY

In the general population, anxiety disorders have been shown to be at least partly familial with varying genetic transmission.[94,101,102] For example, studies examining parents of children with *selective mutism* (mentioned above) found 37% to have lifetime social anxiety compared with 14% of control parents.[97] In addition, a myriad of psychosocial risks in the preschool period have been correlated to later-onset anxiety symptoms and disorders. Empiric literature underscores the higher risks of developing an anxiety disorder in offspring of parents with anxiety and children who exhibit early behavioral inhibition (BI). Another potential contributor may be environmental *fostering of avoidance*, a phrase that refers to situations in which caregivers discourage (or might not encourage) exploration of novel situations or stimuli. This pattern could potentially be targeted for early intervention and prevention of later-onset anxiety disorders.[103,104] Parenting style is commonly suggested as another risk factor for the development of anxiety. However, it accounted for only 4% of the variance in childhood anxiety in a meta-analysis of studies focusing on the role of parenting.[105]

The developmental psychopathology literature has contributed studies of temperament, namely, BI, as it relates to later anxiety disorders.[106,107] BI is a term originally used by Jerome Kagan[106] to describe how a child retreats from a novel situation or stimuli, withdraws, and seeks to remain near the caregiver. Further, BI has also been described as fearfulness exhibited with new people or in new situations.[108] Children with high levels of BI have been shown to have concomitant anxiety disorders;[109] to exhibit unique biologic markers;[107] and to develop higher rates of anxiety disorders in the future. These findings have suggested that BI may be a precursor of later anxiety disorders warranting continued investigation.[90,110] More specifically, BI at 21 months and 6 years of age in the high-risk offspring of parents with affective disorders predicted social anxiety disorder, but no other anxiety disorder 5 years later at follow-up when compared with uninhibited children at baseline (odds ratio, 3.15;

95% CI, 1.16–8.57).[108] Therefore, BI may be a predictor of specific anxiety disorders, most notably, social anxiety disorder and, thus, may be a target for early intervention.[108]

TREATMENT AND PROGNOSIS

Although approximately 60% of parents with preschoolers with anxiety disorders thought they needed help, only 10% reported having been referred for mental health evaluation despite this perceived need.[12] To date, there exists no gold standard or empirically proven treatment for any preschool anxiety disorder other than trauma-related anxiety disorders.[111] Current treatments in use in clinical settings include medication, psychoeducation, and psychosocial and psychotherapeutic treatments, although current empiric support is limited. For example, the extant literature suggests that the number of antidepressant prescriptions given to preschoolers has risen, although their specific indications, efficacy, and safety in long-term studies remain untested.[112] Treatment studies of children with anxiety disorders have specifically included younger children, but caution is still warranted in extrapolation to preschoolers (The Pediatric OCD Treatment Study Team, 2004). For example, three cases of preschool-age-onset OCD, including varied symptoms and signs of contamination fears, repeated hand-washing, and even intrusive thoughts related to being pregnant, have been reported with clinically severe Children's Yale-Brown Obsessive Compulsive Scale[113] scores. These cases were all treated with selective serotonin reuptake inhibitors (SSRIs) as well as augmentation with risperidone with at least temporary remission of symptoms and impairment.[114] In our own clinic, a preschooler with intrusive, obsessional thoughts became suicidal due to the high level of distress these symptoms caused. Due to the paucity of literature on the treatment of preschool disorders overall, and anxiety disorders such as OCD in particular, treatments are often extrapolated from those with proven efficacy over placebo in older children such as the use of SSRIs for OCD.[115] Such extrapolations warrant caution and underscore the need for investigations of preschool-age-specific treatments in anxiety disorders.

A number of educational therapies have been investigated to target early onset BI in the preschool-age group.[104] One intervention, for example, included six teaching sessions for the parents of preschoolers who exhibited BI and withdrawn behaviors. These six, 90-minute educational sessions incorporated psychoeducation on development of anxiety, overprotection and maintenance behaviors, high-risk periods, parent management techniques, gradual exposure techniques, and cognitive restructuring of parental worry. Preschoolers whose parents received this education were compared at 12 months to those preschoolers whose parents did not. Preschoolers whose parents received the educational sessions were less likely to receive an anxiety diagnosis at 12 months posttreatment.[116]

Several variants of cognitive behavioral therapy have been used to target younger children with anxiety disorders as in PTSD,[117,118] but the empiric support is limited overall for other disorders.[119] Also ongoing are investigations of adaptations of Parent Child Interaction Therapy[120,121] validated in preschoolers with disruptive disorders to target those with anxiety disorders.[122]

In addition to medication and other psychotherapies, dyadic play therapy remains the key modality for preschool children in general, although specific studies supporting its efficacy for anxiety disorders are currently lacking. Dyadic play therapy provides opportunities to master fears through play as well as opportunities for scaffolding positive parent-child interactions.[123–125]

EXAMPLE OF A CASE OF AN ANXIOUS/DEPRESSED PRESCHOOLER

L.K. is a 4.5-year-old who first presented to the clinic for symptoms of excessive worry. He worried that his mother would die if he separated from her to attend preschool; he cried excessively and daily at school such that the mother was frequently called to pick him up, affecting her ability to sustain a job. On the few days he stayed at school, he complained of stomachaches to the school nurse, and no medical etiology was found. At night, he could not fall asleep, because he feared that his mother would be taken away by a monster. He began to sulk, and no longer enjoyed playing with the neighborhood children, an activity he once enjoyed. Instead, he insisted on being in physical proximity to his mother, never letting her leave his sight without crying intensely. His affect became globally sad. When in the company of any other caregiver, he would incessantly ask of his mother's safety. Had she died? Was she safe?

There were no reports of developmental delays, abuse, medical illnesses, or other traumas; however, of interest, was a family history of GAD. L.K. was referred for dyadic psychotherapy and responded well to systematic desensitization and exposure to a series of gradual and increasing amounts of time away from his mother without asking for reassurance of her safety. In addition, his mother was coached on how to enact separations more effectively and reassure him that they would be tolerated by both. He was able to resume full-day preschool after several months of therapy.

SUMMARY

It is clear that significant progress has been made in the understanding, validation, and differentiation of internalizing disorders (which include both mood and anxiety disorders) in the preschool period. Advancing earlier models of psychopathology that addressed internalizing symptoms in a global and undifferentiated fashion, the empiric evidence now supports the need to use more nuanced and specific diagnostic distinctions in this domain in young children. Advances in research methodologies that have facilitated the ability to capture young children's internal feeling states, as well as to quantify and interpret observed behavior from which mood and affect can be inferenced, have catalyzed progress in this area. However, as this article elucidates, much work remains to be done in all internalizing disorders in young children. In depression, although there is an emerging body of work validating and describing the disorder in early childhood, further work clarifying the nosology and developing age-appropriate treatments is now needed. In the area of anxiety disorders, there remains a relative paucity of data validating and defining the disorders as they manifest in the preschool period. Along this line, it remains unclear how to differentiate and whether and how to lump or split specific early onset anxiety disorders. At the same time, basic developmental studies have identified early risk factors for later anxiety disorders, which may be helpful to direct studies focused on the definition of internalizing disorders in the preschool period.

REFERENCES

1. Hankin BL, Fraley RC, Lahey BB, et al. Is depression best viewed as a continuum or discrete category? A taxometric analysis of childhood and adolescent depression in a population-based sample. J Abnorm Psychol 2005;114(1):96–110.
2. Lahey BB, Applegate B, Waldman ID, et al. The structure of child and adolescent psychopathology: generating new hypotheses. J Abnorm Psychol 2004;113(3):358–85.

3. Sterba S, Egger HL, Angold A. Diagnostic specificity and nonspecificity in the dimensions of preschool psychopathology. J Child Psychol Psychiatry 2007; 48(10):1005–13.

4. Luby JL, Belden AC, Pautsch J, et al. The clinical significance of preschool depression: Impairment in functioning and clinical markers of the disorder. J Affect Disord 2009;112(1–3):111–9.

5. Achenbach TM, Edelbrock C, Howell CT. Empirically based assessment of the behavioral/emotional problems of 2- and 3- year-old children. J Abnorm Child Psychol 1987;15(4):629–50.

6. Hinshaw SP, Han SS, Erhardt D, et al. Internalizing and externalizing behavior problems in preschool children: correspondence among parent and teacher ratings and behavior observations. J Clin Child Psychol 1992;21(2):143–50.

7. Shaw DS, Keenan K, Vondra JI, et al. Antecedents of preschool children's internalizing problems: a longitudinal study of low-income families. J Am Acad Child Adolesc Psychiatry 1997;36(12):1760–7.

8. Clark LA, Watson D. Distress and fear disorders: an alternative empirically based taxonomy of the "mood" and "anxiety" disorders. Br J Psychiatry 2006;189: 481–3.

9. Zahn-Waxler C, Klimes-Dougan B, Slattery MJ. Internalizing problems of childhood and adolescence: prospects, pitfalls, and progress in understanding the development of anxiety and depression. Dev Psychopathol 2000;12(3):443–66.

10. The Task Force on Research Diagnostic Criteria: infancy and Preschool. Research diagnostic criteria for infants and preschool children: the process and empirical support. J Am Acad Child Adolesc Psychiatry 2003;42(12):1504–12.

11. Warren SL, Umylny P, Aron E, et al. Toddler anxiety disorders: a pilot study. J Am Acad Child Adolesc Psychiatry 2006;45(7):862–6.

12. Egger HL, Angold A. Anxiety disorders. In: Luby JL, editor. Handbook of preschool mental health. New York, London: Guilford Press; 2006. p. 137–64.

13. Warren SL. Anxiety disorders. In: DelCarmen-Wiggins R, Carter A, editors. Handbook of infant, toddler, and preschool mental health assessment. New York: Oxford University Press; 2004. p. 355–76.

14. Eisenberg N, Cumberland A, Spinrad TL, et al. The relations of regulation and emotionality to children's externalizing and internalizing problem behavior. Child Dev 2001;72:1112–34.

15. Mesman J, Bongers IL, Koot HM. Preschool developmental pathways to preadolescent internalizing and externalizing problems. J Child Psychol Psychiatry 2001;42(5):679–89.

16. Mesman J, Koot HM. Early preschool predictors of preadolescent internalizing and externalizing DSM-IV diagnoses. J Am Acad Child Adolesc Psychiatry 2001;40(9):1029–36.

17. Thomas JM, Guskin KA. Disruptive behavior in young children: what does it mean? J Am Acad Child Adolesc Psychiatry 2001;40(1):44–51.

18. Keenan K, Shaw D, Delliquadri E, et al. Evidence for the continuity of early problem behaviors: application of a developmental model. J Abnorm Child Psychol 1998;26(6):441–52.

19. Briggs-Gowan MJ, Carter AS, Bosson-Heenan J, et al. Are infant-toddler social-emotional and behavioral problems transient? J Am Acad Child Adolesc Psychiatry 2006;45(7):849–58.

20. Carter AS, Briggs-Gowan MJ, Jones SM, et al. The infant–toddler social and emotional assessment (ITSEA): factor structure, reliability, and validity. J Abnorm Child Psychol 2003;31(5):495–514.

21. Carter AS, Briggs-Gowan MJ. Manual for the infant-toddler social and emotional assessment. San Antonio (TX); 2006.
22. Murray KT, Kochanska G. Effortful control: factor structure and relation to external-izing and internalizing behaviors. J Abnorm Child Psychol 2002;30(5):503–14.
23. Rothbart MK, Bates JE. Temperament. In: Eisenberg N, editor. 5th edition, Hand-book of child psychology, vol. 3: social, emotional and personality development New York: Wiley 1998. p. 105–76.
24. Kagan J, Snidman N, Zentner M, et al. Infant temperament and anxious symp-toms in school age children. Dev Psychopathol 1999;11(2):209–24.
25. Kerr DC, Lunkenheimer ES, Olson SL. Assessment of child problem behaviors by multiple informants: a longitudinal study from preschool to school entry. J Child Psychol Psychiatry 2007;48(10):967–75.
26. Caron C, Rutter M. Comorbidity in child psychopathology: concepts, issues and research strategies. J Child Psychol Psychiatry 1991;32(7):1063–80.
27. Keiley MK, Lofthouse N, Bates JE, et al. Differential risks of covarying and pure components in mother and teacher reports of externalizing and internalizing behavior across ages 5 to 14. J Abnorm Child Psychol 2003;31(3):267–83.
28. Spitz R. Anaclitic depression: an inquiry into the genesis of psychiatric condi-tions in early childhood. Psychoanal Study Child 1946;1:47–53.
29. Rie HE. Depression in childhood. A survey of some pertinent contributions. J Am Acad Child Psychiatry 1966;5(4):653–85.
30. Denham SA. Emotional development in young children. New York: Guilford Press; 1998.
31. Shonkoff JP, Phillips D. From neurons to neighborhoods: the science of early childhood development. Washington, DC: National Academy Press; 2000.
32. Kashani JH, Ray JS. Depressive related symptoms among preschool-age chil-dren. Child Psychiatry Hum Dev 1983;13(4):233–8.
33. Kashani JH, Holcomb WR, Orvaschel H. Depression and depressive symptoms in preschool children from the general population. Am J Psychiatry 1986;143(9): 1138–43.
34. Kashani JH, Horwitz E, Ray JS, et al. DSM-III diagnostic classification of 100 preschoolers in a child development unit. Child Psychiatry Hum Dev 1986; 16(3):137–47.
35. Kashani JH, Carlson GA. Seriously depressed preschoolers. Am J Psychiatry 1987;144(3):348–50.
36. Kashani JH, Ray JS. Major depression with delusional features in a preschool-age child. J Am Acad Child Adolesc Psychiatry 1987;26(1):110–2.
37. Kashani JH, Carlson GA. Major depressive disorder in a preschooler. J Am Acad Child Psychiatry 1985;24(4):490–4.
38. Zero To Three. Diagnostic classification of mental health and developmental disorders of infancy and early childhood. revised edition (DC:0–3R). Washing-ton, DC: Zero To Three Press; 2005.
39. Luby J, Heffelfinger A, Mrakeotsky C, et al. Preschool major depressive disorder: preliminary validation for developmentally modified DSM-IV criteria. J Am Acad Child Adolesc Psychiatry 2002;41(8):928–37.
40. Shaffer D, Fisher P, Lucas CP. Diagnostic interview schedule for children, version IV [manual]. New York: Division of Psychiatry, Columbia University; 1998.
41. Geller B, Zimerman B, Williams M, et al. Diagnostic characteristics of 93 cases of a prepubertal and early adolescent bipolar disorder phenotype by gender, puberty and comorbid attention deficit hyperactivity disorder. J Child Adolesc Psychopharmacol 2000;10(3):157–64.

42. Luby JL, Mrakotsky C, Heffelfinger A, et al. Modification of DSM-IV criteria for depressed preschool children. Am J Psychiatry 2003;160(6):1169–72.
43. Robins E, Guze SB. Establishment of diagnostic validity in psychiatric illness: its application to schizophrenia. Am J Psychiatry 1970;126(7):983–7.
44. Lesse S. Masked depression. Curr Psychiatr Ther 1983;22:81–7.
45. Luby JL, Heffelfinger AK, Mrakotsky C, et al. The clinical picture of depression in preschool children. J Am Acad Child Adolesc Psychiatry 2003;42(3):340–8.
46. Luby JL, Mrakotsky C, Heffelfinger A, et al. Characteristics of depressed preschoolers with and without anhedonia: evidence for a melancholic depressive subtype in young children. Am J Psychiatry 2004;161(11):1998–2004.
47. Klein DF. Endogenomorphic depression. Arch Gen Psychiatry 1974;31:447–54.
48. Carter AS, Briggs-Gowan MJ, Davis NO. Assessment of young children's social-emotional development and psychopathology: recent advances and recommendations for practice. J Child Psychol Psychiatry 2004;45(1):109–34.
49. Asthana HS, Mandal MK, Khurana H, et al. Visuospatial and affect recognition deficit in depression. J Affect Disord 1998;48(1):57–62.
50. Blumberg SH, Izard CE. Affective and cognitive characteristics of depression in 10- and 11-year-old children. J Pers Soc Psychol 1985;49(1):194–202.
51. McClure E, Rogeness GA, Thompson NM. Characteristics of adolescent girls with depressive symptoms in a so-called "normal" sample. J Affect Disord 1997;42(2–3):187–97.
52. Mrakotsky C. Visual perception, spatial cognition and affect recognition in preschool depressive syndromes [doctoral thesis]. Vienna/St. Louis (MO): Vienna University and Washington University; 2001.
53. Sparrow S, Carter AS, Cicchetti D. Vineland screener: overview, reliability, validity, administration and scoring. New Haven (CT): Department of Psychology, Yale University; 1987.
54. Hodges K. The Preschool and early childhood functional assessment scale (PEC-FAS). Ypsilanti (MI): Department of Psychology, Eastern Michigan University; 1994.
55. Nemeroff C. Neurobiological consequences of childhood trauma. J Clin Psychiatry 2004;65(Suppl 1):18–28.
56. Katz RJ, Roth KA, Carroll BJ. Acute and chronic stress effects on open field activity in the rat: implications for a model of depression. Neurosci Biobehav Rev 1981;5(2):247–51.
57. Rubin RT, Poland RE, Lesser IM, et al. Neuroendocrine aspects of primary endogenous depression–IV. Pituitary-thyroid axis activity in patients and matched control subjects. Psychoneuroendocrinology 1987;12(5):333–47.
58. Plotsky PM, Owens MJ, Nemeroff CB. Psychoneuroendocrinology of depression. Psychiatr Clin North Am 1998;21:293–307.
59. Stokes PE, Stoll PM, Koslow SH, et al. Pretreatment DST and hypothalamic-pituitary-adrenocortical function in depressed patients and comparison groups. A multicenter study. Arch Gen Psychiatry 1984;41(3):257–67.
60. Sachar EJ, Hellman L, Roffwarg HP, et al. Disrupted 24-hour patterns of cortisol secretion in psychotic depression. Arch Gen Psychiatry 1973;28(1):19–24.
61. Halbreich U, Asnis GM, Shindledecker R, et al. Cortisol secretion in endogenous depression. I. Basal plasma levels. Arch Gen Psychiatry 1985;42(9):904–8.
62. Luby JL, Heffelfinger A, Mrakotsky C, et al. Alterations in stress cortisol reactivity in depressed preschoolers relative to psychiatric and no-disorder comparison groups. Arch Gen Psychiatry 2003;60(12):1248–55.
63. Kashani JH, Allan WD, Beck NC Jr, et al. Dysthymic disorder in clinically referred preschool children. J Am Acad Child Adolesc Psychiatry 1997;36(10):1426–33.

64. Jaffee SR, Moffitt TE, Caspi A, et al. Differences in early childhood risk factors for juvenile-onset and adult-onset depression. Arch Gen Psychiatry 2002;59(3): 215–22.

65. Neuman RJ, Geller B, Rice JP, et al. Increased prevalence and earlier onset of mood disorders among relatives of prepubertal versus adult probands. J Am Acad Child Adolesc Psychiatry 1997;36(4):466–73.

66. Goodman SH, Gotlib IH. Risk for psychopathology in the children of depressed mothers: A developmental model for understanding mechanisms of transmission. Psychol Rev 1999;106:458–90.

67. Downey G, Coyne JC. Children of depressed parents: an integrative review. Psychol Bull 1990;108(1):50–76.

68. Weissman MM, Wickramaratne P, Nomura Y, et al. Families at high and low risk for depression: a 3-generation study. Arch Gen Psychiatry 2005;62(1):29–36.

69. Olino TM, Pettit JW, Klein DN, et al. Influence of parental and grandparental major depressive disorder on behavior problems in early childhood: a three-generation study. J Am Acad Child Adolesc Psychiatry 2008;47(1):53–60.

70. Field T, Diego M. Maternal depression effects on infant frontal EEG asymmetry. Int J Neurosci 2008;118(8):1081–108.

71. Schaffer CE, Davidson RJ, Saron C. Frontal and parietal electroencephalogram asymmetry in depressed and nondepressed subjects. Biol Psychiatry 1983; 18(7):753–62.

72. Henriques JB, Davidson RJ. Left frontal hypoactivation in depression. J Abnorm Psychol 1991;100(4):535–45.

73. Davidson RJ, Fox NA. Asymmetrical brain activity discriminates between positive and negative affective stimuli in human infants. Science 1982;218(4578):1235–7.

74. Davidson RJ, Ekman P, Saron CD, et al. Approach-withdrawal and cerebral asymmetry: emotional expression and brain physiology. I. J Pers Soc Psychol 1990;58(2):330–41.

75. Jones NA, Field T, Fox NA, et al. Newborns of mothers with depressive symptoms are physiologically less developed. Infant Behav Dev 1998;21(3):537–41.

76. Dawson G, Frey K, Panagiotides H, et al. Infants of depressed mothers exhibit atypical frontal electrical brain activity during interactions with mother and with a familiar, nondepressed adult. Child Dev 1999;70(5):1058–66.

77. Field T, Diego M, Dieter J, et al. Prenatal depression effects on the fetus and the newborn. Infant Behav Dev 2004;27(2):216–29.

78. Dawson G, Klinger LG, Panagiotides H, et al. Frontal lobe activity and affective behavior of infants of mothers with depressive symptoms. Child Dev 1992;63(3): 725–37.

79. Dawson G, Panagiotides H, Klinger LG, et al. The role of frontal lobe functioning in the development of infant self-regulatory behavior. Brain Cogn 1992;20(1):152–75.

80. Stalets MM, Luby JL. Preschool depression. Child Adolesc Psychiatr Clin N Am 2006;15(4):899–917, viii–ix.

81. Egger HL, Erkanli A, Keeler G, et al. Test-retest reliability of the preschool age psychiatric assessment (PAPA). J Am Acad Child Adolesc Psychiatry 2006; 45(5):538–49.

82. Lavigne JV, Arend R, Rosenbaum D, et al. Psychiatric disorders with onset in the preschool years: I. Stability of diagnoses. J Am Acad Child Adolesc Psychiatry 1998;37(12):1246–54.

83. Campbell SB, Shaw DS, Gilliom M. Early externalizing behavior problems: toddlers and preschoolers at risk for later maladjustment. Dev Psychopathol 2000;12(3):467–88.

84. Campbell S. Behavior problems in preschool children: a review of recent research. J Child Psychol Psychiatry 1995;36(1):113–49.

85. Earls F. Prevalence of behavior problems in 3-year-old children. A cross-national replication. Arch Gen Psychiatry 1980;37(10):1153–7.

86. Macfarlane JW, Allen L, Honzik MP. A developmental study of the behavior problems of normal children between twenty-one months and fourteen years. Publ Child Dev Univ Calif 1954;2:1–222.

87. Richman N, Stevenson J, Graham P. Prevalence of behavior problems in 3-year-old children: an epidemiological study in a London Borough. J Child Psychol Psychiatry 1975;16(4):277–87.

88. Richman N, Stevenson J, Graham P. Preschool to school: a behavioural study. London: Academic Press; 1982.

89. Spence SH, Rapee R, McDonald C, et al. The structure of anxiety symptoms among preschoolers. Behav Res Ther 2001;39(11):1293–316.

90. Warren S. Diagnosis of anxiety disorders in infants, toddlers, and preschool children. In: Narrow W, First M, Sirovatka P, et al, editors. Age and gender considerations in psychiatric diagnosis: a research agenda for DSM-V. Arlington (VA): American Psychological Association; 2007. p. 201–14.

91. Costello EJ, Egger HL, Angold A. The developmental epidemiology of anxiety disorders: phenomenology, prevalence, and comorbidity. Child Adolesc Psychiatr Clin N Am 2005;14(4):631–48, vii.

92. Birmaher B, Ollendick TH. Childhood-onset panic disorder. In: Ollendick TH, March JS, editors. Phobic and anxiety disorders in children & adolescents: a clinician's guide to effective psychosocial and pharmacological interventions. New York: Oxford University Press; 2004. p. 303–33.

93. Hayward C, Killen JD, Hammer LD, et al. Pubertal stage and panic attack history in sixth- and seventh-grade girls. Am J Psychiatry 1992;149(9):1239–43.

94. Eley T, Bolton D, O'Conner T, et al. A twin study of anxiety-related behaviors in preschool children. J Child Psychol Psychiatry 2003;44(7):945–60.

95. Egger HL, Angold A. Common emotional and behavioral disorders in preschool children: presentation, nosology, and epidemiology. J Child Psychol Psychiatry 2006;47(3–4):313.

96. Anstendig KD. Is selective mutism an anxiety disorder? Rethinking its DSM-IV classification. J Anxiety Disord 1999;13(4):417–34.

97. Chavira DA, Shipon-Blum E, Hitchcock C, et al. Selective mutism and social anxiety disorder: all in the family? J Am Acad Child Adolesc Psychiatry 2007; 46(11):1464–72.

98. Vecchio JL, Kearney CA. Selective mutism in children: comparison to youths with and without anxiety disorders. J Psychopathol Behav Assess 2005;27(1): 31–7.

99. Cole DA, Peeke LG, Martin JM, et al. A longitudinal look at the relation between depression and anxiety in children and adolescents. J Consult Clin Psychol 1998;66(3):451–60.

100. Woodward LJ, Fergusson DM. Life course outcomes of young people with anxiety disorders in adolescence. J Am Acad Child Adolesc Psychiatry 2001; 40(9):1086–93.

101. Biederman J, Faraone SV, Hirshfeld-Becker DR, et al. Patterns of psychopathology and dysfunction in high-risk children of parents with panic disorder and major depression. Am J Psychiatry 2001;158(1):49–57.

102. Hettema JM, Neale MC, Kendler KS. A review and meta-analysis of the genetic epidemiology of anxiety disorders. Am J Psychiatry 2001;158(10):1568–78.

103. Hirshfeld-Becker DR, Micco JA, Simoes NA, et al. High risk studies and developmental antecedents of anxiety disorders. Am J Med Genet C Semin Med Genet 2008;148(2):99–117.
104. Rapee RM. The development and modification of temperamental risk for anxiety disorders: prevention of a lifetime of anxiety? Biol Psychiatry 2002;52(10):947–57.
105. McLeod BD, Wood JJ, Weisz JR. Examining the association between parenting and childhood anxiety: a meta-analysis. Clin Psychol Rev 2007;27(2):155–72.
106. Kagan J. Galen's prophecy: temperament in human nature. New York: Basic Books; 1994.
107. Rothbart MK, Ahadi SA, Hershey KL, et al. Investigations of temperament at three to seven years: the children's behavior questionnaire. Child Dev 2001; 72(5):1394–408.
108. Hirshfeld-Becker DR, Biederman J, Henin A, et al. Behavioral inhibition in preschool children at risk is a specific predictor of middle childhood social anxiety: a five-year follow-up. J Dev Behav Pediatr 2007;28(3):225–33.
109. Biederman J, Hirshfeld-Becker DR, Rosenbaum JF, et al. Further evidence of association between behavioral inhibition and social anxiety in children. Am J Psychiatry 2001;158(10):1673–9.
110. Schwartz CE, Snidman N, Kagan J. Adolescent social anxiety as an outcome of inhibited temperament in childhood. J Am Acad Child Adolesc Psychiatry 1999; 38(8):1008–15.
111. Lieberman AF, Van Horn P, Ippen CG. Toward evidence-based treatment: child-parent psychotherapy with preschoolers exposed to marital violence. J Am Acad Child Adolesc Psychiatry 2005;44(12):1241–8.
112. Zito J, Safer D, dosReis S, et al. Trends in the prescribing of psychotropic medications to preschoolers. JAMA 2000;283(8):1025–30.
113. Scahill L, Riddle MA, McSwiggin-Hardin M, et al. Children's Yale-Brown obsessive compulsive scale: reliability and validity. J Am Acad Child Adolesc Psychiatry 1997;36(6):844–52.
114. Oner O, Oner P. Psychopharmacology of pediatric obsessive-compulsive disorder: three case reports. J Psychopharmacol 2008;22(7):809–11.
115. Geller DA, Biederman J, Stewart SE, et al. Which SSRI? A meta-analysis of pharmacotherapy trials in pediatric obsessive-compulsive disorder. Am J Psychiatry 2003;160(11):1919–28.
116. Rapee RM, Kennedy S, Ingram M, et al. Prevention and early intervention of anxiety disorders in inhibited preschool children. J Consult Clin Psychol 2005; 73(3):488–97.
117. Scheeringa MS, Salloum A, Arnberger RA, et al. Feasibility and effectiveness of cognitive-behavioral therapy for posttraumatic stress disorder in preschool children: two case reports. J Trauma Stress 2007;20(4):631–6.
118. Cohen JA, Mannarino AP. A treatment outcome study for sexually abused preschool children: initial findings. J Am Acad Child Adolesc Psychiatry 1996;35(1):42–50.
119. Kendall P, Aschenbrand S, Hudson J. Child-focused treatment of anxiety. In: Kazdin A, Weisz J, editors. Evidence-based psychotherapies for children and adolescents. New York: Guilford Press; 2003. p. 81–100.
120. Eyberg SM, Boggs SR, Algina J. Parent-child interaction therapy: a psychosocial model for the treatment of young children with conduct problem behavior and their families. Psychopharmacol Bull 1995;31(1):83–91.
121. Choate ML, Pincus DB, Eyberg SM, et al. Parent-child interaction therapy for treatment of separation anxiety disorder in young children: a pilot study. Cogn Behav Pract 2005;12(1):126–35.

122. Pincus D, Santucci LC, Ehrenrich JT. The implementation of modified parent-child interaction therapy for youth with separation anxiety disorder. Cognitive Behavioral Practice 2008;15:118–25.

123. Benham AL, Slotnick CF. Play therapy: integrating clinical and developmental perspectives. In: Luby J, editor. Handbook of preschool mental health: development, disorders and treatment. New York: Guilford Press; 2006. p. 331–71.

124. Piaget J. Play, dreams, and imitation in childhood. New York: Norton; 1962.

125. Vygotsky LS. Play and its role in the mental development of the child. Soviet Psychology 1967;5(3):6–18.

Event Trauma in Early Childhood: Symptoms, Assessment, Intervention

Susan Coates, PhD[a],*, Theodore J. Gaensbauer, MD[b]

KEYWORDS

- Early childhood • Trauma • Posttraumatic stress disorder
- Attachment • Assessment • Treatment

A traumatic event is an inherently frightening one that threatens the life or bodily integrity of the person experiencing it. Yet for most of the twentieth century, appreciation that traumatic events could have life-shaping consequences for children, and most especially for very young children such as toddlers and infants, was lacking. This situation has now changed radically. Expanding research over the past two decades has not only documented that young children have essentially similar reactions to traumatic events as do adults, including posttraumatic stress disorder (PTSD), anxiety disorders, and depression, but has suggested that PTSD symptoms in young children may be more unremitting than in adults.[1,2] In addition, several large studies[3,4] have demonstrated that traumatic stress in childhood, and even more so, PTSD in childhood, are risk factors for PTSD in adulthood.

Accordingly, it behooves a clinician working with preschoolers, toddlers, and infants to be attuned to the possibility of trauma in the very young child and to understand its typical and atypical symptomatic presentations. The clinician should be able to elicit a sufficiently careful history such that, if present, a trauma and its effects can be recognized, even if parents for a variety of reasons initially fail to report it. The clinician should also have an appreciation of the unique challenges associated with the treatment of early childhood trauma, given young children's limited capacities and the necessity of maintaining and strengthening ties to their primary caretakers.

In what follows, we first describe the classic triad of symptom clusters in PTSD—reexperiencing, numbing and avoidance, and arousal—as they are manifested in very young children. We then identify three factors that differentiate how a trauma is experienced by young children as compared with older children and adults. Finally, we

[a] Department of Psychology in Psychiatry, College of Physicians and Surgeons, Columbia University, 205 West 89th Street, New York, New York
[b] Department of Psychiatry, University of Colorado Health Sciences Center, 3400 E Bayaud Avenue, Suite 460, Denver, Colorado
* Corresponding author.
E-mail address: swcoates@gmail.com (S. Coates).

Child Adolesc Psychiatric Clin N Am 18 (2009) 611–626
doi:10.1016/j.chc.2009.03.005
1056-4993/09/$ – see front matter © 2009 Elsevier Inc. All rights reserved.

outline approaches to the assessment and treatment of the child in collaboration with his or her caretakers. Our discussion is confined to "event traumas," that is, single, temporally isolated, inherently frightening events that entail actual or perceived risk of great harm either to the child or a principle caretaker.

SYMPTOMATIC MANIFESTATIONS OF EARLY TRAUMA
Overview

Understanding the impact of event traumas in early childhood begins with a recognition that very young children show the same three basic categories of posttraumatic symptoms observed in adults, as defined by the Diagnostic and Statistical Manual of Mental Disorders, fourth edition (DSM-IV),[5] that is, re-experiencing, numbing/avoidance, and hyperarousal.[6–8] These three different clusters of symptoms have consistently been shown to represent independent factors in the traumatic response process. There are now more than 50 published case reports of children younger than the age of 4 years documenting the presence of these three basic symptom patterns[9]—making a very strong prima facie case that the underlying biopsychosocial changes seen in young children are comparable to those seen in older children and adults.

Since systematic long-term studies delineating the symptomatic presentations in very young children over time are lacking, descriptive studies have been influential in the development of contemporary diagnostic criteria for very young children.[7,10] In a series of empirical studies of traumatized infants and young children, Scheeringa and colleagues [7,9,11,12] have found that the DSM-IV criteria are not sensitive enough to adequately diagnose PTSD in very young children. Accordingly, alternative diagnostic criteria have been developed, most notably the clinically based criteria used by the Zero to Three Diagnostic Classification of Mental Health and Developmental Disorders of Infancy and Early Childhood, Revised,[13] and the Research Diagnostic Criteria-Preschool Age (RDC-PA) developed by a task force of the American Academy of Child and Adolescent Psychiatry.[14] For example, the RDC criteria for PTSD, which have received strong empirical support, involve modifications of the DSM-IV wording for four items to make them developmentally sensitive to young children (without changing the essence of the symptoms), lowering the number of items required in the numbing/avoidance category from three to one and lowering the number of arousal items from two to one.[7] Developmentally appropriate criteria that these two diagnostic classifications have in common include the following:

1. Re-experiencing of the traumatic event as evidenced by post-traumatic play or behavior (compulsively driven play or behavior that represents a repetitive reenactment of the trauma), recurrent and intrusive recollections of the traumatic event, repeated nightmares, physiologic distress at exposure to reminders of the trauma, feelings that the traumatic event is recurring, and episodes with features of a flashback or dissociation.
2. Avoidance of activities, places, people, thoughts, feelings, or conversations associated with the trauma and/or numbing of responsiveness that interferes with developmental momentum, revealed by increased social withdrawal, markedly diminished interest in usual activities, restricted range of affect, temporary loss of previously acquired developmental skills, and a decrease or constriction in play.
3. Symptoms of increased arousal, as evidenced by night terrors, difficulty going to sleep, repeated night waking, significant attentional difficulties, increased irritability/temper tantrums, hypervigilance, and exaggerated startle responses.

The youngest case of posttraumatic symptoms reported to date is of a 3-month-old described by Gaensbauer.[15] In addition to the classic triad of symptoms, very young children are vulnerable to developing other new symptoms in the wake of a trauma, such as separation anxiety or other new fears, new forms of aggression, and/or the loss of previously acquired developmental skills. In addition, it is to be noted that in the wake of a severe traumatic event, PTSD may not be the sole expression of traumatic reactions; other reactions, such as anxiety disorder or depression, may also occur with great frequency both in children and adults.[16]

Re-experiencing

Reexperiencing the traumatic event may often involve a distinctive form of repetitive play in toddlers and preschoolers in which themes of the traumatic event are expressed.[17,18] Automatic-appearing, rigidly repetitive play activity that lacks the sense of fun or creative spontaneity inherent in normative play is the hallmark of posttraumatic play.[18,19] Also lacking in posttraumatic play in older toddlers and preschool children will be the burgeoning symbolic capacity that is otherwise typical of this age group. The compulsive forms of play reenactment shown by the traumatized child can take many forms, depending on the child and on his or her developmental capacities. They may closely resemble the traumatic event in content and action, or they may be displaced in content yet contain the affective tone, rhythmicity, or other more abstract features of the event and its associated details. Posttraumatic reenactive play, as a form of reexperiencing, can lead to disorganization and the obfuscation of meaning making in the absence of caregivers who are able to tolerate trauma-associated affects and who are able to reflect on the play's potential meanings. Indeed, the traumatized caregiver's own distress around posttraumatic play, whether it leads to disorganization in the child or not, may in fact be what leads to the initiation of a referral. In a more optimistic vein, as discussed later, the reexperiencing of a traumatic event via play offers an important vehicle for understanding the child's experience and for working therapeutically.

Other important symptomatic forms of reexperiencing include nightmares, eruptions of fears and aggression in the face of traumatic reminders, and in severe cases reenactment in dissociated states.

Avoidance

Avoidance behaviors will depend on the young child's developmental capacities, particularly his or her gross motor abilities.[8] In an office setting, avoidance can sometimes be assessed by the way the child consistently steers clear of any available reminders of the traumatic event. Indeed, the degree to which children avoid traumatic themes during free play coupled with a detailed history of their peritraumatic response and degree of associated dysregulation may be the most important factors in assessing the severity of the condition.[7,20] For an infant up to the age of 12 months, subtle aversion of gaze or turning of the head are common avoidant responses to trauma.[21] An infant who has been abused by an adult will turn away from him or her in distress upon reexposure. In the 6- to 12-month age period, marked anxiety reactions to strange situations and unknown persons may occur following a trauma, with more active attempts to get away from traumatic reminders emerging as the child learns to walk and run. Avoidance behaviors in toddlers and preschoolers may take on extremes of generalization due in part to developmentally based limitations in cognitive capacities.

The symptom cluster around avoidance and numbing will often seriously affect the child's social interactions and thus the consolidation of age-appropriate developmental milestones. Although numbing, social withdrawal, and other dissociative or internalizing symptoms have been observed in very young children, it is thought that children below the age of four may be more likely to exhibit anxious clinging and externalizing behaviors such as tantrums.[9,10]

Hyperarousal

Symptoms of hyperarousal in young children can include generalized changes in psychophysiological self-regulation as well as changes in temperament in the direction of frank fearfulness and/or anger. In infants and toddlers, increased irritability and disruptive behavior, exacerbation of startle responses, increased stranger anxiety, and other manifestations of psychophysiological dysregulation, including disturbances of affect, sleep, and feeding, along with transient loss of developmental milestones (such as bowel/bladder control or speech and language competence), and disorganization of attachment behavior have all been reported.[9] In addition to difficulty falling or staying asleep, traumatized children often have difficulties paying attention, increased hypervigilance, and startle responses, all of which can affect learning. Disturbances of arousal can also often take the form of increased irritability and temper tantrums over minor events.

Other Symptoms

Apart from the analogs of the triad of adult PTSD symptoms, a range of more generalized symptoms can also be seen in very young children following a traumatic event. It is not always easy, or even necessary, to understand how a specific new symptom relates to the traumatic event to deduce that there is a causal relation. Increased separation anxiety, exacerbated specific fears (eg, of the dark, of car noises, or of separation-associated cues), regressive behavior (eg, increased need for pacifier or bottle), and somatoform complaints have all been noted for children aged 1 year and older in the wake of traumatic events.

The case of Katy[22] illustrates the symptomatic impact of a single traumatic event on a very young child. Katy was 3 years of age when the car that she, her mother, and her baby sister were in was hit broadside as they were going through an intersection. Belted in the car seat, Katy experienced a mild whiplash and bruises to her chest. Her baby sister was unhurt. Their mother, however, was knocked unconscious and bled from her head and arm. The mother regained consciousness at the scene and was taken to the hospital by ambulance, whereas Katy and her sister were taken to the hospital by a separate ambulance. In the emergency room, Katy saw her mother briefly before the mother's transfer to the intensive care unit but did not want to approach her.

At the time of an evaluation a few months later, Katy showed symptoms from each of the three PTSD diagnostic categories—reexperiencing, hyperarousal, and numbing, along with other symptoms of avoidance. "She was fearful of riding in the car and was very sensitive to loud noises. She had difficulty going to sleep and described nightmares of monsters trying to hurt her to the point where she hid under the bed. Although she frequently complained of 'owies' following the accident, she would want to be left alone." She also showed additional symptoms affecting her overall adjustment and her relationship with her mother. "Her feelings were easily hurt, and she would refuse to speak and retreat to her room over slight disappointments. She also became uncharacteristically aggressive, slapping and pushing her siblings. Developmental regressions were reflected in constant, almost obsessive use of her pacifier (prior use had been confined to her room and the car) and several bladder accidents in the weeks following the accident…She clung to her father and refused to let her mother comfort her. She would say, 'I don't like you, Mom,' and repeatedly scolded her mother for 'driving on the grass.'"[22]

DIFFERENCES IN THE EXPERIENCING OF TRAUMA IN VERY YOUNG CHILDREN

As in adults, the range of severity of PTSD in children is generally relative to the intensity of the traumatic event. Yet there are notable differences in how a traumatic event impacts an infant, toddler, or preschooler. Here we take up three important factors contributing to these differences: the young child's cognitive immaturity, developmental vulnerability, and dependence on caregivers.

Cognitive Immaturity

The lack of a developed capacity to form and retain verbally mediated memories can make it especially difficult for the child to develop a coherent memory of the trauma, let alone a narrative, and can also lead to unusual generalizations of fears to diverse stimuli that serve as "reminders." Thus little Abby, who at the age of 2 years 4 months was severely traumatized along with her mother[23] during the attack of 9/11, reacted with fright months later to the sight of a new, blue, baby stroller. It brought freshly to mind the green baby stroller that she had been strapped into at the time of the attack. In this case, Abby was able to verbalize the connection; when she would see the new blue stroller she would shout excitedly, "Green stroller, rocks falling, terrible, terrible, terrible!" Sometimes, even when the child cannot verbalize, it is possible to make out the connection to the traumatic event. For example, the behavior of the very young children in Oklahoma City who had had the windows of their classroom blown out during the bombing and who went out of their way to avoid *all* classroom windows thereafter was readily understandable. However, such ready decoding is not always possible. Seemingly inexplicable fears in a young child following a traumatic event may involve "triggers" whose nature appears quite opaque to parents yet are overwhelming to the child. Gaensbauer[24] recounts the case of Stephanie who at the age of 15 months suffered a severe spiral fracture of her leg at her female babysitter's yet subsequently developed a generalized fear of males, and especially of male doctors. The inference was subsequently made that such persons were reminiscent of the hospital personnel who treated her during a painful, 10-day hospitalization.

Cognitive immaturity relates not only to the understanding of the event but also to how it is retained in memory. An issue that has proved fascinating to professionals, and the subject of much controversy and speculation, is whether an infant or toddler can form a reliable memory at ages before he or she has acquired language.[24–26] This controversy has its analog in the sadly widespread and mistaken belief among parents and caretakers that very young children simply do not remember traumatic events — and thus do not need to be talked to about them. Suffice it here to say that there are numerous published cases, perhaps the most dramatic being the 1967 report of a child who at the age of 2 years 4 months verbally recalled details of a medical procedure she had undergone at the age of 3 months,[27] documenting that the retention of very early experiences can and indeed does occur. This kind of anecdotal evidence is in addition to a growing empirical literature documenting the capacity of infants to recall nonverbal experiences as evidenced by some form of behavioral recognition. For example, Perris and colleagues[28] demonstrated that children exposed to an experiment at 6 months could give evidence of having retained information concerning it at follow-up 2 years later. Thus, in addition to the kinds of implicit, procedural memories long associated with infancy, there is growing evidence that young children can also encode memories in more explicit forms, such that at later developmental stages, after language capacity has accrued, they can sometimes demonstrate fragmented but more or less veridical memories, such as through behavioral action or symbolic play.[25] That said, the age of 18 months (when language typically becomes consolidated) remains a noteworthy threshold. Scheeringa and Zeanah have suggested, based on a review of published clinical reports, that children younger than 18 months of age will tend to exhibit less symptomatology in the reexperiencing cluster compared with older children.[9]

A level of complexity is added when one considers that severe traumatic events have been postulated, at least in adults, to be capable of bypassing ordinary systems of memory processing, leading to the formation of "traumatic memories" subserved by distinct neurophysiologic systems.[29] Such "traumatic memories" clearly occur in children. Terr has emphasized in particular that under the age of 28 months powerful and lasting visual images can be created and retained.[30] Gaensbauer has described additional sensory representations beyond the visual, including not only sounds, such as sirens, but also touch and even kinesthesia.[24] Such was the case with Audrey who, subsequent to having witnessed an explosion in which her mother and another adult were killed at the age of 12 ½ months, would repeatedly spin, fall down, and thrash about on the ground. She would also become quite distressed if dust balls or flies landed on her or if she was exposed to a strong wind. Physical sensations also play a role in encoding trauma; "the body keeps the score" as van der Kolk[31] puts it. Such physical sensations can be mystifying to the child who suffers them even when, as with Katy's "owies" after her car accident at the age of 3 described above, they are clear enough to an adult observer.

To be sure, early memories are subject to distortions and elaborations at all subsequent ages, as long emphasized by psychoanalytic theorists and more recently by false-memory critics. However, the possibility of distortion should not distract the clinician from being aware of the likelihood of persistence of memory in some form from before the preverbal period. Sugar[32] has noted that the onset of verbal skills and the ability to make phrases may be crucial to a child's ability to subsequently give a coherent account of the event, especially with regard to time sequences. Before this time, Sugar suggests, echoing Terr,[30] the child may only have comparatively unprocessed visual, auditory, and other sensory memories.

In summary, young children's cognitive immaturity does not preclude them from developing some kind of memory for a traumatic event, though children younger than 18 months of age will tend to have fewer symptoms in the reexperiencing category compared with those in older children. This cognitive immaturity will, however, make it less likely that the child's memories will be coherent or readily understandable, either to the parents or to the child (including, notably, the child who is reexperiencing nonvisual facets of the experience such as tactile sensations). For these reasons, the gathering of detailed information from the parents and other informants about the traumatic event can be crucial to helping the child understand aspects of their experience that may be being remembered only through fragmented images and sensations.

Developmental Derailment

The second great difference in the way very young children react to traumatic events, reflected in the diverse symptoms that can follow afterward, is the vulnerability of the very young child to developmental derailment. When dealing with an infant or toddler younger than 4 years of age, we have a human being whose neurophysiologic regulatory systems, including the stress-management system, are still in the process of formation and stabilization and whose development in general remains inextricably intertwined with, and dependent upon, the caretaking system. A traumatic event not only initiates complex and overwhelming emergency responses internally but can also shatter the child's sense of safety and security with attachment figures—thus removing the scaffolding upon which developmental progression depends. The impact on the psychosocial environment may be as derailing as the impact on the child's trust in his own neurophysiologic self-regulation—daily routines may be disrupted, one or another caretaker may be blamed for allowing the traumatic event, a sense of threat may linger owing not only to the child's fearfulness but also that of the parents, and so on. It is not possible at present to map out how the various known neurophysiologic dysregulations that can follow in the wake of a severe traumatic event will be reflected in behavioral changes. It is even less possible to predict how a traumatic event will intersect with the ongoing life of the family.

In the wake of these complex changes both in the child and in the family system, developmental milestones may be lost or delayed. Since developmental achievements overlap and build on one another, the clinician should be on the lookout for how a traumatic event may be ramifying vis-à-vis later developmental milestones. In infancy, traumatic events may be reflected in "eating and sleeping difficulties, problems with digestion and elimination, inconsolable crying, difficulty being soothed, intense separation anxiety, head banging or other self-injurious behavior, unmodulated affect, and lack of consistent behavioral strategies to derive a sense of safety from the attachment figure."[33] In toddlers, the same kind of dysregulated behaviors may likewise occur, but in addition, difficulties may arise that pertain to the developmental tasks specific to toddlerhood, particularly exploration (symptoms such as recklessness or extreme inhibition) and autonomy (tantrums, rages, aggression toward others, angry noncompliance). Similarly, preschoolers may show any of these foregoing symptoms from earlier stages, but they may also show disturbances in symbolic play (a frequent hallmark of trauma), excessive preoccupation with bodily integrity, difficulties negotiating gender identity, and rivalry with siblings and other children.

Early Trauma and the Caregiver-Child Relationship

The third way in which trauma in very young children differs from that in older children and adults has to do with the nature of the traumatic event itself in the context of the young child's dependency on caregivers.[34] Children absolutely rely on their caretakers to keep them safe—the whole evolution of the system of attachment behavior ("the attachment system") is geared to make the child continually cognizant of this necessity—and what threatens the caretaker, or makes the caretaker unavailable, threatens the child, even if there is no direct threat to the child individually. As Schechter and Tosyali opine, a preschooler who hears his traumatized mother's shrieks may well feel that he is hearing his own death knell, even when there is no tangible threat to self.[8]

When a traumatic event entails a threat both to the child and to the attachment figure, matters are especially grave for the child. In their review of symptom expression in traumatized children younger than 4 years of age, Scheeringa and Zeanah[9] attempted to identify variables that best predicted the severity of the child's reaction; they were able to identify only one—"trauma that occurred when there were threats to the child's caregivers."

Shared or "relational" PTSD has been proposed as a construct for thinking about trauma in very young children that takes into account the various ways in which children take their emotional understanding of an event from their primary caretakers. In their discussion of relational PTSD, Scheeringa and Zeanah conceptualize several variants.[35] In the *moderating effect model*, the child is traumatized directly by an event, but the "mother's relationship with the child (including her ability to read his/her cues and respond effectively to his/her needs)" moderates the degree to which the child will become symptomatic. In the *vicarious traumatization model*, the mother has experienced a trauma and the child has not. In this situation, the impact of the trauma on the mother impinges on her relationship with her child, alters her responsiveness, and thus instigates the child's development of symptoms. In the *compound effect*, the mother and the child are both traumatized, and each exacerbates the symptomatology of the other.

ASSESSMENT AND TREATMENT
Assessment

A "best practices" guideline to assessment, outlined in the Zero to Three diagnostic classification[13] recommends from three to five 45-minute sessions. Typically, the evaluation of a young child will begin with one or more interviews with the child's caregivers. One is concerned not only with specific (PTSD) symptoms in the child but with the full range of disruptive effects that the trauma may be having on the child and the family. In gathering such information, it is helpful to ask parents to assume that any changes that have occurred subsequent to a trauma are related to the trauma until proven otherwise, in order not to miss subtle effects that might otherwise be overlooked. In gathering this information, many opportunities will present themselves to begin to educate the parents about typical traumatic effects—an important goal of treatment—and to facilitate the parents' coming to appreciate the meanings of the specific reactions their child is showing—another important goal of treatment.

We suggest obtaining a detailed, sequential history of every aspect of the child's traumatic experience, including not only the traumatic event itself but all of the events surrounding the trauma that might influence the internal meanings that the trauma has for that particular child. The more detailed the account is, the more it can provide the clinician with important clues as to specific features of the child's fears, nightmares, or reenactment play as well as possibly shed light on possible "triggers" in the environment to which the child is reacting.

In assessing the effects of the trauma on the child in interviews with the parents, one appropriately begins with the expectable posttraumatic symptoms upon which the diagnosis of PTSD is based, including emotional reexperiencing (nightmares, intrusive imagery, and reenactment behavior), avoidance of stimuli associated with the trauma, emotional constriction and other indications of numbing, and autonomic hyperarousal and dysregulation. As discussed earlier, the work of Scheeringa and his colleagues has been instrumental in the establishment of developmentally appropriate criteria for the accurate and reliable diagnosis of PTSD in very young children. A number of semistructured interviews and checklists for PTSD symptoms, which can be used directly in assessment sessions with the parents and the child, are available, most notably the PTSD Semistructured Interview and Observational Record for Infants and Young Children[36] (also see Scheeringa[37] for a further description of various PTSD measures).

Beyond gathering historical data specific to the trauma, one also needs to obtain the kind of detailed developmental and family history typically gathered in any psychiatric evaluation of a young child. Here, too, one must distinguish between development before the trauma and development after the trauma. As illustrated in the example of Katy described above, the child's symptoms and behavioral changes can cause significant disruption in child-caregiver relationships. Inquiring about how the child's symptoms have affected them gives the parents permission and the opportunity to begin to discuss their own difficulties coping with the child. The parents need to feel that they are partners in the unfolding endeavor—as indeed they are—and that the goals are not only to help their child but also to help them directly as well as to help them help the child. Insofar as parental fears about long-term damage to the child can be engaged, and realistically assuaged, this should begin in the assessment process. The parents of preschool children will often be highly mobilized to get help for their child for altruistic reasons and thus may be willing to take emotional risks beyond what they would normally take, provided they feel that the clinician is allied with them and their endeavor.

As long as the parent can manage his or her own reactions, interviews with the child are done most effectively with a parent present. Not only are young children much more comfortable when parents are present, but parents can provide crucial historical information as the session unfolds that help the clinician understand the child's behavior and play. Moreover, direct observations of how the trauma is affecting the child in terms of his or her play and other behaviors help parents to see the need for treatment and promote collaboration with the therapist around interventions both in the office and at home. It is not unusual for parents to react to the child's play as it unfolds with astonishment that the child remembers the event in detail. However, there can be instances when the parents are so upset by the child's play that it is better to see the child individually.

Given their limited verbal abilities and tendencies to express their feelings in action, a particular challenge in working with very young children is to find communicative vehicles that allow them to express their inner thoughts and feelings. Taking advantage of young children's strong propensities for reenactment, the use of toys to create play situations representing the circumstances under which the trauma occurred and then asking the child to demonstrate "what happens next" has long been recognized as an effective therapeutic technique for gaining access to young children's inner world[38,39] and especially for enabling them to convey their understanding of a traumatic event.[17] The presentation of stimulus cues related to a trauma must be done tactfully and with full regard for the child's and parents' ability to manage the feelings that might emerge.

Ideally, in pulling together the kinds of information described here to develop a treatment plan, therapeutic elements are seamlessly intertwined with the evaluative process. Given parent's understandable anxiety and sense of urgency, the provision of educational information about PTSD early in the process can help them make sense of both their and their child's emotional reactions to the trauma and serve to normalize intense responses that can otherwise be experienced as extremely disturbing.[6] Identifying and addressing specific parental concerns, such as anxiety about the child's recovery or guilt about not having been able to protect the child, can help reduce emotional interferences that might otherwise impair their ability to provide the support that the child needs. Conveying a sense of optimism that the child can be helped will also provide important reassurance to worried parents.

Treatment

Different strategies of treatment have been described in the literature depending on the severity of the symptoms, the resources available to parents, and the availability of suitable personnel.[22,33] It is sometimes feasible to treat the child via the parents at home following a consultation; at other times a comparatively brief psychotherapeutic intervention will prove sufficient; at still other times longer-term treatment with both child and parents is clearly warranted.

Treatment approaches to early trauma will almost always involve psychosocial interventions exclusively. Although there are anecdotal reports of the use in traumatized preschoolers of the same kinds of medications prescribed for older children and adults,[17,40,41] and although the use of psychotropic medications in young children has become widespread in recent years,[42] to date there has not been a single systematic study of the use of any medication for PTSD in preschool children. Given the vulnerability of the young nervous system to external influence and the uncertainty about long-term adverse effects, the use of medications in this population for PTSD should be considered only under extreme circumstances.

Within the universe of psychosocial treatments, certain commonalities regularly appear.[33] Here we emphasize especially the therapist's ongoing work with the parents.[43,44] One of the most important contributions that therapists can make to the child's recovery is to help parents provide empathic support and containment within the child's home environment. In the immediate aftermath, the degree to which the parents are able to reinstitute a sense of protection and safety within the home setting will play a crucial role in the child's ability to make use of any subsequent interventions. Reestablishing the daily routine of the home and of the child's life outside the home is an essential part in reinstituting a sense of safety. So, too, is removing reminders of the trauma if that is possible.

Core elements in the treatment of PTSD in young children are the desensitization of traumatic affects in the face of traumatic triggers and the promotion of psychological processing of the trauma. As a prelude to these efforts, therapists can work closely with caregivers to identify effective interventions to reduce autonomic arousal and facilitate calm. With young children and in cases where traumatic triggers are present in the child's everyday environment, desensitization of a child's distress and fearful reliving can occur naturalistically over time as parents provide soothing comfort each time traumatic feelings are triggered. This process can be significantly facilitated, however, if done in a planned and systematic way, such as through the use of graduated or step-wise exposure protocols combined with parental reassurance and self-soothing relaxation techniques.[45,46] To the extent that each exposure results in a successful reduction in distress responses and a new way of experiencing the traumatic stimulus, one can conceptualize that internalized traumatic representations are undergoing cognitive reprocessing, even in the youngest of children. A 12-week manualized treatment protocol using these techniques in combination with close parental involvement, termed Preschool PTSD Treatment, has been developed by Scheeringa and colleagues[47,48] and is currently under study for its clinical efficacy.

With slightly older children, representational expressive vehicles such as language, play, storytelling, and drawing can become the primary modes for desensitization, cognitive reprocessing, and the development of a coherent narrative. At the point that language skills are sufficiently developed, story telling can be a particularly useful vehicle for articulating the child's experience and placing it within the context of a meaningful narrative. It is also a technique that parents do very naturally and well. It offers great flexibility with regard to which aspects of the story are emphasized depending on the needs of the child. Through its creative possibilities and opportunities for child participation, it lends itself to the development of a co-constructed narrative that can become the basis for ongoing dialog between parent and child about the traumatic experience. As long as it does not burden the child, parents can also include themselves in the story. Explaining to the child why they were not able to prevent the trauma and sharing their own reactions can often give the child perspective and help to reduce the child's anger. For example, there was a significant reduction in

Katy's anger (see earlier section) when her mother explained that she had not "driven up on the grass" but that another car had pushed them there.

In terms of treatment goals for the young child, Lieberman and Van Horn[33] and Marmar and colleagues[49] have identified commonalities that can be found among different treatments. Lieberman and Van Horn[33] highlight these commonalities in terms of seven basic goals, which we adapt here to a developmental context appropriate for children younger than 4 years of age:

1. Resuming normal development. This is the primary goal for very young children; it necessarily involves repairing the child's attachment relationship.
2. Fostering a realistic response to threat. For the very young child, this entails not only learning to identify triggers but also to develop strategies, such as seeking Mommy or Daddy out, for handling situations that reawaken the child's fears.
3. Maintaining regular levels of affective arousal. Learning self-soothing techniques, and getting the parents to assist, is particularly useful with very young children. Also invaluable is for the parents to be able to set limits while signaling understanding of the child's emotional upset.
4. Building reciprocity in intimate relationships. In very young children, this means above all restoring the child's sense of safety with and trust in the parents. For the parents, this means not only learning to understand and respond to the child's state of mind but also to work through their own guilt, anxiety, and remorse regarding the child's exposure to the traumatic event.
5. Normalization of the traumatic response. Very young children, no less than older children and adults, need assistance in understanding that their responses to the trauma are inherently normal and expectable—and not "bad," "weird," or unlovable. Their parents similarly need reassurance that the child's symptoms are expectable.
6. Encouraging a differentiation between reliving and remembering. In very young children this will entail reestablishing a sense of safety and reliable continuity on the one hand and helping the child develop the capacity to place narrative meaning on the event on the other.
7. Placing the traumatic experience in perspective. In very young children this will entail not only developing a story about it as development proceeds, but also, importantly, being able to imagine efforts at repair and restoration. Being able to imagine how it might be possible to "fix" or "make better" can be crucial for a very young child.

How best to accomplish these goals will depend on the therapist's skill set and the particular circumstances of the child and family. The choice of a specific modality is less important than its developmental appropriateness. Virtually all practitioners will have recourse to some form of play therapy in their work with the child. As described above, the use of therapist-directed play situations or drawings that recreate the trauma situation and allow the child to play out or describe "what happens next" offers unique opportunities to help the child develop a more accurate and less overwhelming perspective on his or her experience. Within the framework of such therapeutic play recreations, the therapist has a variety of traditional play therapy techniques through which to provide support, guidance, and interpretation. These include direct participation in the play through concrete action or through verbal observations, identification of important affects and motives, provision of narrative commentary regarding sequences and meanings, corrections of distortions and misunderstandings, promotion of mastery through compensatory or reparative play scenarios and constructive action, facilitation of conflicted affects such as anger, and the teaching of strategies for self-protection in the future.[17,50] Two important keys for evaluating how the therapy is progressing are whether affects are coming to be identified with greater specificity and whether the child's play is evolving.

The parents' presence in the child's sessions during reenactment play that mobilizes "relived" traumatic feelings in the child allows them to provide comfort in ways that they were not able to do at the time of the original trauma.[17] This can contribute to a rebuilding of the trust between child and parents that may have been lost as a result of the parents' failure to prevent the trauma in the first place. In collaboration with the therapist, the growing appreciation of how the trauma has been internalized by the child provides a basis for integrating the work that is being done in the office with what is being done in the home environment.

SUMMARY

Trauma in the young child is mediated and moderated by the child's emotional reactions to the traumatizing event and by the primary caretakers' emotional reactions to that event. The child's symptoms in response to a traumatic event and the particular meaning of that event to that child will be, in large part, dependent on the child's developmental capabilities at the time of the trauma and during the subsequent working through of the traumatic experience.

Extensive clinical experience, well supported by research findings[35,51–55] indicates that a traumatic event in the life of a young child must be considered in a relational as well as a developmental context. Attachment, when secure and organized, can be a source of resilience in the face of trauma or, when insecure and disorganized, can be a vehicle for the exacerbation of a trauma's effects as well as for the transmission of those effects across generations. When a prior relational disturbance does exist, it is even more imperative for the clinician to provide support and guidance to the patient's primary caretaker so that he or she can help the child after dealing with his or her own reaction to the trauma.[6] Given this relational context, helping parents to respond empathically to the child's traumatic symptoms and to develop effective behavioral management techniques will be crucial elements in treatment. This is particularly true since many symptoms, such as clinginess and emotional fragility, separation anxiety, sleep disturbances, and temper outbursts, will, because of potential secondary reinforcement, have strong tendencies to persist and even take on a life of their own, depending on how they are handled by parents.

For those children whose traumatic reactions do not subside within the first weeks after a trauma, psychotherapy that is focused on treatment of the posttraumatic stress symptoms is indicated. The time-honored method for treating traumatized children first described by the psychoanalyst David Levy[38] involves controlled exposure to the traumatizing event in structured play situations that are designed to elicit the memory and affective reactions to the traumatic event in a safe environment. Toys such as toy dogs, cars, doctor kits, fire engines, or any item that is associated with the trauma are useful in eliciting the memory of the trauma in the safe environment of the therapist's office.

Particularly for the traumatized young child, meeting a new person, the therapist, in a new environment is likely to initially create anxiety. It is important that the child establish trust in the therapist and that the therapist move slowly enough through the controlled exposure so as not to retraumatize the child. This often takes considerable clinical skill and involves ensuring that the treatment provides a safe, secure base. In addition, the therapist must be active in establishing safety in the present life of the child before addressing past trauma. This can involve collateral efforts such as calling or assisting a nonfamily caregiver such as day-care workers or a nursery school teacher.

Initial consultations with parents should take place before the child is seen and should focus not only on taking a careful history but also on educating the parent about trauma and PTSD and on child development generally and especially on the importance of the relationship to the caregivers in the wake of trauma. We consider it essential that the child and the child's parents develop a coherent narrative together about the traumatic event so that the event can continue to be processed by the family outside of the therapy sessions, both during the course of treatment and into the future. One of the most therapeutic experiences for the child is to know that his or her parent not only holds the traumatic experience in mind but also attempts to hold the *child's experience* of the trauma in mind.[53,56]

REFERENCES

1. Scheeringa MS, Zeanah CH, Myers L, et al. Predictive validity in a prospective follow-up for PTSD in preschool children. J Am Acad Child Adolesc Psychiatry 2005;42:561–70.
2. Meiser-Stedman R, Smith P, Glucksman E, et al. The posttraumatic stress disorder diagnosis in preschool and elementary school-age children exposed to motor vehicle accidents. Am J Psychiatry 2008;165(10):1326–37.
3. Breslau N, Chilcoat HD, Kessler RC, et al. Previous exposure to trauma and PTSD effects of subsequent trauma: results from the Detroit Area Survey of Trauma. Am J Psychiatry 1999;156(6):902–7.
4. Yehuda R, Halligan SL, Grossman R. Childhood trauma and risk for PTSD: relationship to intergenerational effects of trauma, parental PTSD, and cortisol excretion. Dev Psychopathol 2001;13:733–53.
5. Diagnostic and statistical manual of mental disorders. (DSM-IV). 4th Edition. Washington, DC: American Psychiatric Association; 2004.
6. Coates SW, Schechter DS, First E. Brief interventions with traumatized children and families after September 11. In: Coates S, Rosenthal J, Schechter DS, editors. September 11: trauma and human bonds. Hillsdale (NJ): The Analytic Press; 2003. p. 23–49.
7. Scheeringa MS, Zeanah CH, Myers L, et al. New findings on alternative criteria for PTSD in preschool children. J Am Acad Child Adolesc Psychiatry 2003;42(5): 561–70.
8. Schechter DS, Tosyali MC. Posttraumatic stress disorder from infancy through adolescence: a review. In: Essau CA, Petermann F, editors. Anxiety disorders in children and adolescents: epidemiology, risk factors, and treatment. New York: Brunner-Routledge; 2001. p. 285–322.
9. Scheeringa MS, Zeanah CH. Symptom expression and trauma variables in children under 48 months of age. Infant Ment Health J 1995;16:259–70.
10. Gurwitch RH, Sullivan MA, Long PJ. The impact of trauma and disaster on young children. Child Adolesc Psychiatr Clin N Am 1998;7(1):19–32.
11. Scheeringa MS, Zeanah CH, Drell MJ, et al. Two approaches to the diagnosis of posttraumatic stress disorder in infancy and early childhood. J Am Acad Child Adolesc Psychiatry 1995;34:191–200.
12. Scheeringa MS, Wright MJ, Hunt JP, et al. Factors affecting the diagnosis and prediction of PTSD symptomatology in children and adolescents. Am J Psychiatry 2006;163:644–51.

13. Zero To Three. Diagnostic classification of mental health and developmental disorders of infancy and early childhood. (DC: 0-3R). Revised edition. Washington, DC: ZERO TO THREE Press; 2005.
14. Task force on research diagnostic criteria: Infancy and preschool. Research diagnostic criteria for infants and preschool children: the process and empirical support. J Am Acad Child Adolesc Psychiatry 2003;42(12):1504–12.
15. Gaensbauer TJ. The differentiation of discrete affects: a case report. Psychoanal Study Child 1982;37:29–66.
16. Hoven CW, Mandell DJ, Duarte CS. Mental health of New York City public school children after 9/11. In: Coates SW, Rosenthal J, Schechter DS, editors. September 11: trauma and human bonds. Hillsdale (NJ): The Analytic Press; 2003. p. 51–74.
17. Gaensbauer TJ, Siegel CH. Therapeutic approaches to posttraumatic stress disorder in infants and toddlers. Infant Ment Health J 1995;16(4):292–305.
18. Terr LC. Childhood psychic trauma. Advances and new directions. In: Noshpitz JD, editor, Basic handbook of child psychiatry, vol. 5. New York: Basic Books; 1987. p. 262–72.
19. Coates SW, Moore MS. The complexity of early trauma: representation and transformation. Psychoanalytic Inquiry 1997;17:286–311.
20. Pfefferbaum B. The impact of the Oklahoma City bombing on children in the community. Mil Med 2001;166(12 Suppl):49–50.
21. Beebe B, Lachmann FM. Representation and internalization in infancy: three principles of salience. Psychoanalytic Psychology 1994;11(2):127–65.
22. Gaensbauer TJ. Traumatized young children: assessment and treatment processes. In: Osofsky J, editor. Young children and trauma: intervention and treatment. New York: Guilford Press; 2004. p. 194–216.
23. Coates SW, Schecter DS. Preschoolers' traumatic stress post 9/11: relational and developmental perspectives. Psychiatr Clin North Am 2004;17(3):473–89.
24. Gaensbauer TJ. Trauma in the preverbal period: symptoms, memories and developmental impact. Psychoanal Study Child 1995;50:122–49.
25. Gaensbauer TJ. Representations of trauma in infancy: clinical and theoretical implications for the understanding of early memory. Infant Ment Health J 2002; 23:259–77.
26. Gaensbauer TJ. Telling their stories: representation and reenactment of traumatic experiences occurring in the first year of life. In: Tortora S, editor. The multisensory world of the infant. Journal of ZERO TO THREE: National Center for Infants, Toddlers, and Families 2004;25(5):25–31.
27. Bernstein AE, Blacher RS. The recovery of a memory from three months of age. Psychoanal Study Child 1967;22:156–67.
28. Perris EE, Myers NA, Clifton RK. Long-term memory for a single infancy experience. Child Dev 1990;61:1769–807.
29. LeDoux JE. The emotional brain. New York: Touchstone; 1996.
30. Terr LC. What happens to early memories of trauma: a study of twenty children under age five at the time of documented traumatic events. J Am Acad Child Adolesc Psychiatry 1988;27:96–104.
31. Van der Kolk B. The body keeps the score: memory and the evolving psychobiology of post traumatic stress. Harv Rev Psychiatry 1994;1(5):253–65.
32. Sugar M. Toddlers' traumatic memories. Infant Ment Health J 1992;13:245–51.
33. Lieberman AF, Van Horn P. Assessment and treatment of young children exposed to traumatic events. In: Osofsky J, editor. Young children and trauma: intervention and treatment. New York: Guilford Press; 2004. p. 111–38.

34. Coates SW. Introduction: trauma and human bonds. In: Coates S, Rosenthal J, Schechter DS, editors. September 11: trauma and human bonds. Hillsdale (NJ): The Analytic Press; 2003. p. 1–14.
35. Scheeringa MS, Zeanah CH. A relational perspective on PTSD in early childhood. J Trauma Stress 2001;14:799–815.
36. Scheeringa MS, Zeanah CH. Posttraumatic stress disorder semi-structured interview and observational record for infants and young children. New Orleans: Tulane University; 1994.
37. Scheeringa MS. Posttraumatic stress disorder: clinical guidelines and research findings. In: Luby JL, editor. Handbook of preschool mental health: development, disorders, and treatment. New York: Guilford Press; 2006. p. 165–85.
38. Levy D. Release therapy. Am J Orthopsychiatry 1939;9:713–36.
39. Emde RN, Wolf DP, Oppenheim D. Revealing the inner worlds of young children: the MacArthur Story Stem Battery and parent-child narratives. New York: Oxford University Press; 2003.
40. Harmon RJ, Riggs PD. Clonidine for posttraumatic stress disorder in preschool children. J Am Acad Child Adolesc Psychiatry 1996;35:1247–9.
41. Thomas JM. Traumatic stress disorder presents as hyperactivity and disruptive behavior: case presentation, diagnoses, and treatment. Infant Ment Health J 1995;16:306–17.
42. Zito JM, Safer DJ, dos Reis S, et al. Trends in the prescribing of psychotropic medications to preschoolers. JAMA 2000;283:1025–30.
43. Lieberman AF, Van Horn P. Psychotherapy with infants and young children: repairing the effect of stress and trauma on early attachment. New York: The Guilford Press; 2008.
44. Lieberman AF. Child-parent psychotherapy: a relationship-based approach to the treatment of mental health disorders in infancy and early childhood. In: Sameroff A, McDonough SC, Rosenblum K, editors. Treating parent-infant relationship problems: strategies for intervention. New York: Guilford Press; 2004. p. 97–122.
45. Wallick MM. Desensitization therapy with a fearful two-year-old. Am J Psychiatry 1979;136:1325–6.
46. Chatoor I. Eating and nutritional disorders of infancy and early childhood. In: Wiener J, editor. Textbook of child and adolescent psychiatry. Washington, DC: Academy of Child and Adolescent Psychiatry Press; 1991. p. 352–61.
47. Scheeringa MS, Amaya-Jackson L, Cohen J. Preschool PTSD Treatment; 2002.
48. Scheeringa MS, Salloum A, Arnberger RA, et al. Feasibility and effectiveness of cognitive-behavioral therapy for posttraumatic stress disorder in preschool children: two case reports. J Trauma Stress 2007;20:631–6.
49. Marmar C, Foy D, Kagan B, et al. An integrated approach for treating posttraumatic stress. In: Oldham JM, Talman A, editors, American Psychiatric Association review of psychiatry, vol. 12. New York: Guilford Press; 1993. p. 238–72.
50. Gaensbauer TJ, Kelsay K. Situational and story stem scaffolding in psychodynamic play therapy with very young children. In: Schaefer C, Kelly-Zion P, McCormick J, Ohnogi A, editors. Play therapy for very young children. Lanham (MD): Rowman and Littlefield; 2008. p. 173–98.
51. Lyons-Ruth K, Block D. The disturbed caregiving system: relations among childhood trauma, maternal caregiving, and infant affect and attachment. Infant Ment Health J 1996;17:257–75.
52. Schechter DS. Intergenerational communication of maternal violent trauma: understanding the interplay of reflective functioning and posttraumatic

psychopathology. In: Coates SW, Rosenthal J, Schechter DS, editors. September 11: trauma and human bonds. Hillsdale (NJ): The Analytic Press; 2003. p. 115–42.

53. Schechter DS, Coates SW, First E. Observations from New York on young children's and their families' acute reactions to the World Trade Center attacks. Journal of Zero to Three: National Center for Infants, Toddlers, and Families 2001; 22(3):9–13.
54. Schechter DS, Coots T, Zeanah CH, et al. Maternal mental representations of the child in an inner-city clinical sample: violence-related posttraumatic stress and reflective functioning. Attach Hum Dev 2005;7(3):313–31.
55. Cornely P, Bromet E. Prevalence of behavior problems in three-year-old children living near Three Mile Island: a comparative analysis. J Child Psychol Psychiatry 1986;27:489–98.
56. Coates SW. Having a mind of one's own and holding the other in mind. Psychoanalytic Dialogues 1998;8(1):115–48.

Viewing Preschool Disruptive Behavior Disorders and Attention-Deficit/ Hyperactivity Disorder Through a Developmental Lens: What We Know and What We Need to Know

Anil Chacko, PhD[a],*, Lauren Wakschlag, PhD[b], Carri Hill, PhD[b],
Barbara Danis, PhD[b], Kimberly Andrews Espy, PhD[c]

KEYWORDS

• Disruptive behavior • ADHD • Preschool
• Psychopathology • Nosology

There is now little doubt that Diagnostic and Statistical Manual of Mental Disorders, fourth edition (DSM-IV), behavior disorders are present and are identifiable during the preschool years.[1,2] With only minor modifications to DSM-IV disruptive behavior disorders (DBDs) and attention-deficit/hyperactivity disorder (ADHD) nosology,

During preparation of this paper, Dr. Chacko was supported through a Klingenstein Third Generation ADHD Fellowship. Dr. Wakschlag, Dr. Hill, and Dr. Danis were supported by NIMH grants R01 MH68455 and MH62437 as well as by the Shaw and Children's Brain Research Foundations. Dr. Espy was supported in part by R01 MH065668, R01 DA014661, P01 HD 038051, and R01 HD050399.
[a] Department of Psychology, Queens College, City University of New York, 65-30 Kissena Boulevard, Flushing, NY 11367, USA
[b] Department of Psychiatry, Institute for Juvenile Research, University of Illinois at Chicago 1747 W. Roosevelt Road, MC 747 (Room 155), Chicago, IL 60608, USA
[c] Department of Psychology, University of Nebraska-Lincoln, 303 Canfield Administration Building, Lincoln, NE 68588-0433, USA
* Corresponding author.
E-mail address: anil.chacko@qc.cuny.edu (A. Chacko).

Child Adolesc Psychiatric Clin N Am 18 (2009) 627–643
doi:10.1016/j.chc.2009.02.003
1056-4993/09/$ – see front matter © 2009 Elsevier Inc. All rights reserved.

multiple, independent studies have shown similar prevalence rates and correlates as in older children.[1] In the preschool-age range, these disorders also have modest stability.[3–6] It is clear that the behaviors that comprise DBDs and ADHD (eg, noncompliance, rule breaking, aggression, destruction of property, hyperactivity, inattention, and impulsivity) impair children's functioning and that caregivers of young children often experience considerable difficulty in managing children who exhibit high levels of these behaviors. Increasingly, preschoolers are being referred to mental health clinics for DBDS and ADHD,[7] with escalating rates of pharmacologic treatments.[8] Thus, the "real-world" consequences of behavior disorders are substantial for young children and their families and often mark the onset of long-term developmental maladaptation that marks psychopathology.[9] Concerted efforts to characterize the clinical manifestations of these disorders in early childhood more precisely will maximize our ability to intervene effectively in the lives of young children affected with DBDs and ADHD and, ultimately, to reduce their long-term health burden.

The increasing consensus that these syndromes exist in young children also comes with growing concern that these disorders may be developmentally misspecified, particularly for young children who are not at the extremes.[10] In this article, we review the extant empirical evidence through a "developmental lens," with an eye to analyzing how the absence of a developmental approach may hinder accurate identification. Further, we show how integrating evidence from developmental science provides useful guideposts for generating and testing a developmentally specified nosology. Together with the plethora of work on preschool psychopathology during the past decade, this provides a strong foundation for charting a course for the next generation of more refined efforts in early childhood.

DISRUPTIVE BEHAVIOR DISORDERS AND ATTENTION-DEFICIT/HYPERACTIVITY DISORDER: WHAT WE KNOW

Although multiple, overlapping terms have been used for capturing behavioral syndromes, for the sake of clarity here, we will use the terms DBDs and ADHD when specifically referring to these clinical syndromes and the term "behavior disorders" to refer to the two syndromes collectively. The study of behavior disorders, has taken on two, somewhat distinct, lines. There is a long history of studies of "preschool behavior problems" that have generally used checklist ratings of externalizing behaviors, which combine disruptive attention/hyperactivity behaviors.[9] Collectively, studies that have emphasized the dimensional classifications of disorders have informed the field tremendously by enhancing our understanding of the developmental nature of behavior problems in young children, the co-occurrence of various problems (eg, impulsivity, noncompliance, aggression), the longitudinal course of these problems, and potential underlying mechanisms of these problems.[9,11] More recently, DSM-IV nosology has been applied to preschoolers.[2] Although the categorical approach of the DSM is not without limitations, we focus our review on *DSM-defined DBDs and ADHD* as a means of highlighting issues related to categorical identification, clinical significance, and service provision. Studies were included in this review if the following criteria were met: (1) DSM DBDs (oppositional defiant disorder (ODD) and/or conduct disorder [CD]) and/or ADHD were assessed, (2) the majority of the sample was preschool age (3–5 years), and (3) data were reported on the prevalence, convergent validity or correlates, and/or predictive validity of these disorders. We extend beyond existing reviews[1,12] by incorporating more recent work with developmentally validated instruments, attempting to bridge preschool studies of DBDs and ADHD that come from somewhat different traditions and heretofore have proceeded along fairly separate lines, highlighting developmental limitations of existing work and linking to extant developmental science.

DISRUPTIVE BEHAVIOR DISORDERS
Prevalence

In the absence of validated diagnostic instruments for use in this age period, a variety of instruments have been used for diagnosis in preschoolers. Early studies often used nonstandardized, relatively minor modifications of existing diagnostic instruments to determine diagnosis[13,14] or determined diagnosis through clinical consensus using multiple and varied assessment information.[15] Most recently, interviews specifically validated for the preschool period have been employed, including the Preschool Age Psychiatric Assessment (PAPA; [3]), in addition to other diagnostic tools (Kiddie Disruptive Behavior Disorders Schedule), which have been evaluated using clinical samples.[16] Across community samples, prevalence rates of ODD have ranged from 4% to 16.6%, which is similar to that found in older children.[17] Importantly, although Lavigne and colleagues[15] found the highest rates of ODD (ie, 16.6%), this rate was reduced in half when impairment associated with the symptoms was required for the diagnosis (ie, 8.1%). Thus, the presence of symptoms of DBDs alone is misleading, and interpreting the presence of symptoms as disorder likely results in higher prevalence of DBDs when impairment resulting from these symptoms is not taken into account. Assessment of impairment, however, is notably absent from most preschool DBD studies. To our knowledge, only two studies have assessed CD as a separate disorder in community samples of preschoolers,[3,18] with rates somewhat lower than ODD (3.9%–6.6%), again, without considering impairment.

Age differences within the preschool period have received little attention. Although some studies[3] have reported no age differences in prevalence rates, Lavigne and colleagues[15] found a modest linear age trend in the prevalence of ODD during the preschool period. The prevalence of ODD as defined by the presence of four symptoms was 22.5% in 3-year-old children but was only 15% in 5-year-old children.

Validity

Determining the validity of a psychiatric diagnosis in multifaceted. Here, we focus on two important aspects: concurrent validity and predictive validity. Concurrent (also termed convergent) validity represents the extent to which a test or measure correlates highly with other variables with which it should theoretically correlate, whereas predictive validity is the extent to which a measured construct demonstrates a predictive relation to the same or a similarly measured construct over time (ie, longitudinal stability of diagnostic status; 1). Predictive validity of a disorder, however, is a particularly challenging issue in young children, as substantial behavioral shifts occur from 3 to 5 years, and thus, normative frequencies may shift, making the determination of stability complex. Thus, if manifestation or frequencies of symptoms vary with age, the predictive validity (stability) of a disorder may be obscured. On the other hand, the rapid developmental shifts of this period may reduce stability.

Studies have demonstrated that key aspects of the family environment, parent psychopathology, parenting behavior, parent-child interactions, observed child behavior, child neuropsychological functioning, and social information processing differ among children with DBDs compared with typically developing children.[18–31] These correlates are similar to those found in older youth with disruptive disorders. Not surprisingly, children who meet symptom criteria for DBDs also experience substantial impairment in these domains.[3,16]

Several investigators have also assessed predictive validity. Wakschlag and colleagues[6] found that 55% of their clinically enriched sample retained DBD status at one-year follow-up. Speltz and colleagues[20] assessed the 2-year stability of ODD and found that that the vast majority of children in their clinic-based sample (76%) continued to meet criteria for ODD diagnosis 2 years later. In two papers, Lavigne and colleagues[29,31] report on the 2-year and 5-year follow-up results within their preschool, community-based sample. They reported that the 2-year stability of any behavior disorder (ODD, CD, and/or ADHD) or a combination of the three was moderate. Stability was higher for older preschoolers (65% for 4- to 5-year-olds) than younger preschoolers (50% for 2- 3-year-olds). It is not clear whether this is a true difference in stability, more "noise" in terms of transient variability in behavior at the younger preschool age, or due to the absence of developmentally specified cutoff points at these different ages. The diagnostic stability of ODD dropped substantially with longer follow-up—with stability of 43%, 27%, and 24% at 3-, 4-, and 5-year follow-ups, respectively. Thus, the probability of a diagnosis of ODD during the school-age period was substantial if ODD was present during the preschool years. On the other hand, these data also demonstrate that most of the preschoolers (nearly half of the preschoolers with an ODD diagnosis at baseline) do not persist in meeting clinical criteria at school age. Similar patterns were reported by Kim-Cohen and colleagues[18] on the 2-year stability of CD in a community sample of children followed from 5 to 7 years of age. Meeting criteria for CD at age 5 years significantly increased the odds of a CD diagnosis at age 7 years (odds ratio = 20.6), with more boys retaining the CD diagnoses than girls. On the other hand, half of these children did not exhibit *any* CD symptoms at age 7 years, with 60% of these children failing to exhibit any CD symptoms at the subsequent age 10 years follow-up.[32] Despite this relatively poor diagnostic stability, Kim-Cohen and colleagues[18,32] report significant impairment in behavioral and academic functioning in these children. Collectively, although the short-term reliability of DBDs appears robust, the longer-term (2–5 year) stability of DBDs is questionable. As we discuss in greater detail in the second half of this paper, it is likely that the downward extension of DSM symptoms largely derived for school-age children to preschool children misspecifies the symptom presentation of DBDs in preschool children. Greater attention to this issue may assist in better defining DBDs in young children, which will result in more accurate identification and greater stability over time.

This lack of clear stability is a particularly critical issue for those interested in preventing poor long-term outcomes in children. As prevention and early intervention efforts are increasingly recognized as key to altering the often poor trajectories of youth with mental health disorders,[33] identifying children who will have persistent disorder is essential. Providing often costly services to children whose difficulties are developmentally transient and who are not experiencing current distress or suffering does not maximize the use of valuable resources. Likewise, not identifying children who are likely to develop persistent problems and ultimately poor outcomes is equally, if not more, problematic. Reviews of the literature[34] suggest that substantial misclassification results when the criterion of early onset symptoms of behavioral disorder assessed through parent and/or teacher self-report is applied to predict long-term development of disorder. Moreover, including pervasiveness or persistence does not result in improved identification of high-risk children.[35] Although incorporating data from other key areas of risk that are associated with problematic longer-term outcomes (eg, parental psychopathology) may prove useful in identifying children with the highest-risk, one potential avenue to pursue is improving on the developmental appropriateness of the symptoms used to capture behavioral disorders in young children.

Lastly, diagnostic differentiation between ODD and CD in young children has rarely been investigated. Keenan and colleagues[16] observed that virtually all preschoolers who met criteria for CD also met criteria for ODD. The one study that has examined the "fit" of this DSM diagnostic differentiation in preschoolers did not provide support for the ODD/CD distinction but rather for a unidimensional DBD construct.[36] Taken together with the low stability of preschool-age CD symptoms[18] and the attenuation of parent-reported CD symptoms over a 1-week period,[3] these data suggest that although multiple independent studies support the presence of DBDs at preschool age, considerably more work is needed to determine the validity of CD as a distinct diagnostic entity in young children.

ADHD
Prevalence

Estimating prevalence rates of DSM-defined ADHD in preschoolers is often challenging, as an ADHD diagnosis requires symptoms to be present in more than one setting, but many young children are not in school. Thus, assessing for ADHD depends on the extent to which preschoolers spend a considerable portion of their day outside of parental care. Prevalence rates from community and pediatric clinic samples of preschoolers for ADHD range from 2% to 18.2%,[3,12–15,37–39] with a range from 2% to 9.5% in pediatric samples, which are in line with prevalence rates for older youth.[17] Clearly, differences in prevalence rates of preschool ADHD between studies are a function of the type of assessment conducted, with clinical consensus and structured interviews resulting in lower prevalence rates. The use of DSM-referenced symptom checklists resulted in higher prevalence rates, which is not surprising given that these checklists typically do not assess additional DSM criteria necessary for a diagnosis (eg, presence of impairment; pervasiveness across settings). These additional criteria for an ADHD diagnosis may pose a significant issue in early childhood. For instance, the issue of pervasiveness across settings as a criterion is a good example of the extent to which "downward" extensions of existing criteria may obscure meaningful patterns in young children, because they do not reflect the "context" of early childhood. Although this issue has received scant attention in the preschool period, more recent instruments do incorporate developmentally appropriate consideration of the context. For example, the PAPA has adapted criteria for pervasiveness across settings by requiring that ADHD symptoms to occur in at least 2 activities and be, at least sometimes, uncontrollable by the child or by adult admonition.

Prevalence data are relatively sparse regarding specific ADHD subtypes in young children.[3,12,37–39] First, the hyperactive/impulsive type is most commonly observed in preschool children, followed by ADHD combined type. Studies suggest that ADHD inattentive type is relatively rare in the preschool-age range; however, again this raises issues of the developmental sensitivity of symptoms as most of the inattentive symptoms in the current nosology focus on school-based tasks. When significant inattentive symptoms are endorsed, these symptoms usually co-occur with hyperactive-impulsive symptoms. To our knowledge, only one study has assessed age effects on ADHD diagnosis, with results demonstrating that the combined type ADHD was more commonly diagnosed in older preschool children.[12]

Validity

Numerous studies have assessed the convergent validity of DSM-defined ADHD in preschoolers.[13,40–47] Similar to what is observed in older youth with ADHD, preschoolers with ADHD have poorer social skills, more difficulties with their peers, greater academic difficulties, and poorer cognitive and neuropsychological functioning. Moreover, their parents often have greater levels of psychopathology and stress, negative parenting behavior, feel less competent in their role as parent, and have poorer coping styles.

To date, Lahey and colleagues[5,47] have conducted the most extensive studies of stability of DSM ADHD and ADHD subtypes. Lahey and colleagues[47] found that 75% to 85% of 4- to 6-year-old preschool children meeting ADHD criteria initially retained this diagnosis during the following three subsequent years. Over the course of an 8-year follow-up, the proportion of youth who retained an ADHD diagnosis decreased in a pattern similar to that observed in older children.[48] Additionally, children who initially met criteria for either the inattentive or hyperactive/impulsive subtype alone were more likely not to meet ADHD diagnosis at follow-up assessment compared with children who initially met criteria for ADHD combined type. For those children who continued to meet ADHD diagnosis, there was considerable instability in DSM ADHD subtypes. Collectively, these findings call into question the reliability and utility of the DSM nominal categories of ADHD in young children. As Lahey and colleagues[5] note, "the subtypes cannot be viewed as discrete (nominal) categories that are permanent over time". Perhaps, as the authors state, continuous measures of ADHD symptoms, particularly the hyperactive/impulsive symptoms that appear to vary considerably over time, would be an appropriate diagnostic qualifier to classifying ADHD subtypes. It is clear that although the broad ADHD diagnosis has utility as a diagnostic entity in young children, further study must be conducted on the longer-term outcomes of preschool children with ADHD to best determine the utility of DSM ADHD subtypes. Alternatively, as we discuss later, an approach that includes a more developmentally specified definition of ADHD symptoms may better capture the presentation of ADHD in young children. Ultimately, greater precision in our conceptualization of ADHD symptoms for younger children is needed to clarify issues of subtypes and stability.

DBDs AND ADHD: APPLYING A DEVELOPMENTAL ANALYSIS

Does the extant literature suggest that the road ends here for our understanding of DBDs and ADHD in early childhood? We have suggested that it does not.[10,49,50] The early approach of "adhering as closely as possible to DSM-IV" with only minor developmental modifications[2] was a critical first step in broadly establishing syndromal coherence that extends down to early childhood. This process has demonstrated that young children can experience clinically relevant and pervasive behavior problems, which warrant attention and further investigation. With this accomplished, however, narrowly constraining the conceptualization of behavior disorder phenomenology to the existing nosology may contribute to misspecification in early childhood. We have suggested that accurate identification during this developmental period requires a developmentally specified approach to establish the critical features of behavior disorders that distinguish symptoms from the normative misbehavior of early childhood.[6,10] This developmentally specified approach would include elements such as identifying unique criterial features of behavior disorders in young children, establishing duration and symptom criteria cutoff points to generate maximally sensitive and specific thresholds, and defining symptom parameters in a manner that sharpens the typical: atypical distinction. In the following section, we apply a developmental lens to elucidate this approach.

DEVELOPMENTALLY IMPRECISE, IMPOSSIBLE, IMPROBABLE AND INAPPROPRIATE

Many DBD and ADHD symptoms overlap substantially with the normative misbehaviors of early childhood (eg, often interrupts, loses temper, defies adults; 51). For instance, Egger, Kondo, and Angold[12] found that many preschoolers met school-age cutoff criteria for the symptoms of "often loses temper" (30%), "often interrupts or intrudes" (47%), and "often actively defies" (57%), respectively. Moreover, Pavuluri and colleagues[51] found that parents rated 48% and 65% of preschoolers as "often easily distracted" and "often talking excessively," respectively. Although this is particularly true for ODD and ADHD, even some CD symptoms that are generally defined as more serious, low-incidence behaviors may be prevalent in young children. For example, Keenan and colleagues[16] found that a significant number of nonreferred preschool children without behavioral concerns met DSM-IV symptom criteria for "uses object to harm" (14%) and "often lies" (20%). Further, these symptoms are defined solely by frequency ("ie, often") during a period in which the presence of these behaviors per se is not pathognomonic.[49] In addition to developmental specification of frequency cutoff points, the *quality* of behavior (eg, its intensity, responsivity to environmental modification) may be important for such typical: atypical distinctions during the preschool period.[10,49] Symptoms that overlap with commonly occurring misbehaviors of young children without specification of how frequently they must occur in order for these behaviors to be of clinical concern and/or critieral clinically defining features beyond frequency are *developmentally imprecise*. Developmental imprecision is likely to contribute to *overidentification*, because normative misbehaviors (such as temper tantrums and defiance) may be mistakenly considered symptoms.

In contrast, many DSM symptoms (CD in particular) are *developmentally impossible* for young children (eg, truancy).[10] Others are *developmentally improbable:* although preschoolers may be capable of these behaviors (ie, stealing with confrontation), they represent extreme forms of behavior that are unlikely to occur and are not likely to be the critical defining features at this young age.[10] Thus, reformulating these symptoms to capture the underlying construct being assessed in a manner that better reflects the preschool-age period is necessary. In addition, some symptoms, particularly those for ADHD, are *developmentally inappropriate* (eg, often fails to give close attention to details or makes careless mistakes in schoolwork, work, or other activities; does not follow through on instructions and fails to finish schoolwork, chores, or duties in the workplace; often loses things necessary for tasks or activities). Developmental inappropriateness occurs when constructs that are more easily assessed in school-age children versus preschool children are included in the psychiatric nosology. For instance, for DSM ADHD symptoms of inattention, the inattentive symptoms focus on distraction, which is too diffuse and may be more challenging to measure precisely in young children. Thus, this "developmental inappropriateness" may lead to under-identification of inattentive subtypes during early childhood.

Although no studies to date have examined patterns of sensitivity and specificity of the existing DSM-IV nosology for preschoolers (eg, false positives, false negatives, subsequent onsetters, remitters), it is likely that developmentally impossible, improbable, and inappropriate symptoms contribute to *underidentification of certain children as well as entirely missing children who may have a disorder*. This is because (a) dropping *"impossible"* symptoms leads to a restricted item pool; (b) *"improbable"* symptoms are likely to capture only a small number of preschoolers with extreme manifestations and (c) *"inappropriate"* symptoms are not likely to effectively capture these behaviors in the manner they are present in most young children. For instance, conclusions that the ADHD-inattentive type does not occur (or is not a meaningful subtype) in preschoolers may be premature in the absence of developmentally appropriate operationalization of symptoms.

Given the rapid growth young children experience during early childhood in language, cognitive skills, executive functioning, moral reasoning, and self-regulation,[52] elucidating the parameters, presentation, meaning, and occurrence of the behaviors that define disruptive and attentional syndromes during this developmental period is particularly complex. Fortunately, major strides in developmental science over the past few decades have provided substantial evidence of the sequenced unfolding of these capacities in early childhood.[53–57] Although a comprehensive review is beyond the scope of this article,[10,50] the following sections briefly describe the developmental underpinnings of core processes that underlie the defining behaviors of DBDs and ADHD. These "clues" from developmental science provide a critical foundation toward the goal of a developmentally specified nosology for preschool behavior disorders.

AGGRESSION

As posited by Tremblay and colleagues,[58] aggression during early childhood peaks during the toddler period but is "unlearned," resulting in a normative decline of aggression over time, as self-control, language, and adaptive problem-solving skills are acquired with maturation. Thus, persistently high levels of aggression across early childhood are not normative. This suggests that mere frequency of aggression during early childhood is likely not informative—moving beyond subjective frequency (ie, "often") to determine normative frequency patterns within this developmental period is critical for demarcating the clinical threshold as well as for determining whether this differs at various ages across early childhood.

TEMPER LOSS

The quality of tantrums has also been identified as clinically discriminating both in distinguishing disruptive from normative behavior and in distinguishing DBDs from other disorders.[59] These qualities, including intensity of anger expressions, destructive tantrums, and difficulty recovering, have been linked to clinical problems in young children.[10,59–61] Frequency, although important, is not in and of itself a key indicator of disorder in young children. Likely a combination of both developmentally inappropriate frequency of tantrums (determined across the preschool-age range) in addition to the quality of the tantrum can best help determine whether a tantrum of particular preschool child is concerning.

NONCOMPLIANCE

As in the case of tantrums, developmental studies have focused on *quality* of noncompliance as a key distinction between typical and atypical manifestations.[62–64] Normative noncompliance is characterized by affectively regulated, goal-directed, adaptive behaviors, which are responsive to adult redirection. In contrast, problematic noncompliance has been defined as active resistance to control and refusal that is often associated with negative affect.[61,64,65] This includes "doing the opposite" of what was asked, an automatic, reflexive "no," and noncompliance in the context of angry outbursts.[50]

The clinical implications of these developmental patterns for both tantrums and noncompliance are that taking quality of misbehavior into account is likely to be critical to developing empirically based parameters for distinguishing disruptive behavior symptoms in a developmentally sensitive manner in early childhood. Identifying the interactional context of normative misbehaviors may also be clinically discriminating.[49]

Attention

Disruptive behaviors are discrete and relatively easily defined (eg, loses control of temper, hits another child). Although there are issues in how the construct of disruptive behavior varies with development, there is little question as how to define the problem behaviors in question. In contrast, the two main constructs of ADHD, inattention and impulsivity/hyperactivity, both involve "control" and are mixed to include cognitive and behavioral aspects. For example, attention is typically considered a cognitive ability, and yet in ADHD it is defined behaviorally by distractibility, poor persistence across time, and so on. Impulsivity includes both acting without thinking and reward-driven disinhibition, whereas hyperactivity typically is considered to reflect increased motor activity level, although it is rarely measured objectively in clinical settings. Not surprisingly, these measurement issues have precluded adequate specification of the key control processes across early development.

Attention is a basic cognitive construct, which is surprisingly difficult to define. Although aspects of focused, obligatory attention are evident in infancy,[66] there are marked developmental changes in the control of attention during the preschool years.[67,68] Ruff, Capozzoli, and Weissberg[69] conducted a series of seminal studies on the development of sustained visual attention in preschool children. Importantly, the set of studies attempted to determine developmental trends in attention in several different situations (ie, free play, television viewing, and reaction time task), to assess attention, consistency within, and stability across situations. Attention is typically considered a biologically based cognitive skill that is "endogenous" and thus should be highly consistent across contexts. In fact, however, attention is no different from compliance and temper behaviors in its dependence on context. Attention across different contexts is not as stable within individuals as attention measured in the same context across time. Clinically, these results highlight that individual differences in attention during the preschool period observed by assessment in one setting may be problematic for capturing clinically relevant attention problems.

Furthermore, it is not clear how actively sustaining attention differs from executive control. Indeed, a single latent factor has recently been found to underlie performance in inhibitory and working memory tasks[70] in typically developing preschool children, although preschoolers diagnosed with ADHD show deficits across task conditions when it is manipulated experimentally to load on motor inhibition (Go-No-Go Task) or sustained attention (Continuous Performance Task;[71]). Most studies to date in preschoolers with ADHD have shown deficits in control processes, some more in attention, some more in motor, and some in control in light of reward.[72] Collectively, it is clear that in the preschool-age range, children with ADHD have difficulty controlling behavior or cognition in light of expectation or instructions, although whether this difficulty is related to "attention," "executive function," or 'motivation" is not clear.

Impulsivity and Activity Level

Impulsivity is most often defined at the behavioral level as the inability to delay, inhibit, or control behavior in light of reward or direction. At the behavioral level, developmentally, these behaviors have been lumped under the rubric of self-regulation or effortful control. Kochanska and colleague's[73–76] studies of effortful control (ie, low levels of impulsivity, although Kochanska's conceptualization of effortful control also includes effortful attention and control of motor activity) demonstrated significant developmental progress in effortful control across the preschool period such that by 45 months, effortful control was highly stable and appeared to be a trait-like characteristic of young children. Thus, effortful control (ie, impulsivity), unlike attention in young children, appears to be less affected by setting or context.

Activity level has been less studied but also shows similar developmental patterns. In one of the few studies on the development of hyperactivity, Romano and colleagues[77] in a large national survey of parents of young children found that there were 4 trajectories depicting hyperactivity in children from the age of 2 to 6/7 years. Data indicated that a small proportion of the children (4.5%; n = 132) exhibited very few initial hyperactive symptoms, which decreased to zero over time. A significant number of children (42.0%; n = 1237) also exhibited few initial hyperactive symptoms, which remained at a low level over time. An equally substantial number of children (46.3%; n = 1365) exhibited moderate initial levels of hyperactivity, which declined slightly over time. Finally, a small number of children (7.2% n = 212) exhibited high initial levels of hyperactivity at age 2 years, and this level increased slightly over time. The data clearly demonstrate that hyperactivity, even in young children, is not uniformly high. In fact, 90% of young children have low to moderate levels of hyperactivity, which decrease over time. Clearly more data are necessary on understanding the presentation of hyperactivity in young children beyond the assessment of frequency.

CHARTING A DEVELOPMENTALLY REFINED NOSOLOGY FOR DBDs AND ADHD

As we have discussed at several points throughout this paper, there is an opportunity to better capture the phenomena of DBDs and ADHD as manifested in the early childhood period, particularly by applying a more "bottom-up," developmentally driven approach to the specification of symptoms, with an emphasis on quality of the behavior (intensity, expectability in context, flexibility, and organization of behavior). For instance, although "is often angry and resentful" is a symptom of ODD, a more developmentally sensitive specification of the underlying construct of anger in young children may include "Gets angry or mad for no reason," "loses control when angry," and/or "has trouble calming down when angry."[10] These multiple definitions of temper loss are derived from incorporating the developmental literature on the *quality* of anger in young children as pathognomic rather than just frequency of anger outbursts. Thus, these developmentally driven definitions of temper loss may more precisely capture the specific facets of temper loss that are clinically discriminating in young children. Likewise, current ADHD symptoms of inattention (eg, often has difficulty sustaining attention in tasks or play activities), hyperactivity (eg, often talks excessively) and impulsivity (often interrupts or intrudes on others) could alternatively be captured by symptoms of dyscontrol, such as "difficulty with controlling attention to the relevant rule in one-to-one play activities," "cannot control talking in situations when remaining quiet is expected (eg, story book reading) over short periods of time," and "cannot desist in interrupting others when provided structure and support to participate in engaging activities," respectively. These alternative symptoms define clinical patterns in reference to developmentally expectable tasks and capabilities in early childhood. Although these examples represent potential developmentally sensitive specifications of DBD and ADHD symptoms for young children, to date these are theoretically derived and will require systematic linkage to distributional characteristics of these behaviors within this developmental period and empirical validation of the incremental utility of a developmentally specified approach.

Do Developmentally Specified Refined Symptoms of DBDs and ADHD Add Value and How Would We Know?

Revision of existing DBD and ADHD criteria specifically for young children requires strong justification. As Moffitt and colleagues[78] contend, altering an established nosology may alter "patient's access to health care and educational services, confuse the use of diagnosis on the courts and undermine the cumulative nature of scientific research into mental disorders." Thus, there must be substantial evidence that a change in symptom specification leads to incremental benefits compared with the standard specification documented in the DSM. We propose that developmental specification will provide substantial incremental value, but, of course, this requires empirical validation.[10] First, developmental specification of symptoms is likely to substantially enhance accurate identification, thus increasing sensitivity, specificity, and stability of symptoms. As Bennett and colleagues[34,35] contend, our ability to provide intervention to those in greatest need depends greatly on accurate identification of children who are on the beginnings of a chronic disruptive behavior trajectory. Currently, relatively poor prediction from preschool disruptive behavior does not provide adequate targeted, prevention efforts.

TREATMENT

Over the past 2 decades, there has been an increasing evidence base for both psychosocial and pharmacologic interventions for DBDs and ADHD in preschoolers.[79–81] Although a comprehensive review of this literature is beyond the scope of this article (see articles in this issue), we highlight here some key findings of the primary psychosocial intervention for which there is substantial evidence of validity in preschoolers, specifically, Behavioral Parent Training (BPT;[79,82,83]).

BPT has been evaluated as a treatment for ODD, CD, and ADHD in children as young as 2 years old, demonstrating significant reductions in observed and parent-reported behavioral problems[84–89] and inattentive and hyperactive behavior.[84,90] Moreover, beyond statistical significance, studies demonstrate that some preschool children attain clinically significant (ie, normalization of behavior) benefits from BPT.[91,92] BPT has also been shown to reduce punitive parenting behavior[86,89,92] and parenting stress[84,93] increase positive parenting behavior[91] and parenting sense of competence.[86,91] Furthermore, maintenance of treatment gains for some preschool children has been seen for periods ranging from a few months[84,86] to a year[94] or more.[87,89,95] Some studies have demonstrated continued improvement for these children after termination of treatment.[87] Moreover, studies have shown that BPT for preschool children with ODD/CD has a broader impact for targeted children and their families. For example, studies have demonstrated effects of BPT on the school behavior of targeted preschool children[85] as well as improving the behavior of nontargeted siblings.[91,96] Collectively, the evidence suggests that BPT should be a first-line treatment for preschool-aged children who are at risk for or are diagnosed with ODD, CD, or ADHD.

The clear evidence for BPT for DBDs and ADHD must also be kept in light of the fact that a substantial minority of children do not respond to BPT.[97,98] Although multiple reasons have been posited, we note that the lack of developmental specification of DBD and ADHD symptoms potentially undermines the efficacy of BPT and other interventions (eg, stimulant medication). For example, we noted earlier that noncompliance per se is not pathognomic but can be adaptive and developmentally appropriate for preschoolers. However, developmentally, certain expressions of noncompliance, in particular the reflexive "no" and noncompliance in the context of angry outbursts, are problematic. Thus, if we only target BPT to those children who, developmentally, have *maladaptive noncompliance*, we are likely maximizing the effectiveness of BPT. Likewise, implementing BPT for children with developmentally appropriate expressions of noncompliance is a misuse of costly services. Similarly, when multiple expressions of developmentally maladaptive behavior exist, such as noncompliance as reflexive "no" versus noncompliance in the context of anger, developing targeted interventions based on the varying expression of the behavior can lead to better-tailored treatment. For instance, a reflexive "no" may be considered more temperamentally/biologically driven and thus perhaps more responsive to pharmacologic intervention, whereas noncompliance in the context of anger may suggest the utility of implementing psychosocial interventions that focus on assisting parents to support emotional regulation in their child. Although space prohibits further elaboration of the treatment implications of developmental specifications of DBD and ADHD symptoms, we believe that this approach has great potential to obtaining a greater understanding of how best to treat young children with DBDs and ADHD.

SUMMARY

Although DSM-defined DBDs and ADHD manifest during early childhood in meaningful ways, the emphasis of extending the DBD and ADHD nosology, which is based on studies of older youth, to younger children potentially limits the utility of these symptoms. Given that it is clear that DBDs and ADHD often emerge during early childhood and that early intervention is most efficacious, developing a more refined understanding of the clinical phenomenology of behavior disorders in early childhood is a critical next step. We contend that an approach that emphasizes the developmental specification of symptoms has the potential to address several long-standing issues in the literature, including enhancing the specificity, sensitivity, and stability of DBD and ADHD symptoms. Moreover, progress toward developmentally specified symptoms may inform our understanding of which type of treatment works best for whom. Answers to these questions are critical if we are to ultimately intervene to improve the lives of young children affected with DBDs and ADHD.

REFERENCES

1. Keenan K, Wakschlag L. Can a valid diagnosis of disruptive behavior disorder be made in preschool children? Am J Psychiatry 2002;159:351–8.
2. Task Force on Research Diagnostic Criteria: Infancy and Preschool. Research diagnostic criteria for infants and preschool children: The process and empirical support. J Am Acad Child Adolesc Psychiatry 2003;42(12):1504–12.
3. Egger H, Erkanli E, Keelr G, et al. Test-retest reliability of the Preschool Age Psychiatric Assessment (PAPA). J Am Acad Child Adolesc Psychiatry 2006; 45(5):538–49.
4. Lahey B, Pelham W, Stein M, et al. Validity of DSM-IV attention-deficit/hyperactivity disorder for young children. J Am Acad Child Adolesc Psychiatry 1998; 37:695–702.
5. Lahey B, Pelham W, Loney J, et al. Instability of DSM-IV subtypes of ADHD from preschool through elementary school. Arch Gen Psychiatry 2005;62:896–902.
6. Wakschlag L, Briggs-Gowan M, Hill C, et al. Observational assessment of preschool disruptive behavior, part II: validity of the Disruptive Behavior Diagnostic Observation Schedule (DB-DOS). J Am Acad Child Adolesc Psychiatry 2008;47(6):632–41.

7. Wilens T, Biederman J, Brown S, et al. Psychiatric comorbidity and functioning in clinically referred preschool children and school-age youths with ADHD. J Am Acad Child Adolesc Psychiatry 2002;41:262–8.

8. Zito J, Safer D, dosReis S, et al. Trends in the prescribing of psychotropic medications to preschoolers. JAMA 2000;283:1025–30.

9. Campbell SB. Behavior problems in preschool children: clinical and developmental issues. New York: Guilford; 2002.

10. Wakschlag L, Tolan P, Leventhal B. Research review: 'ain't misbehavin': towards a developmentally-sensitive nosology for preschool disruptive behavior. Invited review, forthcoming. J Child Psychol Psychiatry 2008, in press.

11. Shaw D, Gilliom M, Ingoldsby E, et al. Trajectories leading to school age conduct problems. Dev Psychol 2003;39(2):189–200.

12. Egger H, Kondo D, Angold A. The epidemiology and diagnostic issues in preschool attention-deficit/hyperactivity disorder. Infants Young Child 2006; 19(2):109–22.

13. Keenan K, Shaw DS, Walsh B, et al. DSMIII-R disorders in preschool children from low-income families. J Am Acad Child Adolesc Psychiatry 1997;36:620–7.

14. Briggs-Gowan M, Horowitz S, Schwab-Stone M. Mental health in pediatric settings: distribution of disorders and factors related to service use. J Am Acad Child Adolesc Psychiatry 2000;39(7):841–9.

15. Lavigne J, Gibbons R, Christoffel K, et al. Prevalence rates and correlates of psychiatric disorders among preschool children. J Am Acad Child Adolesc Psychiatry 1996;35(2):204–14.

16. Keenan K, Wakschlag L, Danis B, et al. Further evidence of the reliability and validity of DSM-IV ODD and CD in preschool children. J Am Acad Child Adolesc Psychiatry 2007;46:457–68.

17. American Psychiatric Association. Diagnostic and statistical manual for mental health disorders. Washington, DC: APA Press; 2000.

18. Kim-Cohen J, Arseneault L, Caspi A, et al. Validity of DSM-IV conduct disorder in 4 1/2-5 year-old children: a longitudinal epidemiological study. Am J Psychiatry 2005;162:1108–17.

19. Speltz M, DeKlyen M, Greenberg M. Clinic referral for oppositional defiant disorder: relativeness significance of attachment and behavioral variables. J Abnorm Child Psychol 1995;23:487–507.

20. Speltz M, McLellan J, DeKlyen M, et al. Preschool boys with oppositional defiant disorder: clinical presentation and diagnostic change. J Am Acad Child Adolesc Psychiatry 1999;38:838–45.

21. Coy K, Speltz M, DeKlyen M. Social cognitive processes in boys with and without oppositional defiant disorder. J Abnorm Child Psychol 2001;29(2): 107–19.

22. Greenberg M, Speltz M, DeKlyen M. Correlates of clinic referral for early conduct problems: variable- and person-oriented approaches. Dev Psychopathol 2001; 13:255–76.

23. Schwebel D, Speltz M, Jones K. Unintentional injury in preschool boys with and without early onset of disruptive behavior. J Pediatr Psychol 2002;27(8):727–37.

24. Wakschlag L, Keenan K. Clinical significance and correlates of disruptive behavior symptoms in environmentally at risk preschoolers. J Clin Child Adolesc Psychol 2001;30:262–75.

25. Webster-Stratton C. Early-onset conduct problems: does gender make a difference? J Consult Clin Psychol 1996;64(3):540–51.

26. Webster-Stratton C, Lindsay D. Social competence and conduct problems in young children: issues in assessment. J Clin Child Adolesc Psychol 1999; 28(1):25–43.

27. Keenan K, Wakschlag L. More than the terrible twos: the nature and severity of behavior problems in clinic-referred preschoolers. J Abnorm Child Psychol 2000;28:33–46.

28. Keenan K, Wakschlag L. Are ODD and CD symptoms normative behaviors in preschoolers? A comparison of referred and non-referred children. Am J Psychiatry 2004;161:356–8.

29. Lavigne J, Arend R, Rosenbaum D, et al. Psychiatric disorders with onset in the preschool years: I. Stability of diagnoses. J Am Acad Child Adolesc Psychiatry 1998;37:1246–54.

30. Lavigne J, Arend R, Rosenbaum D, et al. Psychiatric disorders with onset in the preschool years: II. Correlates and predictors of stable case status. J Am Acad Child Adolesc Psychiatry 1998;37(12):1255–61.

31. Lavigne J, Cicchetti C, Gibbons R, et al. Oppositional defiant disorder with onset in preschool years: longitudinal stability and pathways to other disorders. J Am Acad Child Adolesc Psychiatry 2001;40:1393–400.

32. Kim-Cohen J, Arseneault L, Newcombe R, et al. Five-year predictive validity of DSM-IV conduct disorder research diagnosis on 4 ½ –5-year-old children. Eur Child Adolesc Psychiatry, in press.

33. Surgeon General, 2000 U.S. Public Health Service. Report of the Surgeon General's Conference on Children's Mental Health: a National Action Agenda. Washington, DC: Department of Health and Human Services; 2000.

34. Bennett K, Lipman E, Racine Y, et al. Annotation: do measures of externalizing behavior in normal populations predict later outcome? Implications for targeted interventions to prevent conduct disorder. J Child Psychol Psychiatry 1998; 39(8):1059–70.

35. Bennett K, Lipman E, Brown S, et al. Predicting conduct problems: can high-risk children be identified in kindergarten and grade 1? J Consult Clin Psychol 1999; 67(4):470–80.

36. Sterba S, Egger H, Angold A. Diagnostic specificity and nonspecificity in the dimensions of preschool pathology. J Child Psychol Psychiatry 2007;48(10): 1005–13.

37. Pineda D, Ardila A, Rosselli M, et al. Prevalence of attention-deficit/hyperactivity disorder symptoms in 4–17 year old children in the general population. J Abnorm Child Psychol 1999;27(6):455–62.

38. Gimpel G, Kuhn B. Maternal report of attention-deficit/hyperactivity disorder symptoms in preschool children. Child Care Health Dev 2000;26:163–79.

39. Gadow K, Sprafkin J, Nolan E. DSM-IV symptoms in community and clinical preschool children. J Am Acad Child Adolesc Psychiatry 2001;40:1383–92.

40. Dewolfe N, Byrne J, Bawden H. ADHD in preschool children: parent-rated psychosocial correlates. Dev Med Child Neurol 2000;42:825–30.

41. Byrne J, DeWolfe N, Bawden H. Assessment of attention deficit hyperactivity disorder in preschoolers. Child Neuropsychol 1998;4:49–66.

42. DuPual G, MCgoey K, Eckert T. Preschool children with attention-deficit/hyperactivity disorder: impairments in behavioral, social, and school functioning. J Am Acad Child Adolesc Psychiatry 2001;40(5):508–15.

43. Hartung C, Willcutt E, Lahey B. Sex differences in young children who meet criteria for attention-deficit/hyperactivity disorder. J Clin Child Adolesc Psychol 2002;31(4):453–64.

44. Chronis A, Lahey B, Pelham W, et al. Psychopathology and substance use in parents of young children with attention-deficit/hyperactivity disorder. J Am Acad Child Adolesc Psychiatry 2003;42:1424–32.
45. Lee S, Lahey B, Owens E, et al. Few preschool boys and girls with ADHD are well-adjusted during adolescence. J Abnorm Child Psychol 2008;36:373–83.
46. Massetti G, Lahey B, Pelham W, et al. Academic achievement over 8 years among children who met modified criteria for attention-deficit/hyperactivity disorder at 4–6 years of age. J Abnorm Child Psychol 2008;36:399–410.
47. Lahey B, Pelham W, Loney J, et al. Three-year predictive validity of DSM-IV attention-deficit/hyperactivity disorder in children diagnosed at 4–6 years of age. Am J Psychiatry 2004;161:2014–20.
48. Barkley R, Fischer M, Smallish L, et al. The persistence of attention-deficit/hyperactivity disorder as a function of reporting source and definition of disorder. J Abnorm Psychol 2002;111:279–89.
49. Wakschlag L, Leventhal B, Thomas B. Disruptive behavior disorders & ADHD in preschool children: characterizing heterotypic continuities for a developmentally informed nosology for DSM V. In: Narrow W, First M, Sirovatka P, et al, editors. Age and gender considerations in psychiatric diagnosis: a research agenda for DSM-V. Arlington (VA): American Psychiatric Association; 2007. p. 243–58.
50. Wakschlag L, Danis B. Characterizing early childhood disruptive behavior: enhancing developmental sensitivity. In: Zeanah C, editor. Handbook of infant mental health, 3rd edition. New York: Guilford. In press.
51. Pavuluri M, Luk S, McGee R. Parent reported preschool attention deficit hyperactivity: measurement and validity. Eur Child Adolesc Psychiatry 1999;8(2):126–33.
52. National Research Council and Institute of Medicine. From neurons to neighborhoods: the science of early childhood development. Washington, DC: National Academy Press; 2000.
53. Baillargeon R, Normand C, Seguin J, et al. The evolution of problem and social competence behaviors during toddlerhood: a prospective population based study. Infant Ment Health J 2007;28:12–38.
54. Brownell D, Kopp M, editors. Socioemotional development in the toddler years: transitions and transformations. New York Guilford.
55. Espy K, Bull R, Martin J, et al. Measuring the development of executive control with the shape school. Psychol Assess 2006;18(4):373–81.
56. Kochanska G, Aksan N. Children's conscience and self-regulation. J Pers 2006; 74:1587–617.
57. Tremblay R. The development of aggressive behaviour during childhood: what have we learned in the past century? Int J Behav Dev 2000;24(2):129–41.
58. Côté S, Vaillancourt T, LeBlanc J, et al. The development of physical aggression during childhood: a nation wide Joint development of physical and indirect aggression 53 longitudinal study of Canadian children. J Abnorm Child Psychol 2006;34:71–85.
59. Belden A, Thompson N, Luby J. Temper tantrums in healthy versus depressed and disruptive preschoolers: defining tantrum behaviors associated with clinical problems. J Pediatr 2008;152:117–22.
60. Needleman R, Stevenson J, Zuckerman B. Psychosocial correlates of severe temper tantrums. J Dev Behav Pediatr 1991;12:77–83.
61. Crockenberg S, Litman C. Autonomy as competence in 2 year olds: maternal correlates of child defiance, compliance, and self assertion. Dev Psychol 1990; 26:961–71.

62. Dirks M, Henry D, Hill C, et al. Contextual variations in preschoolers' social skills during laboratory observations: Implications for real world functioning.

63. Drabick D, Strassberg Z, Kees M. Measuring qualitative aspects of preschool boys' noncompliance: the response style questionnaire (RSQ). J Abnorm Child Psychol 2001;29:129–40.

64. Kuczynski L, Kochanska G. Development of children's noncompliance strategies from toddlerhood to age five. Dev Psychol 1990;26:398–408.

65. Bates J, Petit G, Dodge K, et al. Interaction of temperamental resistance to control and restrictive parenting in the development of externalizing behavior. Dev Psychol 1998;34:982–95.

66. Sheese B, Rothbart M, Posner M, et al. Executive attention and self-regulation in infancy. Infant Behav Dev 2008;31:501–10.

67. Reuda M, Posner M, Rothbart M. The development of executive attention: Contributions to the emergence of self-regulation. Dev Neuropsychol 2005;28(2): 573–94.

68. Ruff H, Rothbart M. Attention in early development: themes and variations. New York: Oxford University Press; 1996.

69. Ruff H, Capozzoli M, Weissberg R. Age, individuality, and context as factors in sustained visual attention during the preschool years. Dev Psychol 1998;34(3): 454–64.

70. Wiebe S, Andrews K, Charak D. Using confirmatory factor analysis to understand executive control in preschool children: I. Latent structure. Dev Psychol 2008; 44(2):575–87.

71. Berwid O, Kera E, Marks D, et al. Sustained attention and response inhibition in young children at risk for attention-deficit/hyperactivity disorder. J Child Psychol Psychiatry 2005;46(11):1219–29.

72. Sonuga-Barke E, Auerbach J, Campbell S, et al. Varieties of preschool hyperactivity: multiple pathways from risk to disorder. Dev Sci 2005;8(2):141–50.

73. Kochanska G, Coy K, Murray K. The development of self-regulation in the first four years of life. Child Dev 2001;72(4):1091–111.

74. Kochanska G, Murray K, Harlan E. Effortful control in early childhood: continuity and change, antecedents, and implications for social development. Dev Psychol 2000;36:220–32.

75. Kochanska G, Knaack A. Effortful control as a personality characteristic of young children: antecedents, correlates, and consequences. J Pers 2003;71(6): 1087–112.

76. Murray K, Kochanska G. Effortful control: factor structure and relation to externalizing and internalizing behavior. J Abnorm Child Psychol 2002;30:503–14.

77. Romano E, Tremblay R, Abdeljelil F, et al. Development and prediction of hyperactive symptoms from 2-7 years in a population-based sample. Pediatrics 2006; 117:2101–11.

78. Moffitt T, Arseneault L, Jaffee S, et al. Research review: DSM-IV conduct disorder: research needs for an evidence base. J Child Psychol Psychiatry 2008;49(1): 3–33.

79. Nixon R. Treatment of behavior problems in preschoolers: a review of parent training programs. Clin Psychol Rev 2002;22:525–46.

80. McGoey KE, Eckert T, DuPual G. Early intervention for preschool-age children with ADHD: a literature review. J Emot Behav Disord 2002;10(1):14–30.

81. Greenhill LL, Posner K, Vaughan BS, et al. Attention deficit hyperactivity disorder in preschool children. Child Adolesc Psychiatr Clin N Am 2008;17:347–59.

82. Eyberg S, Nelson M, Boggs S. Evidence-based psychosocial treatments for children and adolescents with disruptive behavior. J Clin Child Adolesc Psychol 2008;37(1):215–37.
83. Pelham WE, Fabiano GA. Evidence-based psychosocial treatments for attention-deficit/hyperactivity disorder. J Clin Child Adolesc Psychol 2008;37(1):184–214.
84. Eisenstadt TH, Eyberg S, McNeil CB, et al. Parent-child interaction therapy with behavior problem children: relative effectiveness of two stages and overall treatment outcome. J Clin Child Adolesc Psychol 1993;22(1):42–51.
85. McNeil CB, Eyberg S, Eisenstadt TH, et al. Parent-child interaction therapy with behavior problem children: generalization of treatment effects to the school setting. J Clin Child Adolesc Psychol 1991;20(2):140–51.
86. Schuhmann EM, Foote RC, Eyberg SM, et al. Efficacy of parent-child interaction therapy: interim report of a randomized trial with short-term maintenance. J Clin Child Adolesc Psychol 1998;27(1):34–45.
87. Webster-Stratton C. The effects of father involvement in parent training for conduct problem children. J Child Psychol Psychiatry 1985;26(5):801–10.
88. Webster-Stratton C. Enhancing the effectiveness of self-administered videotape parent training for families with conduct-problem children. J Abnorm Child Psychol 1990;18(5):479–92.
89. Webster-Stratton C, Hammond M. Predictors of treatment outcome in parent training for families with conduct problem children. Behav Ther 1990;21:319–37.
90. Sonuga-Barke EJS, Daley D, Thompson M, et al. Parent-based therapies for preschool attention-deficit/hyperactivity disorder: a randomized controlled trial with a community sample. J Am Acad Child Adolesc Psychiatry 2001;40:402–12.
91. Eyberg SM, Boggs SR, Algina J. New developments in psychosocial, pharmacological, and combined treatments of conduct disorders in aggressive children. Psychopharmacol Bull 1995;31:83–91.
92. Webster-Stratton C, Hammond M. Treating children with early-onset conduct problems: a comparison of child and parent training interventions. J Consult Clin Psychol 1997;35:93–108.
93. Pisterman S, Firestone P, McGrath P, et al. The role of parent training in treatment of preschoolers with ADHD. Am J Orthop 1992;62:397–408.
94. Funderburk BW, Eyberg S, Newcomb K, et al. Parent-child interaction therapy with behavior problem children: maintenance of treatment effects in the school setting. Child Fam Behav Ther 1998;20(2):17–39.
95. Webster-Stratton C. Long-term follow-up of families with young conduct problem children: from preschool to grade school. J Clin Child Adolesc Psychol 1990;19:144–9.
96. Brestan EV, Eyberg SM, Boggs SR, et al. Parent-child interaction therapy: parents' perceptions of untreated siblings. Child Fam Behav Ther 1997;19:13–29.
97. Chacko A, Wymbs BT, Flammer-Rivera L, et al. A pilot study of the feasibility and efficacy of the strategies to enhance positive parenting program for single mothers of children with ADHD. J Atten Disord 2008;12(3):270–80.
98. Chacko A, Wymbs BT, Arnold FW, et al. Enhancing traditional behavioral parent training for single-mothers of children with ADHD. J Clin Child Adolesc Psychol in press.

Autism Spectrum Disorders in Young Children

Frances de L. Martínez-Pedraza, BA, Alice S. Carter, PhD*

KEYWORDS

• Autism • Young children • Early diagnosis
• Early intervention • Family

The focus of this review is on the early identification, assessment, and treatment of young children (0–5 years of age) with autism spectrum disorders (ASDs). ASDs are diagnosed in approximately 1 out of 150 children in the United States,[1,2] and given the increasing evidence that early intervention improves outcomes for children with ASD, there is an urgent need to enhance early detection and intervention efforts.[3] Retrospective parent reports,[4,5] early home videotapes,[6,7] and newer prospective studies of younger siblings of children with ASD who are at elevated risk [8,9] provide converging evidence that the age at onset for the majority of cases of ASD is the second year of life. We first review the early signs and symptoms of ASD, then describe some of the measures that can be employed for screening and diagnosis, discuss the family context with respect to both adaptation to diagnosis and treatment, and conclude with a brief review of interventions for young children with ASD.

Traditionally, the term pervasive developmental disorders (PDDs) has been employed in the Diagnostic and Statistical Manual of Mental Disorders, fourth edition, text revision (DSM-IV-TR), referring to autistic disorder, Asperger's disorder, PDD not otherwise specified (PDD-NOS), childhood disintegrative disorder, and Rett Disorder.[10] In this article, we use the term ASDs to refer to the diagnostic category of PDDs. Specifically, we focus on the diagnosis of autistic disorder (AD) and PDD-NOS, as the majority of research on young children has focused on these conditions. Our preference for the term ASD reflects recognition that along with restrictive interests and repetitive behaviors, the primary developmental perturbations that characterize ASDs are social and communicative in nature. Moreover, the term ASD reflects an understanding that symptoms and behaviors in these three domains are best quantified as continuous phenomena.[11]

This work was supported by a grant to A. Carter from Autism Speaks.

Graduate Clinical Psychology Program, Department of Psychology, University of Massachusetts, 100 Morrissey Boulevard, Boston, MA 02125, USA

* Corresponding author.

E-mail address: alices.carter@umb.edu (A.S. Carter).

Child Adolesc Psychiatric Clin N Am 18 (2009) 645–663
doi:10.1016/j.chc.2009.02.002
1056-4993/09/$ – see front matter © 2009 Elsevier Inc. All rights reserved.

Although these behaviors lie on a continuum in the general population, individuals with ASD are characterized by severe and pervasive impairments in reciprocal social interaction and communication and exhibit stereotyped behaviors, as well as restricted interests, and activities. To meet full criteria for a DSM-IV diagnosis of AD, a child must demonstrate the following symptoms (**Table 1**):

1. Qualitative impairment in social interaction as manifested by two of the following: impairment in the use of multiple nonverbal behaviors (eg, eye gaze, facial expression, body postures), failure to develop peer relationships, lack of sharing of enjoyment, or lack of social or emotional reciprocity.
2. Qualitative impairment in communication in at least one of the following areas: delay or total lack of spoken language, marked impairment in the ability to initiate or sustain a conversation with others, stereotyped or repetitive use of language, or lack of varied spontaneous play.
3. Restricted repetitive and stereotyped patterns of behaviors, interests, and activities as manifested by preoccupation with one or more restricted patterns of interests, inflexible adherence to nonfunctional routines or rituals, repetitive motor mannerisms, or preoccupation with parts of objects.

A diagnosis of PDD-NOS is assigned when the child does not meet full criteria for AD or any other ASD but has marked severe and pervasive impairment in the development of reciprocal social interaction skills and in communication skills or exhibits stereotyped behaviors.[10]

Particularly before the age of 3 years, distinctions between AD and PDD-NOS may be less meaningful due to low stability across these two disorders.[12,13] Thus, when children receive a diagnosis of PDD-NOS or AD prior to age 3 years, they are likely to remain on the spectrum (albeit less likely than older children), but there is little specificity across these 2 conditions. A study suggests that up to 50% of PDD-NOS cases could have been overdiagnosed, whereas around 22% of cases were underdiagnosed.[12] By the age of 4 years, the stability of diagnostics has shown to improve significantly (80%–88% stability rate) and is comparable to that observed in older children and adolescents.[14,15]

Prior to evaluating a young child, it is essential to be knowledgeable about normative infant and toddler development as well as other early emerging psychopathological conditions. This is particularly important with children under the age of 2 years, as

Table 1	
Diagnostic criteria for autistic disorder	
Domains Involved in ASD Symptomatology	**Related Areas Impaired or Delayed**
Social interaction	Nonverbal behaviors Peer relationships Sharing of enjoyment Social and emotional reciprocity
Communication	Spoken language Conversation abilities Spontaneous play
Restricted and repetitive behaviors	Preoccupation with restricted interests Motor mannerisms Preoccupation with parts of objects Nonfunctional routines and rituals

delays or losses of age-appropriate social and communicative skills are often central to making a differential diagnosis of ASD.[16–18] In addition, young children with extreme temperamental inhibition, other regulatory challenges, or anxiety disorders or those who have been exposed to trauma may be socially reticent in a novel setting with a new evaluator. Thus, they may evidence unusual eye contact and restricted pretend play and may even engage in repetitive behaviors. Therefore, in addition to learning the signs of ASD in young children, a firm grounding in normative development and infant-toddler mental health is requisite to reliable differential diagnosis.

SIGNS OF ASD IN YOUNG CHILDREN

In this section, we discuss research conducted on very young children that highlights the early age at onset and specific signs that can be observed before age 2 years in children diagnosed with ASD. Such a research review is limited, however, and we strongly recommend reading case presentations of children diagnosed before 18 months of age[19,20] as well as reviewing the *ASD Video Glossary* of early signs, now available through Autism Speaks (http://www.autismspeaks.org/video/glossary.php). This website offers examples of red flags and diagnostic features of ASD.

Although the DSM-IV criteria acknowledge the importance of development in assigning criteria, no specific developmental guidelines are offered for applying criteria to young children. For example, when evaluating a 16-month-old child, an age at which typically developing children are expected to engage in parallel, rather than reciprocal play with peers, adaptation of the peer criteria is required. The 16-month-old (as well as a 12-month-old) would be expected to show interest in other children and their play, even though they have not yet acquired the social and emotional skills to develop reciprocal peer relationships or identify other children who they relate to as special friends. Similarly, it can be very challenging to determine whether children under 30 months of age and/or children with significant delays in the acquisition of language evidence atypical language and communication patterns and/or if they are atypical in a manner that is consistent with an ASD. For example, during the normative explosion in word learning in the second year of life, it is normative for children to repeat the last word or phrase that they hear (ie, mirroring the ASD symptom of echolalia). Attending to the intonation of word repetition can sometimes aid in clarifying normative from atypical word repetition. Specifically, young children with ASD who evidence echolalia, or atypical word repetition, will most often repeat words with exactly the same intonation used by the individual they are mimicking. Thus, the repetition of "cookie" following the query, "Do you want a cookie?" has a questioning intonation rather than an emphatic declarative intonation, which would be the more typical expression (ie, "Cookie?" versus "Cookie!"). Odd intonation can also be heard in nonword utterances, such as unusual screeching and crying.

Such behavioral distinctions are crucial, for in the absence of any reliable, specific, physical markers for ASD, clinicians must rely on behavioral signs for assigning diagnoses. Although not a reliable bio-marker, an early increase in head circumference in the first year of life, leading to macrocephaly, appears to be evident in some children with autism.[21,22] In recent years, research on the early emergence of ASD has expanded beyond reliance on parental retrospective reports and early home videos of children later diagnosed with ASD[6,7,23] to include newer prospective studies of high-risk infants with an older sibling with ASD.[4,8,9,24] These studies have greatly informed understanding of the earlier signs and symptoms of ASD and provide critical insights into the developmental unfolding of these disorders.

Retrospective studies provided important early clues regarding the emergence of ASD signs and symptoms. Although some parents recalled developmental differences, such as their infants preferring to feed facing away from them in early infancy, the majority of parents of children later diagnosed with ASD first became concerned about their children's developmental differences in the second year of life.[25,26] Several studies document that the mean age at which parents first report concerns to a professional, usually the pediatric health provider, is between 18 and 24 months of age.[25,27,28] Most parents first report concerns in the area of speech and language,[25] with other concerns, including extreme sensory over- or underreactivity and disturbances in the acquisition of social communication, play, and motor development.[28,29] A significant percentage of parents (10%–50%) retrospectively report a significant loss or regression in language and/or social-emotional relatedness in the middle of the second year of life.[30,31] Parents also report concerns regarding sleep and eating, which may be associated with sensory sensitivities and/or with insistence on sameness.[32–35] These findings highlight the importance of attending to parental concerns[36–38] as well as to the early emergence of ASD signs.

Analyses of home videos from first birthday parties indicate that many (80%–93% of children), but not all, children later diagnosed with ASD evidence social and communication signs, such as atypical patterns of social orienting (eg, failing to respond to their name being called), limited imitation, greater negative affectivity, and ambiguous affective expressions.[6,39–45] These findings are not due to global cognitive delays; one early video study revealed that the play and gestures of children later diagnosed with ASD was limited with respect to flexibility and variety and was less likely to be employed in a contextually appropriate manner when compared with children later diagnosed with mental retardation.[46] Finally, there is evidence of early unusual repetitive or stereotypical behaviors that have been interpreted as atypical sensory or perceptual responses,[47] including unusual visual inspection of objects,[6] hand and whole body posturing, repetitive motor behaviors (with and without objects), and excessive mouthing and babbling.[6]

A very exciting area of work that is informing our understanding of the earliest signs of ASD is prospective studies of siblings of children with ASD.[9,48,49] This design capitalizes on family genetic data supporting a first-degree relative recurrence risk of approximately 5%–10%.[50–52] Typically, researchers first compare the entire group of at-risk siblings to siblings who do not have an older sibling with ASD and then look within the group of at-risk siblings to compare siblings who are later diagnosed with an ASD to those who do not develop an ASD. As summarized by Zwaigenbaum and colleagues,[53] using innovative experimental and clinical tasks, ASD siblings of children with ASD evidence impairments and/or delays in the following 4 areas by 12 to 18 months of age compared with those of siblings of ASD children who do not develop ASD: (1) Social communication, with reduced, unusual, or limited eye contact, limited or delayed orienting to name being called, deficits in imitation, reduced social smiling and responding to reciprocal social games (not including those that involve physical activity such as tickling), limited or unusual social interest, and increased expression of negative and decreased expression of positive emotion;[9,24,48] (2) Language, communication, and general cognition, with delays in cognitive development, language comprehension and production, and in gesturing;[4,8,49,54] (3) Visual, including atypical patterns of visual tracking of objects and longer periods of fixation on objects;[54] and (4) Motor, with decreased activity levels,[55] delayed fine and gross motor skills[4] and atypical motor mannerisms.[56]

It is critical to note that from the first years of life through the lifespan, individuals with ASD show a great deal of heterogeneity with respect to the severity, onset, course, and constellation of ASD symptoms exhibited; cognitive, linguistic, and communication impairments; social-emotional, behavioral, and regulatory problems; and sensory sensitivities. Consistent with heterogeneity, there is diversity in early expression. In early development, it is often the absence or loss of typical social development markers that signal the beginning of the ASD diagnosis rather than the presence of atypical behaviors. However, some young children do manifest atypical behaviors, such as repetitive and rigid play, odd body postures and motor mannerisms (eg, rocking, hand flapping, finger flicking), or visually inspecting objects at unusual angles, out of the corner of their eyes, and/or for a prolonged period of time.[16,18] Therefore, it is critical to use assessments that press for social behaviors, such as social smiling and delight in simple reciprocal play (eg, rolling a ball back and forth), and joint attention behaviors, such as following a parent or examiner's gaze and/or point, pointing to show an object that is far away (protodeclarative pointing), integrating gaze with a vocalization or gesture to request, showing an object of interest by raising it up, vocalizing and looking at the parent or examiner, or looking at the parent or examiner to share pleasure or distress (ie, directing a range of facial expressions).

Assessment of cognitive and linguistic functioning is also critical, as one does not expect to see these adaptive social responses and joint attention behaviors in children with a mental age that is lower than the age at which these developmental attainments appear in typical development. Thus, it can be very challenging to determine whether a child with marked cognitive delays has ASD. In addition to delays or deficits in social and communicative behaviors, the presence of unusual prosody or intonation in word or nonword utterances, repetitive movements (with or without objects), and perseveration in play with objects are red flags that can aid in identifying very young children with ASD.

A very promising measure of the earliest symptoms, developed within the context of the infant sibling work, is the Autism Observational Scale for Infants (AOSI), a semi-structured play-based assessment, which comprises items that assess multiple markers of risk in visual, social, communication, motor, and affective domains.[57] Twelve risk markers are rated for presence and severity, which yields both a total score and a sum of the severity of scores.

SCREENING AND EARLY DETECTION

As awareness of ASD prevalence, early emergence of symptoms, and the value of early detection and intervention for enhanced long-term outcomes have increased, screening initiatives have been developed to increase early detection in the general population. For example, the American Academy of Pediatrics now recommends routine ASD screening to be included as part of a general developmental assessment during regular well-child visits at 18 and 24 months of age.[58] However, there is still debate about whether autism-specific screeners or screeners for general developmental delays should be used, and more research is needed to determine optimal methods and measures for screening for ASD.

Screening is often approached as a staged process[59] in which a brief, relatively inexpensive screener is followed by a more comprehensive observational tool, interview, or referral to a specialty evaluation provider or clinic. In addition, screening can focus on identifying autism-specific behaviors or can be more general, using screening tools that will be sensitive to a wide range of developmental disorders and psychopathology. Within autism-specific screening, a distinction is made between measures that are designed to identify ASD within the general population (level 1) versus measures that are designed to identify ASD within a sample of children for whom developmental concerns have been raised (level 2).

With respect to level 1, the Checklist for Autism in Toddlers (CHAT),[60,61] the Modified Checklist for Autism in Toddlers (M-CHAT),[62,63] and the Pervasive Developmental Disorders Screening Test-II (PDDST-II)[64] have been employed. Of these, only the CHAT has been assessed in a geographically defined cohort, and data on diagnostic status at follow-up were collected for both screen-positive and screen-negative children.[65] Using the original criteria, which required the absence of gaze monitoring, pointing to show, and pretend play (as measured by parental questionnaire and direct observation), only 18% of children diagnosed with ASD between 20 and 84 months of age were detected by the CHAT at 18 months of age.[66] With less-stringent criteria (absence of pointing to show), the proportion of children with ASD detected by the CHAT at 18 months of age (ie, sensitivity) was only 38%.

The M-CHAT is a parent questionnaire that is followed by an interview if responses suggest the presence of ASD. Available on the Internet, the M-CHAT includes a list of behavioral signs and covers a wider age range (18–30 months) than the CHAT. The M-CHAT (based on the use of both questionnaire and interview) is estimated to detect 85% of children later diagnosed with ASD. However, follow-up of the original test cohort was of a short duration of 2 years, and ascertainment of ASD diagnoses among the screen-negative cases was limited.[63] In addition, only screen-positive children were formally evaluated, providing more evidence for the positive predictive value of the M-CHAT than for the instrument's overall sensitivity, which requires formal evaluation of both screen-positive and a subset of screen-negative children.

The PDDST-II [64] is a parent questionnaire that surveys a wide range of early relevant behaviors in nonverbal communication, temperament, sensory responses, play, attachment, and social interaction. It is used with children under 6 years of age, and level 1 and level 2 screener versions were developed. To date there are no published studies regarding the sensitivity and specificity of the PDDST-II.

A relatively new potential level 1 screener, the First Year Inventory, is a parent report instrument that was developed to differentiate very young children (12 months old) who are at risk for atypical development, with a special focus on infants with ASD-related risk patterns.[67] Parents are asked to respond to 63 items that describe their children on two dimensions: (1) social and communicative behaviors and (2) sensory and regulatory behaviors.

A measure designed as a level 2 screener is the Screening Tool for Autism in Two-Year-Olds (STAT).[68] This direct assessment of the child is a play-based, interactive set of items that provide the opportunity for observation of social-communicative behaviors, including directing attention, requesting, reciprocal and pretend play, and motor imitation. This measure has been found to have high specificity, sensitivity, and predictive validity in 2-year-old children with developmental delays later diagnosed with ASD.[69] One concern about this measure is that it has had limited availability for clinical use.[70]

The Communication and Symbolic Behavior Scales Developmental Profile (CSBS DP) [71] integrates general first-stage developmental screening with a second-stage screening that meets the criteria for a level 2 screener, in that it is possible to detect many ASD symptoms. The CSBS DP measures prelinguistic skills (eg, emotion, eye gaze, communication, gestures, sounds, words, object use, and understanding) to identify children at risk for developmental delays. It consists of a general developmental screener, the Infant Toddler Checklist that is completed by the parent, a follow-up caregiver questionnaire, and a behavior sample that is videotaped and later analyzed. The researchers have reported that nine CSBS DP behavioral items distinguish children later diagnosed with

ASD from children later diagnosed with other developmental disabilities.[72] In addition, four behaviors differentiated children with ASD from typically developing children but not from children later diagnosed with other developmental disabilities. These findings suggest that failing many of these 13 behavioral items, called "red flag" items, indicate the need for referral to comprehensive evaluation for ASD.

Given the wide range of developmental, emotional, and behavioral problems that can impair the lives of infants and toddlers as well as their families, we advocate the use of broader first-stage screeners at the population level (eg, in pediatric clinics) that target language and/or developmental functioning (eg, Ages and Stages Questionnaire [ASQ], Infant Toddler Checklist)[73,74] paired with a social-emotional/behavior problem screener (eg, ASQ-Social Emotional, Brief Infant Toddler Social Emotional Assessment),[75–77] rather than employing autism-specific level 1 screeners. Of course, it is critical to determine the specificity of the broader screeners in detecting ASD, and it is preferable to use a broader screener that includes items that are specific red flags for ASD. Given the time pressure in pediatric practice, a single tool that can detect a wide range of problems in the earliest stages of screening is advantageous. Once a child screens positive, the health care provider will need to have a conversation with the parent to determine whether a level 2 screener is appropriate, referral to early intervention or a mental health service is most appropriate, or if the problem can be addressed within the pediatric office. This discussion is essential, as a wide range of factors, including cultural beliefs, can influence how parents complete the initial parent questionnaires.[78] When a child appears to have an ASD, employing a second-stage screener, such as the STAT or CSBS DP, ideally by a trained staff person in the pediatric office, could streamline diagnostic practice and improve parents' experience. When the child fails a level 2 screener, it is critical to refer for a comprehensive diagnostic and developmental evaluation.

DIAGNOSTIC ASSESSMENT

In light of the greater instability in diagnoses prior to 3 years of age, assessments of young children often focus on establishing or confirming diagnosis, whereas assessments at later ages typically focus on measuring skills.[79] However, both accurate diagnosis and identifying strengths and weaknesses of the child's developed skills are central to inform treatment planning for young children, whether they are newly diagnosed or being seen for reevaluation.

The gold standard diagnostic tools in research and clinical assessment of ASD are the Autism Diagnostic Observational Schedule (ADOS)[80] and the Autism Diagnostic Interview-Revised (ADI-R).[81] These instruments alone do not determine diagnostic status. Rather, results obtained guide clinical decision making for assigning an ASD diagnosis. The ADOS is a semistructured assessment of communication, social interaction, and play that presents a variety of semistructured situations that are designed to "press" for social and communicative behaviors. Children can be assessed with one of four modules, depending on the particular developmental and language level of the individual. The ADOS performs best in children with a nonverbal mental age of 15 months or higher.[82,83] In younger children, the sensitivity of the instrument is excellent, but its specificity decreases.[12,82,83] Recently, the ADOS has undergone important revisions to include a toddler module that can guide in the diagnosis of children as young as 12 months (ADOS-Toddler Module [ADOS-T]).[84] The ADOS-T does not have cutoff points that indicate diagnostic categories. It rather indicates ranges of concern for ASD. High sensitivity and specificity of the instrument were found in a sample of high-risk infants.

The ADI-R has been suggested as a complementary instrument to the Autism Observational Schedule in diagnostic assessments of children and adults for ASD.[85] The ADI-R is a standardized caregiver interview for use in the differential diagnosis of ASDs.[86] When the ADI-R is administered to parents of children younger than 4 years, items that measure imaginative play, imaginative play with peers, and group play are not considered.[81] Items related to the child's reciprocal friendships or circumscribed interests are administered only for children older than 10 years.

At present, there are no clinical instruments available for use in the first year of life. This may be appropriate, as to date, the infant sibling studies have not revealed consistent markers for ASD before 12 months of age. In addition to the ADOS-T, the AOSI, a semistructured, play-based assessment was developed to identify early signs of autism in infants at high-risk, which has been defined as infants with older siblings diagnosed with ASD.[57] Currently a research tool, this instrument shows promise for use in clinical applications.

In many regions of the United States, obtaining a diagnosis of ASD is essential for receipt of high-intensity, ASD-specific interventions. However, a diagnosis alone is insufficient to make treatment recommendations. At a minimum, a comprehensive assessment must include a detailed developmental history, including the range of settings and caregivers that the child has experienced, as well as standardized assessments of language and communication, intellectual functioning, adaptive functioning, and co-occurring social-emotional (eg, anxiety), behavioral (eg, aggression), and regulatory problems (eg, sleep and eating problems) that are not specific to ASD. Although it is beyond the scope of this paper to review specific assessment tools in these relevant domains, Goldstein and colleagues[87] present a comprehensive review of assessment instruments that are uniquely suited for the assessment of individuals with ASD, with detailed recommendations for young children.

FAMILY CONSIDERATIONS

All young children are embedded in family relationships. When a child is diagnosed with ASD, families are affected in different ways. Elevated parenting stress and depressive symptom scores have often been reported among parents raising children with ASD, whether they are compared with parents raising typically developing children or to parents of children with other developmental delays.[88] This finding has been replicated among parents raising young children with ASD.[89,90]

There are several stressors that families of young children with ASD may confront that affect their psychological adjustment.[91] Families of young children are typically in the early phases of reacting and adjusting to the news that their child meets criteria for a diagnosis of an ASD, particularly if this is the first child in the family receiving a diagnosis. Parental stress is particularly high when there is no confirmed diagnosis, but either parents, early intervention, or health care providers suspect that an ASD diagnosis may be present. Parents report being less satisfied and more frustrated when delays are long and the diagnosis less clear.[92] Uncertainty about diagnostic status may be due in part to any and all of the following: (1) long waiting lists to see ASD diagnostic specialists; (2) expectations of rapid developmental changes, which may lead parents and health care providers to delay formal evaluation; and (3) inconsistent child symptom presentations, in which very young children with ASD may appear to have age-adequate social skills in limited contexts (eg, during familiar routines). The unusual and uneven course of development of children with ASD also contributes to parents' confusion and frustration about the diagnosis. It could be challenging for parents to follow a period of little developmental variation or regression that was preceded by an apparently normal period of early development. Children with ASD also exhibit variability in skills across domains, which at times lead parents to over- or underestimate their child's capacities and can influence parents' perceptions and expectations of their child's development. Certain delays (eg, language, imitation, and play) can be overlooked due to perceived strengths in other developmental areas (eg, visual spatial skills and motor skills) or due to expectations that deficits are developmental lags, which are temporary. Indeed, the use of the term developmental "delay" rather than deficit may implicitly suggest to parents that the child will catch up to his or her peers. Further, parents may hear the ASD diagnosis but not understand that a child also has significant cognitive and linguistic delays/deficits that accompany the ASD diagnosis. Indeed, this is particularly challenging for parents and professionals, as there are no biological or behavioral markers to predict who will respond to early intensive interventions.

When a child is diagnosed with ASD, parents might experience stress as a result of a feeling of losing the life they expected for their children, for themselves as parents, and for their family.[93,94] Several changes and modifications to their lives are also very likely to occur. Efforts for coordinating, advocating for, and making decisions related to treatment, as well as acquiring skills to foster their child's development, are only a few examples of challenges parents of children diagnosed with ASD face.[95] Parents also have the responsibility of choosing treatments for their children from a wide range of options despite limited data to guide decision making. The redirection of parents' efforts to meet the needs of their child often times affects families' finances, as many parents stop working to coordinate their children's treatment, either by choice or because their employers do not allow them the flexibility to attend the necessary appointments. Some parents spend additional money for treatments beyond those provided by the state-financed programs (eg, more hours of same treatment or other treatments). When parents stop working, their previous expectations, identities, and desires of pursuing their own careers are also affected.

Parents of young, newly diagnosed children also report elevated parenting stress associated with behavior difficulty and severity of deficits and delays in children's social relatedness.[89] Families, and particularly parents and siblings, experience stressors related to specific child behaviors.[96] Parents might feel frustrated when their child responds inconsistently across settings, people, and time. They question whether their child cannot, does not want to, or will not be able to carry out certain actions. Child-related stress in parents is also reported with regard to (1) children's lack of reciprocity to their parents[97] and (2) children's disruptive or embarrassing acts, especially in public places. These behaviors could also place restrictions on family activities and interactions with others.[98] In addition, parents of children with ASD could experience stress, anxiety, and isolation related to their inability to control their child, who in most cases appears to be physically normal to others. Child behaviors have been shown to differentially impact parenting stress depending on the parent's gender. Maternal stress shows stronger relation to child regulatory problems, whereas paternal stress is more related to child externalizing behaviors.[89] Some studies have demonstrated that mothers of children with ASD report more stress and other negative effects than fathers do.[99,100]

A more systemic assessment approach has been helpful to understand family functioning variables and interrelations within families with children with ASD. From a systems analysis standpoint, maternal stress is not only predicted by the severity of the preschool child's behavioral symptoms but also by the partner's depressive symptoms, whereas paternal stress was found to be predicted only by maternal depressive symptoms.[101] This model recognizes that family members affect one another. However, further incorporation of how siblings' stress could be related to other family members or of how maternal and paternal stress might affect the child with ASD should be considered. Several studies have suggested that characteristics of parent-child relationships are associated with gains in language for children with ASD.[102] In addition, maternal interaction style has been observed to be influenced by the mother's acceptance of the child's diagnosis and her sense of resolution.[95] For these reasons, it might be relevant to identify and develop strategies to reduce parental stress, negative emotions, and negative cognitions for the benefit of both parents and their children. Such models exist, as several intervention approaches include parents as co-therapist for their children. Increases in parent confidence and self-efficacy due to learning techniques have been observed to decrease parent stress levels.[103,104] However, parents may also feel increased stress associated with role demands of providing direct services to their children.[105] Coping strategies,[106] having informal social support sources, and holding positive beliefs about the effects or impact of interventions in their children [88] have also been shown to decrease parenting stress.

INTERVENTIONS

In concert with efforts to enhance earlier detection of ASD, there has been a great deal of work to improve early interventions for young children with ASD. This work has been informed by our deepening understanding of the earliest signs and relationships between deficits in joint attention, play, social communication, and language.[18,107] The existing studies document that early intervention improves later communication and adaptive outcomes,[108] but there are many questions regarding early intervention efficacy that have yet to be addressed. Specifically, few completed studies provide evidence regarding the efficacy of different treatment interventions that young children with ASD receive, particularly for children under the age of 2 years. In addition, even for treatments for which evidence exists, there is limited empirical information available to guide decisions regarding treatment intensity, intervention settings, integration of parents and other caregivers, and different intervention approaches. Further, critical outcome variables and individual responses to interventions still need to be addressed.[109]

Interventions for young children with ASD that are designed to provide optimal learning opportunities must be individualized to meet the child's current learning and developmental characteristics. For example, for 12- to 24-month-olds, social interaction contexts must almost always give priority to caregiving rather than peer interactions; communication patterns require a focus on nonverbal communication, gestures, and joint attention; and learning approaches need to address exploration of objects and developing imitation and play skills in a manner that is quite distinct from the approaches that are appropriate for older children.[110] For these reasons, interventions for older children cannot be simply extrapolated to younger children without first addressing key developmental and contextual factors. The purpose of discussing several interventions for young children with ASD is to provide a brief review that does not intend to be exhaustive or conclusive about best intervention approaches. First, examples of home-based and school-based intervention programs are described, followed by a review of several interventions that teach specific skills relevant to children with ASD (eg, language interventions). It should be noted that for children under 2 years of age, ASD-specific interventions might not be widely available. Yet families and their children could benefit from other early intervention services such as speech-language therapy, and providers should seek opportunities for further training.

Many young children diagnosed with ASD receive home-based interventions, such as Applied Behavior Analysis (ABA). ABA has a body of data that supports it.[111–113] This intervention emphasizes systemic teaching of new skills, reinforcement of adaptive and acquired skills, imitation, discrimination learning (ie, rewarding behaviors in the presence of specific stimuli or activities but not rewarding the same behaviors when these conditions are not met), and control of interfering/maladaptive behaviors, among other aspects.[114] A second home-based program that is based on ABA principles is Pivotal Response Training.[115] This intervention offers a naturalistic approach, in which parents learn to teach their children different skills and to motivate them to perform these skills when engaging in daily routines. Skills include responding to more than one cue, initiating behaviors such as help seeking and requesting, and responding to prompts.[116] Research suggests that children who are able to learn these social-communication skills will have better long-term outcomes, with respect to social, communication, and academic functioning.[117] Finally, Floortime is a developmentally based intervention designed to facilitate social communication.[118,119] There has been very limited systematic study of the efficacy of Floortime, but several published case studies have reported improvements in language development and other areas of functioning.[119,120]

School-based programs intend to provide services to preschoolers within the traditional school context as opposed to specialized schools or the home-based services that are more typical before 3 years of age. The Treatment and Education of Autistic and Related Communication Handicapped Children (TEACCH)[121] is a school-based program developed at the University of North Carolina, which focuses on structured teaching, visual spatial understanding, and object manipulation, all of which seem to be relevant learning principals for children with ASD. The program also emphasizes development of communication skills through incidental teaching, and use of alternative communicative technique. Parent-delivered TEACCH intervention for preschoolers was found to be effective for improving developmental areas, such as cognition and nonverbal perception, when compared with a behavioral-education-only control group.[122]

A second school-based program is the Denver Model, developed at the University of Colorado. The Denver Model is based on a developmental model of ASD that emphasizes the development of play skills, positive affect, interpersonal relationships, and language development.[123] This model integrates treatment techniques such as behavioral teaching, language therapy, and occupational therapy. The Early Start Denver Model is the early intervention component of this model, which targets parents of children from 14 months to 3 years of age.[124] Studies have shown that children who participate in the Denver Model intervention demonstrate significant gains in symbolic play and receptive and expressive language; notably, gains were not influenced by symptom severity.[27]

Some interventions for children with ASD target specific ASD impairments/ behaviors. For example, certain interventions target behaviors such as joint attention (eg, Joint Attention [JA]).[125,126] The JA intervention has shown to be effective for initiating joint attention and responding to joint attention but not for other developmental domains such as symbolic play.[125] Still other interventions focus instead on different aspects of language (eg, the Picture Exchange Communication System [PECS] and the Responsive Education and Prelinguistic Milieu Teaching [RPMT]).[127] The JA intervention has shown to be effective for initiating joint attention and responding to joint attention but not for other developmental domains such as symbolic play.[125] Language interventions for young children also focus on children's prelinguistic pragmatic functions for intentional communication (eg, initiating joint attention, requesting, and turn taking). RPMT teaches object exchange as a means of turn taking, whereas PECS teaches requesting through picture exchange in young children. In a randomized, controlled trial that compared PECS and RPMT, (1) PECS was found to facilitate more generalized requests in children with little initiating joint attention, whereas (2) RPMT was found to facilitate turn taking and initiating joint attention for children with some initiating joint attention before the intervention.[127]

These results suggest that certain interventions might be more appropriate for specific individuals at specific stages of development or based on a specific level of skill acquisition. To date, little research has been conducted to address which specific intervention will best meet the needs of specific children. In light of the heterogeneity of symptom presentation and strengths and weaknesses observed among young children with ASD, research that informs how to tailor treatments to individual children is greatly needed.

SUMMARY

There is now clear evidence that the first signs and symptoms of ASD are evident for most children by 12 to 18 months of age. This knowledge, coupled with emerging evidence that early intervention that targets social-communicative behaviors improves long-term outcomes, has led to increased early detection efforts. Families who are confronted with a diagnosis of ASD often experience significant parenting stress and strain as they must navigate complex intervention decisions and learn to adapt to their child's unique set of challenges. The severity of social and communication deficits, along with sensory sensitivities and behavioral difficulties, appears to exacerbate parenting stress. Helping parents of very young children learn how to facilitate their children's social and communicative behaviors is the goal of several relatively new interventions for young children (eg, Early Denver Model, Floortime). Such approaches, which show great promise for children's long-term adaptation, are also likely to increase parenting efficacy and reduce stress. Earlier detection and intervention efforts are improving the long-term functioning of children with ASD. This is an extremely exciting moment for research on young children with ASD. In addition to many novel experimental approaches, important questions regarding intervention are being studied, including dismantling studies that illuminate which intervention may be most efficacious for which children and families.

REFERENCES

1. Centers for Disease Control and Prevention. Prevalence of the autism spectrum disorders in multiple areas of the United States, surveillance years 2000 and 2002. Available at: http://www.cdc.gov/ncbddd/dd/addmprevalence.htm. 2007. Accessed November 11, 2008.
2. Rice CE, Baio J, Van Naarden Braun K, et al. A public health collaboration for the surveillance of autism spectrum disorders. Blackwell Publishing Limited. Paediatr Perinat Epidemiol 2007;21:179–90.
3. Woods JJ, Wetherby AM. Early identification of and intervention for infants and toddlers who are at risk for autism spectrum disorder. Lang Speech Hear Serv Sch 2003;34:180–93.
4. Landa R, Garrett-Mayer E. Development in infants with autism spectrum disorders: a prospective study. J Child Psychol Psychiatry 2006;47:629–38.
5. Watson LR, Baranek GT, Crais ER, et al. The first year inventory: retrospective parent responses to a questionnaire designed to identify one-year-olds at risk for autism. J Autism Dev Disord 2007;37:49–61.

6. Baranek GT. Autism during infancy: a retrospective video analysis of sensory-motor and social behaviors at 9-12 months of age. J Autism Dev Disord 1999; 29:213–24.
7. Clifford S, Young R, Williamson P. Assessing the early characteristics of autistic disorder using video analysis. J Autism Dev Disord 2007;37:301–13.
8. Mitchell S, Brian J, Zwaigenbaum L, et al. Early language and communication development of infants later diagnosed with autism spectrum disorder. J Dev Behav Pediatr 2006;27:S69–78.
9. Zwaigenbaum L, Thurm A, Stone W, et al. Studying the emergence of autism spectrum disorders in high-risk infants: methodological and practical issues. J Autism Dev Disord 2007;37:466–80.
10. American Psychiatric Association. Diagnostic and statistical manual of mental disorders. Text rev. 4th edition. Washington, DC: American Psychiatric Association; 2000.
11. Volkmar FR, Carter A, Sparrow SS, et al. Quantifying social development in autism. J Am Acad Child Adolesc Psychiatry 1993;32:627–32.
12. Chawarska K, Klin A, Paul R, et al. Autism spectrum disorder in the second year: stability and change in syndrome expression. J Child Psychol Psychiatry 2007; 48:128–38.
13. Lord C, Richler J. Early diagnosis of children with autism spectrum disorders. In: Charman T, Stone W, editors. Social & communication development in autism spectrum disorders: early identification, diagnosis, intervention. New York: Guilford Press; 2006. p. 35–59.
14. Moss J, Magiati I, Charman T, et al. Stability of the autism diagnostic interview-revised from pre-school to elementary school age in children with autism spectrum disorders. J Autism Dev Disord 2008;38:1081–91.
15. Turner LM, Stone WL, Pozdol SL, et al. Follow-up of children with autism spectrum disorders from age 2 to age 9. Autism 2006;10:243–65.
16. Charman T, Baird G. Practitioner review: diagnosis of autism spectrum disorder in 2- and 3-year-old children. J Child Psychol Psychiatry 2002;43:289–305.
17. Mundy P, Sigman M. Specifying the nature of the social impairment in autism. In: Dawson G, editor. Autism: nature, diagnosis, and treatment. New York: Guilford Press; 1989. p. 3–21.
18. Mundy P, Sigman M. The theoretical implications of joint-attention deficits in autism. Dev Psychopathol 1989;1:173–83.
19. Dawson G, Osterling J, Meltzoff AN, et al. Case study of the development of an infant with autism from birth to two years of age. J Appl Dev Psychol 2000;21: 299–313.
20. Klin A, Chawarska K, Paul R, et al. Autism in a 15-month-old child. Am J Psychiatry 2004;161:1981–8.
21. Courchesne E, Carper R, Akshoomoff N. Evidence of brain overgrowth in the first year of life in autism. JAMA 2003;290:337–44.
22. Courchesne E. Brain development in autism: early overgrowth followed by premature arrest of growth. Ment Retard Dev Disabil Res Rev 2004;10:106–11.
23. Palomo RN, Belinchón M, Ozonoff S. Autism and family home movies: a comprehensive review. J Dev Behav Pediatr 2006;27:S59–68.
24. Sullivan M, Finelli J, Marvin A, et al. Response to joint attention in toddlers at risk for autism spectrum disorder: a prospective study. J Autism Dev Disord 2007; 37:37–48.
25. De Giacomo A, Fombonne E. Parental recognition of developmental abnormalities in autism. Eur Child Adolesc Psychiatry 1998;7:131–6.

26. Gray KM, Tonge BJ. Are there early features of autism in infants and preschool children? J Paediatr Child Health 2001;37:221–6.
27. Rogers SJ, DiLalla DL. Age of symptom onset in young children with pervasive developmental disorders. J Am Acad Child Adolesc Psychiatry 1990;29:863–72.
28. Young RL, Brewer N, Pattison C. Parental identification of early behavioural abnormalities in children with autistic disorder. Autism 2003;7:125–44.
29. Charman T, Swettenham J, Baron-Cohen S, et al. An experimental investigation of social-cognitive abilities in infants with autism: clinical implications. In: Muir D, Slater A, editors. Infant development: the essential readings. Malden (MA): Blackwell Publishing; 2000. p. 343–63.
30. Hoshino Y. Early symptoms of autism in children and their diagnostic significance. Jpn J Child Adolesc Psychiatr 1980;21:284–99.
31. Luyster R, Richler J, Risi S, et al. Early regression in social communication in autism spectrum disorders: a CPEA study. Dev Neuropsychol 2005;27:311–36.
32. Ledford JR, Gast DL. Feeding problems in children with autism spectrum disorders: a review. Focus Autism Other Dev Disabl 2006;21:153–66.
33. Malow BA, Marzec ML, McGrew SG, et al. Characterizing sleep in children with autism spectrum disorders: a multidimensional approach. Sleep 2006;29:1563–71.
34. Goodlin-Jones BL, Tang K, Liu J, et al. Sleep patterns in preschool-age children with autism, developmental delay, and typical development. J Am Acad Child Adolesc Psychiatry 2008;47:930–8.
35. Johnson CR, Handen BL, Mayer-Costa M, et al. Eating habits and dietary status in young children with autism. J Dev Phys Disabil 2008;20:437–48.
36. Glascoe FP. Using parents' concerns to detect and address developmental and behavioral problems. J Soc Pediatr Nurs 1999;4:24–35.
37. Glascoe FP, Macias MM, Wegner LM, et al. Can a broadband developmental-behavioral screening test identify children likely to have autism spectrum disorder? Clin Pediatr (Phila) 2007;46:801–5.
38. Glascoe FP. Screening for developmental and behavioral problems. Ment Retard Dev Disabil Res Rev 2005;11:173–9.
39. Adrien JL, Perrot A, Hameury L, et al. Family home movies: identification of early autistic signs in infants later diagnosed as autistics. Brain Dysfunction 1991;4:355–62.
40. Osterling J, Dawson G. Early recognition of children with autism: a study of first birthday home videotapes. J Autism Dev Disord 1994;24:247–57.
41. Maestro S, Muratori F, Barbieri F, et al. Early behavioral development in autistic children: the first 2 years of life through home movies. Psychopathology 2001;34:147–52.
42. Maestro S, Muratori F, Cavallaro MC, et al. Attentional skills during the first 6 months of age in autism spectrum disorder. J Am Acad Child Adolesc Psychiatry 2002;41:1239–45.
43. Maestro S, Muratori F, Cavallaro MC, et al. How young children treat objects and people: an empirical study of the first year of life in autism. Child Psychiatry Hum Dev 2005;35:383–96.
44. Maestro S, Muratori F, Cesari A, et al. Course of autism signs in the first year of life. Psychopathology 2005;38:26–31.
45. Dawson G, Toth K, Abbott R, et al. Early social attention impairments in autism: social orienting, joint attention, and attention to distress. Dev Psychol 2004;40:271–83.
46. Colgan SE, Lanter E, McComish C, et al. Analysis of social interaction gestures in infants with autism. Child Neuropsychol 2006;12:307–19.

47. Dahlgren SO, Gillberg C. Symptoms in the first two years of life: a preliminary population study of infantile autism. Eur Arch Psychiatry Neurol Sci 1989;238: 169–74.

48. Landa RJ, Holman KC, Garrett-Mayer E. Social and communication development in toddlers with early and later diagnosis of autism spectrum disorders. Arch Gen Psychiatry 2007;64:853–64.

49. Yirmiya N, Ozonoff S. The very early autism phenotype. J Autism Dev Disord 2007;37:1–11.

50. Ritvo ER, Jorde LB, Mason-Brothers A, et al. The UCLA-University of Utah epidemiologic survey of autism: recurrence risk estimates and genetic counseling. Am J Psychiatry 1989;146:1032–6.

51. Bailey A, Phillips W, Rutter M. Autism: towards an integration of clinical, genetic, neuropsychological, and neurobiological perspectives. J Child Psychol Psychiatry 1996;37:89–126.

52. Sumi S, Taniai H, Miyachi T, et al. Sibling risk of pervasive developmental disorder estimated by means of an epidemiologic survey in Nagoya, Japan. J Hum Genet 2006;51:518–22.

53. Zwaigenbaum L, Bryson S, Carter A, et al. Clinical assessment and management of toddlers with suspected ASD: Insights from studies of high-risk infants. Pediatrics, in press.

54. Bryson SE, Zwaigenbaum L, Brian J, et al. A prospective case series of high-risk infants who developed autism. J Autism Dev Disord 2007;37:12–24.

55. Zwaigenbaum L, Bryson S, Rogers T, et al. Behavioral manifestations of autism in the first year of life. Int J Dev Neurosci 2005;23:143–52.

56. Loh A, Soman T, Brian J, et al. Stereotyped motor behaviors associated with autism in high-risk infants: a pilot videotape analysis of a sibling sample. J Autism Dev Disord 2007;37:25–36.

57. Bryson SE, Zwaigenbaum L, McDermott C, et al. The autism observation scale for infants: Scale development and reliability data. J Autism Dev Disord 2008;38: 731–8.

58. Johnson CP, Myers SM. Identification and evaluation of children with autism spectrum disorders. Pediatrics 2007;120:1183–215.

59. Carter A. Assessing social-emotional and behavior problems and competencies in infancy and toddlerhood: available instruments and directions for application. In: Zuckerman B, Lieberman A, Fox N, editors. Emotion regulation and developmental health: infancy and early childhood. New York: Johnson & Johnson Pediatric Institute; 2002. p. 277–99.

60. Baron-Cohen S, Allen J, Gillberg C. Can autism be detected at 18 months? The needle, the haystack, and the chat. Br J Psychiatry 1992; 161:839–43.

61. Baron-Cohen S, Cox A, Baird G, et al. Psychological markers in the detection of autism in infancy in a large population. Br J Psychiatry 1996;168: 158–63.

62. Robins DL, Fein D, Barton ML, et al. The modified checklist for autism in toddlers: an initial study investigating the early detection of autism and pervasive developmental disorders. J Autism Dev Disord 2001;31:131–44.

63. Kleinman JM, Robins DL, Ventola PE, et al. The modified checklist for autism in toddlers: a follow-up study investigating the early detection of autism spectrum disorders. J Autism Dev Disord 2008;38:827–39.

64. Siegel B. Pervasive developmental disorders screening test-ii (pddst-ii). San Antonio (TX): Harcourt; 2004.

65. Baird G, Charman T, Baron-Cohen S, et al. A screening instrument for autism at 18 months of age: a 6-year follow-up study. J Am Acad Child Adolesc Psychiatry 2000;39:694–702.

66. Baird SM, Campbell D, Ingram R, et al. Young children with cri-du-chat: genetic, developmental and behavioral profiles. Infant-Toddler Intervention: transdisciplinary journal 2001;11:1–14.

67. Reznick JS, Baranek GT, Reavis S, et al. A parent-report instrument for identifying one-year-olds at risk for an eventual diagnosis of autism: the first year inventory. J Autism Dev Disord 2007;37:1691–710.

68. Stone WL, Coonrod EE, Ousley OY. Screening tool for autism two-year-olds (stat): development and preliminary data. J Autism Dev Disord 2000;30:607–12.

69. Stone WL, Coonrod EE, Turner LM, et al. Psychometric properties of the stat for early autism screening. J Autism Dev Disord 2004;34:691–701.

70. Bryson SE, Rogers SJ, Fombonne E. Autism spectrum disorders: early detection, intervention, education, and psychopharmacological management. Can J Psychiatry 2003;48:506–16.

71. Wetherby AM, Prizant BM. Communication and symbolic behavior scales: developmental profile. 1st normed edition. Baltimore (MD): Paul H Brookes Publishing; 2002.

72. Wetherby AM, Woods J, Allen L, et al. Early indicators of autism spectrum disorders in the second year of life. J Autism Dev Disord 2004;34:473–93.

73. Squires J, Bricker D, Potter L. Revision of a parent-completed developmental screening tool: ages and stages questionnaires. J Pediatr Psychol 1997;22:313–28.

74. Wetherby AM, Brosnan-Maddox S, Peace V, et al. Validation of the infant-toddler checklist as a broadband screener for autism spectrum disorders from 9 to 24 months of age. Autism 2008;12:487–511.

75. Squires J, Bricker D, Heo K, et al. Identification of social-emotional problems in young children using a parent-completed screening measure. Early Child Res Q 2001;16:405–19.

76. Squires J, Bricker D, Twombly E. Parent-completed screening for social emotional problems in young children: the effects of risk/disability status and gender on performance. Infant Ment Health J 2004;25:62–73.

77. Briggs-Gowan MJ, Carter AS, Irwin JR, et al. The brief infant-toddler social and emotional assessment: screening for social-emotional problems and delays in competence. J Pediatr Psychol 2004;29:143–55.

78. Carter AS, Briggs-Gowan MJ, Davis NO. Assessment of young children's social-emotional development and psychopathology: recent advances and recommendations for practice. J Child Psychol Psychiatry 2004;45:109–34.

79. Shea V, Mesibov G. Age-related issues in the assessment of autism spectrum disorders. In: Goldstein S, Naglieri J, Ozonoff S, editors. Assessment of autism spectrum disorders. New York: The Guilford Press; 2009. p. 117–37.

80. Lord C, Risi S, Lambrecht L, et al. The autism diagnostic observation schedule–generic: a standard measure of social and communication deficits associated with the spectrum of autism. J Autism Dev Disord 2000;30:205–23.

81. Lord C, Rutter M, Le Couteur A. Autism diagnostic interview-revised: a revised version of a diagnostic interview for caregivers of individuals with possible pervasive developmental disorders. J Autism Dev Disord 1994;24:659–85.

82. Lord C, Risi S, Wetherby AM, et al. Diagnosis of autism spectrum disorders in young children. In: Wetherby AM, Prizant BM, editors. Autism spectrum disorders: a transactional developmental perspective. Baltimore (MD): Paul H Brookes Publishing; 2000. p. 11–30.

83. Risi S, Lord C, Gotham K, et al. Combining information from multiple sources in the diagnosis of autism spectrum disorders. J Am Acad Child Adolesc Psychiatry 2006;45:1094–103.

84. Luyster R, Guthrie W, Gotham K, et al. The autism diagnostic observation schedule-toddler module: preliminary findings using a modified version of the ADOS, in International meeting for autism research. London, England, May 15–17, 2008.

85. Le Couteur A, Haden G, Hammal D, et al. Diagnosing autism spectrum disorders in pre-school children using two standardized assessment instruments: the ADI-R and the ADOS. J Autism Dev Disord 2008;38:362–72.

86. Lord C, Storoschuk S, Rutter M, et al. Using the ADI-R to diagnose autism in preschool children. Infant Ment Health J 1993;14:234–52.

87. Goldstein H, Naglieri J, Ozonoff S, editors. Assessment of autism spectrum disorders. New York: The Guildford Press; 2009. p. 384.

88. Hastings RP, Johnson E. Stress in UK families conducting intensive home-based behavioral intervention for their young child with autism. J Autism Dev Disord 2001;31:327–36.

89. Davis NO, Carter AS. Parenting stress in mothers and fathers of toddlers with autism spectrum disorders: associations with child characteristics. J Autism Dev Disord 2008;38:1278–91.

90. Cassidy A, McConkey R, Truesdale-Kennedy M, et al. Preschoolers with autism spectrum disorders: the impact on families and the supports available to them. Early Child Dev Care 2008;178:115–28.

91. Marcus LM, Kunce LJ, Schopler E, et al. Working with families. In Handbook of autism and pervasive developmental disorders, vol. 2: Assessment, interventions, and policy (3rd edition). Hoboken (NJ): John Wiley & Sons Inc.,; 2005. p. 1055–86

92. Howlin P, Moore A. Diagnosis in autism: a survey of over 1200 patients in the UK. Autism 1997;1:135–62.

93. Gombosi PG. Parents of autistic children: some thoughts about trauma, dislocation, and tragedy. Psychoanal Study Child 1998;53:254–75.

94. Avdi E, Griffin C, Brough S. Parents' construction of the 'problem' during assessment and diagnosis of their child for an autistic spectrum disorder. J Health Psychol 2000;5:241–54.

95. Wachtel K, Carter AS. Reaction to diagnosis and parenting styles among mothers of young children with ASDs. Autism 2008;12:575–94.

96. Herring S, Gray K, Taffe J, et al. Behaviour and emotional problems in toddlers with pervasive developmental disorders and developmental delay: associations with parental mental health and family functioning. J Intellect Disabil Res 2006; 50:874–82.

97. Tobing LE, Glenwick DS. Relation of the childhood autism rating scale-parent version to diagnosis, stress, and age. Res Dev Disabil 2002;23:211–23.

98. Larson E. Caregiving and autism: how does children's propensity for routinization influence participation in family activities? OTJR 2006;26:69–79.

99. Hastings RP, Brown T. Behavior problems of children with autism, parental self-efficacy, and mental health. Am J Ment Retard 2002;107:222–32.

100. Hastings RP. Child behaviour problems and partner mental health as correlates of stress in mothers and fathers of children with autism. J Intellect Disabil Res 2003;47:231–7.

101. Hastings RP, Kovshoff H, Ward NJ, et al. Systems analysis of stress and positive perceptions in mothers and fathers of pre-school children with autism. J Autism Dev Disord 2005;35:635–44.

102. Siller M, Sigman M. The behaviors of parents of children with autism predict the subsequent development of their children's communication. J Autism Dev Disord 2002;32:77–89.
103. McConachie H, Diggle T. Parent implemented early intervention for young children with autism spectrum disorder: a systematic review. J Eval Clin Pract 2007; 13:120–9.
104. Kuhn JC, Carter AS. Maternal self-efficacy and associated parenting cognitions among mothers of children with autism. Am J Orthop 2006;76:564–75.
105. Plant KM, Sanders MR. Predictors of care-giver stress in families of preschool-aged children with developmental disabilities. J Intellect Disabil Res 2007;51: 109–24.
106. Smith LE, Seltzer MM, Tager-Flusberg H, et al. A comparative analysis of well-being and coping among mothers of toddlers and mothers of adolescents with ASD. J Autism Dev Disord 2008;38:876–89.
107. Rutherford MD, Young GS, Hepburn S, et al. A longitudinal study of pretend play in autism. J Autism Dev Disord 2007;37:1024–39.
108. Rogers SJ, Vismara LA. Evidence-based comprehensive treatments for early autism. J Clin Child Adolesc Psychol 2008;37:8–38.
109. Rogers SJ. Empirically supported comprehensive treatments for young children with autism. J Clin Child Psychol 1998;27:168–79.
110. Rogers SJ, Reddy LA, Files-Hall TM, et al. Play interventions for young children with autism spectrum disorders. In: Reddy LA, Files Hall TM, Schaefer CE, editors. Empirically based play interventions for children. Washington, DC: American Psychological Association; 2005. p. 215–39.
111. Lovaas OI. Behavioral treatment and normal educational and intellectual functioning in young autistic children. J Consult Clin Psychol 1987;55:3–9.
112. Smith T, Groen AD, Wynn JW. Randomized trial of intensive early intervention for children with pervasive developmental disorder. Am J Ment Retard 2000;105: 269–85.
113. Smith T, Buch GA, Gamby TE. Parent-directed, intensive early intervention for children with pervasive developmental disorder. Res Dev Disabil 2000;21: 297–309.
114. Steege MW, Mace FC, Perry L, et al. Applied behavior analysis: beyond discrete trial teaching. Psychol Sch 2007;44:91–9.
115. Koegel LK, Koegel RL, Harrower JK, et al. Pivotal response intervention I: overview of approach. J Assoc Pers Sev Handicaps 1999;24:174–85.
116. Koegel LK, Koegel RL, Fredeen RM, et al. Naturalistic behavioral approaches to treatment. In: Chawarska K, Klin A, Volkmar FR, editors. Autism spectrum disorders in infants and toddlers: diagnosis, assessment, and treatment. New York: Guilford Press; 2008. p. 207–42.
117. Koegel RL, Koegel LK. Pivotal response treatments for autism: communication, social, academic development. Baltimore (MD): Paul H Brookes Publishing; 2006.
118. Greenspan SI, Wieder S. Engaging autism: using the floortime approach to help children relate, communicate, and think. Cambridge (ME): Da Capo Press; 2006.
119. Greenspan SI, Wieder S, Hollander E, et al. The developmental individual-difference, relationship-based (dir/floortime) model approach to autism spectrum disorders. In: Hollander E, Anagnostou E, editors. Clinical manual for the treatment of autism. Arlington (VA): American Psychiatric Publishing, Inc.; 2007. p. 179–209.

120. Solomon R, Necheles J, Ferch C, et al. Pilot study of a parent training program for young children with autism: the play project home consultation program. Autism 2007;11:205–24.
121. Schopler E, Mesibov GB, Hearsey K, et al. Structured teaching in the teach system. In: Schopler E, Mesibov GB, editors. Learning and cognition in autism. New York: Plenum Press; 1995. p. 243–68.
122. Ozonoff S, Cathcart K. Effectiveness of a home program intervention for young children with autism. J Autism Dev Disord 1998;28:25–32.
123. Rogers SJ, DiLalla DL. A comparative study of the effects of a developmentally based instructional model on young children with autism and young children with other disorders of behavior and development. Top Early Child Spec Educ 1991;11:29–47.
124. Rogers SJ, Hayden D, Hepburn S, et al. Teaching young nonverbal children with autism useful speech: a pilot study of the Denver model and prompt interventions. J Autism Dev Disord 2006;36:1007–24.
125. Kasari C, Freeman S, Paparella T. Joint attention and symbolic play in young children with autism: a randomized controlled intervention study. J Child Psychol Psychiatry 2006;47:611–20.
126. Kasari C, Paparella T, Freeman S, et al. Language outcome in autism: randomized comparison of joint attention and play interventions. J Consult Clin Psychol 2008;76:125–37.
127. Yoder P, Stone WL. Randomized comparison of two communication interventions for preschoolers with autism spectrum disorders. J Consult Clin Psychol 2006;74:426–35.

Disturbances of Attachment and Parental Psychopathology in Early Childhood

Daniel S. Schechter, MA, MD[a,b,]*, Erica Willheim, PhD[c,d]

KEYWORDS

- Disturbances of attachment • Secure-base distortions
- Reactive attachment disorder • Parental PTSD
- Parental psychopathology • Mutual regulation

PART I: PERSPECTIVES ON THE CHILD AND RELATIONAL PSYCHOPATHOLOGY
Origins of Attachment Theory

The study of "attachment" now spans 4 decades and multiple domains; theory, research, psychobiology, and clinical application. This ever-expanding field of study owes its inception to Bowlby. Synthesizing object-relational and ethological perspectives, Bowlby theorized that the evolutionary interests of the species are best served by a biobehavioral caregiver-infant system that ensures the safety of the vulnerable human infant.[1,2] To that end, the human infant is biologically predisposed to engage in proximity seeking behaviors toward the caregiver in times of distress. In this conceptualization, Bowlby radically departed from the Freudian paradigm of primary

This work was financially supported by the Bender-Fishbein Fund, the Sackler Institute for Developmental Psychobiology at Columbia University, and an NIH grant to the first author (K23-MH68405).

[a] Consult-Liaison and Parent-Infant Research Units, Division of Child and Adolescent Psychiatry, University Hospitals of Geneva, 51 Boulevard de la Cluse, 2nd Floor, Geneva 1205, Switzerland
[b] Columbia University College of Physicians and Surgeons, 1051 Riverside Drive, Unit 40, New York, NY 10029, USA
[c] Department of Psychiatry, Columbia University College of Physicians & Surgeons; Parent-Infant Psychotherapy Training Program, Columbia University Center for Psychoanalytic Training & Research, 1051 Riverside Drive, Unit 63, New York, NY 10032, USA
[d] Early Childhood Mental Health Consultation and Treatment Program, New York Center for Child Development, 2082 First Avenue, New York, NY 10029, USA
* Corresponding author. Daniel S. Schechter, MD, Pediatric Psychiatry Consult-Liaison and Parent-Infant Research Units, Division of Child and Adolescent Psychiatry, University Hospitals of Geneva, 51 Boulevard de la Cluse, 2nd Floor, Geneva 1205, Switzerland.
E-mail address: daniel.schechter@hcuge.ch (D.S. Schechter).

Child Adolesc Psychiatric Clin N Am 18 (2009) 665–686
doi:10.1016/j.chc.2009.03.001
1056-4993/09/$ – see front matter © 2009 Elsevier Inc. All rights reserved.

drives (eg, the pleasure principle) that operate independently of the object. By contrast, attachment theory was based on "a new type of instinct theory",[1] one that viewed the formation of relational bonds as a primary human instinct. Attachment theory additionally departed from traditional psychoanalytic models in its attention to the direct observation of caregiver-infant interaction rather than adult retrospection and fantasy concerning childhood experience (eg, the "seduction theory").

Bowlby proposed that infant motivation operates according to 4 principle systems; attachment, exploration, affiliation, and fear/wariness.[3] The attachment and exploratory systems are understood to operate inversely to maintain a homeostatic goal of felt security. Proximity seeking attachment behaviors are activated and exploratory behaviors deactivated by fear or distress. Upon the reestablishment of felt security, attachment behaviors deactivate and exploratory behaviors can once again emerge. Bowlby suggested that based on the caregiver's actual history of providing comfort and safety, the infant constructs an internal working model (IWM) of self and the attachment figure that will subsequently guide the infant's behavior and expectations of attachment figures, most significantly in times of stress. This internal mental representation, termed "object constancy" by Mahler and colleagues,[4] is theorized to remain stable over time, but it may be susceptible to alteration later in life through ameliorative attachment relationships.[5,6]

Observable attachment behaviors change phenotypically as development proceeds over the first years of life. In early infancy, behaviors such as crying, clinging, and smiling are mechanisms by which the infant seeks proximity. The emergence of stranger wariness and separation protest, beginning at approximately 7 to 9 months of age and consolidating by the end of the first year of life, signals the establishment of the attachment system with its discrimination of, and preference for, the primary attachment figure. Following the attainment of mobility beginning at approximately 12 months, attachment behaviors are reflected in the toddler's balancing of proximity seeking and exploration, returning to the caregiver as a "secure base" or "safe haven" when external or internal factors become stressful or frightening.[1]

The core component of attachment theory, that the quality of infant attachment is directly related to the quality of experienced caregiving (the provision of felt security), was operationalized by Ainsworth and colleagues in a laboratory paradigm known as the Strange Situation Procedure (SSP).[7] Observing 12-month-old infants in a structured series of eight standardized episodes, which included separations and reunions between caregiver and infant, Ainsworth coded and categorized infant behavioral adaptations in response to the reintroduction of the attachment figure during the reunion episode. Ainsworth delineated three attachment classifications: (1) Secure (B) in which the infant actively seeks and effectively derives felt security from proximity to and interaction with the attachment figure, (2) Insecure-Avoidant (A) in which the infant "conspicuously" avoids proximity seeking or interaction with the attachment figure, and (3) Insecure-Resistant (Ambivalent) (C) in which the infant simultaneously seeks and resists proximity and interaction with the attachment figure.

Attachment Organization and Disorganization

The secure and insecure attachment classifications first identified by Ainsworth represent behavioral strategies related to the IWM (internal representation) the infant holds of the availability, reliability, and responsivity of the attachment figure in times of distress. Whether optimal or not, the B, A, and C strategies are adaptive and, indeed, organized. Over repeated interactions with the caregiver, the infant has learned what he or she may reliably expect in terms of comfort and security and has modified his or her attachment behavior accordingly. For example, the avoidant infant appears to have learned that very little or nothing will be offered by the caregiver and adaptively suppresses overt proximity seeking behaviors.

As attachment research progressed, investigators observed that a subset of infants exhibited reunion behaviors that did not fit into any of the extant categories.[8,9] Main and Solomon[10,11] added the classification "Disorganized-Disoriented" (subtype D) for these children and described their behavior as odd, chaotic, interrupted, mistimed, and incoherent with respect to stress and separation during reunion with their parents. In addition to discrete behaviors characteristic of the other subtypes, upon reunion such infants exhibited fearful responses, contradictory but simultaneous movements (eg, approaching a parent while moving in circles), or freezing in place with a "trance-like" expression. Main and Hesse[12,13] have suggested that the source of this behavioral presentation may be caregivers who display frightening and/or frightened behavior, creating an impossible bind for the infant. Proximity seeking and avoidance/flight are simultaneously activated, because the caregiver is the source of both fear and comfort. Main[14] has termed this bind "fright without solution" such that any and all strategies are rendered ineffective, and the attachment behavioral system is effectively derailed.

Correlates of Attachment

In her original study of nonclinical middle-class infants, Ainsworth found attachment distributions of 66% secure (B) and 34% insecure (A and C). Early meta-analytic reviews of infant attachment studies using the SSP showed distributions of 62% secure and 38% secure in US samples[15] and 65% secure and 35% insecure internationally.[16] Subsequent reviews continued to find only up to 40% insecure attachment in general population samples.[17] However, the rate of insecure attachment was found to rise dramatically in samples of maltreated infants, with insecurity ranging from 70% to 100%.[18] The development and use of the type D classification confirmed a robust association between maltreatment and disorganized attachment, with disorganized attachment rates as high as 82% found in maltreated infant samples.[19]

Security of attachment has been found to predict personal and interpersonal competence in early childhood[20–22] and middle childhood.[23,24] Insecure attachment has been generally associated with factors such as increased dependence, impaired social competence, and decreased ego resilience in later childhood.[24,25] Given the association between maltreatment and disorganized attachment, however, the well-documented negative sequelae of maltreatment alone become of particular interest. These impairments span the domains of development, self-perception, social interaction, internalizing, and externalizing behaviors.[26–32]

The research findings that link (a) insecure attachment, particularly disorganized-disoriented attachment, with maltreated populations and (b) maltreatment with negative outcomes raise the question of the relationship between attachment and early childhood psychopathology. At such a juncture, it is critical to remember that the construct of attachment belongs to the field of developmental psychology. Classifications of secure and insecure attachment, including disorganized-disoriented, were conceived as descriptive, *not* diagnostic, categories.[33] Zeanah and Smyke[34] warn against the tendency to relate attachment classifications directly to pathology: "there is no clear association between classifications of attachment and specific psychiatric sequelae". Attachment classifications are better thought of as risk and protective factors for concurrent or later pathologic disorders.[35] Indeed, strong evidence continues to mount for the risk-conferring nature of the disorganized classification.

Investigators have documented associations between disorganized attachment and internalizing, externalizing, anxiety, and dissociative disorders.[36–42]

Disorders of Attachment—Historical Background

In contrast to the plethora of research on correlates of attachment classifications, until very recently scant research existed regarding actual psychiatric "disorders of attachment." Early descriptive studies by Bowlby,[43] Robertson,[44] and Spitz[45] indicated that "extreme" or "pathogenic" caregiving environments, such as those found in cases of maltreatment or institutional settings, were necessary precipitants of attachment disturbances. Yet the problem with diagnosis of infant psychopathology is unusually complicated by several factors specific to infancy and early childhood. Infants and young children are inherently changing entities, their range of behaviors are limited relative to developmental age, they cannot report on their experiences, observers often know them only in certain contexts, infant behavior exists within a relational context, and attachment is a normative developmental pathway.[46] Thus, progress in delineating and validating criteria for disorders of attachment has been a "slow" and "limited" process.[33]

The first formal inclusion of criteria for a disorder of attachment occurred with the publication of the *Diagnostic and Statistical Manual of Mental Disorders III* (DSM-III).[47] Criteria were based on the research of Tizard and Rees[48] on attachment abnormalities in 4-year-olds raised since birth in residential nurseries in England. Tizard and Rees had found that most of the children exhibited either withdrawn/unresponsive behaviors *or* indiscriminate/attention seeking behaviors. The original DSM-III version also included failure to thrive, lack of social responsivity, and onset before 8 months of age as criteria. In the DSM-III-R edition,[49] failure to thrive was removed and the age of onset expanded to within the first 5 years of life. Additionally two subtypes were formalized: Inhibited and Disinhibited.

The nomenclature, definition, and criteria for these subtypes were maintained through DSM-IV[50] and the International Classification of Diseases, 10th revision (ICD-10),[51] with slight variations existing between DSM-IV and ICD-10 regarding social relatedness across contexts. Importantly, both DSM-IV and ICD-10 continued to recognize the disorder as a reaction to pathogenic caregiving and excluded children meeting criteria for pervasive developmental disorder (PDD).[33] They differed in that DSM-IV grouped both subtypes and a mixed subtype under reactive attachment deprivation (RAD), whereas in ICD-10, RAD referred to the inhibited subtype only, with the disinhibited subtype termed "Disinhibited Attachment Disorder." DSM-IV-TR[52] maintained the centrality of abnormal social relatedness across contexts—which is not accounted for by PDD or developmental delay—and the etiology of pathogenic care.

Boris and Zeanah.[53] noted that the development and revision of these criteria were performed independent of substantiating research, since no published data existed on the topic between 1980 and 1994. In a critique concerning the state of attachment disorder diagnoses at the time, Zeanah and colleagues[54] suggested that the DSM-IV's characterization of RAD as a disturbance of *nonattachment* did not properly take into account children who have observable, focused attachment relationships, albeit ones that are highly disturbed. Moreover, in more recent work with a Romanian orphanage sample, Zeanah and colleagues[55] have pointed out that traditional measures of attachment behavior such as the SSP, among other measures, are ill suited to assess relational behavior in children who have never discriminated a preferred attachment figure due to institutional care.

In 1994, the Zero to Three National Center for Clinical Infant Programs published the *Diagnostic Classification: 0 to 3* (DC: 0-3)[56] in an attempt to provide a more developmentally based and comprehensive classification system for mental health and developmental disturbances of early childhood. DC: 0-3 termed its version of RAD "Reactive Attachment Deprivation/Maltreatment Disorder of Infancy and Early Childhood" with an emphasis on the association between early abuse or neglect and later relational disturbance. The revised version (DC: 0-3R)[57] included criteria based on the work of Boris and Zeanah,[53] removed the term "reactive attachment," and defined "Deprivation/Maltreatment Disorder" as follows:

> *This disorder occurs in the context of deprivation or maltreatment, including persistent and severe parental neglect or documented physical or psychological abuse. The disorder may develop when a child has limited opportunity to form selective attachments because of frequent changes in primary caregiver(s) or the marked unavailability of an attachment figure, as in institutional settings. (DC: 0-3R).[57]*

An alternative model of attachment disorders has been proposed,[33,58] one that more closely reflects both developmental research into attachment and clinical descriptions of "secure-base distortions."[59] The model delineates three types of attachment disorders: (1) Disorders of Nonattachment (similar to DSM and ICD), (2) Secure-Base Distortions, and (3) Disrupted Attachment Disorder. Where the psychiatric perspective of a one-person (one-child) pathology characterizes the first of these categories, the second and third are intended to capture pathology that may exist within a two-person context, pathology that is relationship (attachment) specific.[34]

Reactive Attachment Disorder: Disorders of Nonattachment

In times of distress or uncertainty, typically developing young children desire proximity to their preferred caregiver, accept the overtures of that caregiver, and are effectively comforted. Disorders of nonattachment are principally characterized by the absence of any preferred attachment figure and any attachment behaviors directed toward such a figure. According to the suggested alternative criteria,[33] nonattached children must have a mental age of at least 10 months and show no variability in attachment behaviors across relationships or contexts. Additionally, a proven history of pathogenic care should not be required for the diagnosis, since early histories are often unreliable or unavailable at the time of initial evaluation.

Emotionally Withdrawn/Inhibited

In this pattern, the child does not seek comfort from a preferred caregiver, does not respond, or may even resist, when comfort is offered,[60–62] and is not easily soothed. Such children exhibit severe restrictions or an absence of affectionate displays, cooperative or collaborative interaction, reciprocal response to the social overtures of others, and reliance on a preferred caregiver for assistance or reassurance. Children with this subtype are also characterized by disturbances in emotional regulation.[53] The pattern has been found in populations of institutionalized children,[63] neglected children,[64] and children in foster care.[60,61]

The matter of differential diagnosis is especially pertinent to this subtype. Withdrawn and inhibited behavior may also be characteristic of early childhood depressive or anxiety disorders. It is important to note that although depressive symptoms inherently accompany nonattachment, the reverse is not the case.[33] The clinician must similarly be alert to the possibility that inhibited functioning may actually be related to hyperarousal, possibly brought on by early trauma.[64,65] Questions of differential diagnosis are further complicated by the fact that institutionalization has been associated with a quasi-autistic disorder that looks similar to PDD as well as with the RAD inhibited subtype, the two disorders sharing a lack of social responsivity.[66] Although PDD has been found to occur in environments that are considered adequate, RAD is singularly found in environments of extreme deprivation.[34] Additionally, unlike PDD, a substantial proportion of children with quasi-autism improve after placement in an adequate caregiving environment.[67]

Indiscriminate/Disinhibited

In this pattern, the child displays "indiscriminate sociability" toward unfamiliar adults, without the developmentally appropriate reticence young children typically exhibit around strangers. The literature has described these children as "attention seeking," "shallow," and "interpersonally superficial."[53] In interaction with unknown adults, such children will seek comfort, accept comfort when offered, and even protest upon the departure of the strange adult. The indiscriminate child will wander away from their caregiver without checking back. There is even recent evidence that these children are at particularly high risk for "going off with a stranger."[68] In a comparative study using the "Stranger at the Door" Procedure, the investigators found that institutionalized children were the most likely to go off with a stranger, and children in foster care were "intermediate," and the least likely were the control sample children who belonged to neither group. The indiscriminate subtype has been found in children who have experienced frequent placement changes while in foster care or institutionalization.[63,69]

Course and Amelioration of RAD

The preponderance of research into attachment disorders conducted over the past decade has concerned the outcomes of children reared in institutions. Data from studies following children adopted from Romanian orphanages has lead to new insights concerning the nature and variations of RAD. The data from these studies do not appear to support the notion of a critical period in the formation of human attachment bonds.[53] Romanian children initially assessed as nonattached were found to develop attachment behaviors with their British adoptive parents, assuming that the new caregiving environment was normative.[70,71] Among both British and Canadian adoption studies no children were found to meet criteria for the withdrawn/inhibited subtype following adoption, although the quality of their attachments could be atypical, insecure, and/or disorganized.[72,73] Additional data from foster care studies[74] support the conclusion that remediation of the emotionally withdrawn/inhibited subtype is possible.

By contrast, studies specifically focused on the course of indiscriminate sociability have yielded the fascinating outcome that this feature appears to persist regardless of child placement into adoptive homes, return to biologic families, or continued institutionalization.[75] Romanian children adopted by Canadians continued to exhibit indiscriminate friendliness at both 11 months and 39 months postadoption, despite increases in attachment security with their caregiver during the same time frame.[72,76] Zeanah and Boris[33] conclude that the persistence of indiscriminate sociability in children adopted from institutions may be a "long-term complication" of early institutionalization.

Although the overall prevalence of RAD is extremely low (less than 1%),[77] as many as 38% of children in foster care studies have been found to exhibit symptoms of RAD,[78] and 40% of institutionalized Romanian children were found to meet criteria for RAD, with an additional 33% evidencing features of RAD.[62,79] The Romanian studies have further suggested that the presentations of the two subtypes may not be as mutually exclusive as initially identified and as defined in DSM-IV-TR. Rather, institutionalized children may display features of both subtypes.[62,79]

Secure-Base Distortions

Although validation for the disorders of attachment known as secure-base distortions is not well established,[53] these relational pathologies may be more closely related to what clinicians encounter in referred populations. In fact, the behaviors described in this category are reminiscent of childhood disturbances described by Fraiberg and colleagues as early as 1975.[80] The presentation of these symptoms is observed almost exclusively in the context of a specific attachment relationship. The subtypes are Attachment Disorder with: Self-Endangerment, Clinging/Inhibited Exploration, Vigilance/Hypercompliance, and Role Reversal.[33] It is of interest that the subtypes for secure-base distortions are remarkably similar to behaviors observed among peer-reared primates who did form attachment bonds, but problematic ones.[81]

The *Self-Endangering* subtype refers to behaviors in which the child impulsively engages in exploratory behaviors unfettered and unmodulated by the opposing activation of attachment behaviors (eg, proximity seeking, checking back). Aggression toward the self or caregiver is often present as is significant risk-taking or self-endangering behavior (eg, running away from the caregiver in a public place, running into traffic, climbing to dangerous heights). Such children frequently come from homes where interpersonal violence has occurred, and their behavior suggests an attempt to activate the protective instincts of a caregiver who may be preoccupied, dissociative, passive, or unavailable in some other manner.[58,59,82]

The *Clinging/Inhibited Exploration* subtype describes a child for whom the attachment system is hyperactivated, to the detriment of the exploratory system. These children stick close to the parent but particularly when in unfamiliar settings. It remains unclear at what point such behavior constitutes an actual disorder rather than a temperamental disposition.[33] The subtype of *Vigilance/Hypercompliance* describes a pattern in which the child is hypervigilant regarding the caregiver, hypercompliant with caregiver requests, and emotionally constricted. The child impresses one as frightened of displeasing or provoking the caregiver. This pattern has been previously described as "frozen watchfulness"[83] in the literature on child abuse.

In the *Role Reversal* subtype the child is observed to be preoccupied with the caretaking of the parent. In a manner that is developmentally inverted, the child seems to take on the responsibility of managing the parent's emotional wellness, providing nurturance, empathy, even protection. In studies of children at age 6, role reversed controlling behaviors, frequently with an aggressive or threatening quality, were associated with disorganized-disoriented attachment classifications in infancy.[23,84]

Disrupted Attachment Disorder

The third alternative criteria for attachment disorders proposed by Lieberman and Zeanah[85] addresses the sudden loss of an important attachment figure during early childhood. It was James and Joyce Robertson[86] who first described a sequence of protest, despair, and detachment in children experiencing prolonged separations from their caregivers. This subtype is intended to acknowledge the centrality and profound impact of such a loss for very young children. The clinical literature is rich with descriptions concerning the deleterious effects of the death of a parent[87] and of the attachment disruptions inherent in foster care placement.[88] Questions regarding risk and protective factors as well as empiric validation efforts remain regarding this disorder.[33]

Attachment-Based Interventions for Disturbances of Attachment

A number of interventions have been developed over the past several years with the explicit intent of addressing disturbances of child-parent attachment. Several of these interventions are reviewed elsewhere in this volume: see Child-Parent Psychotherapy[89]; Interaction Guidance,[90] Clinician Assisted Video feedback Exposure Session,[91] and Circles of Security (COS).[92] In addition to those already described in this volume, some additional interventions that are specifically targeted at attachment disorders include the following.

Minding the Baby[93,94] is a relationship-based weekly home-visiting program for young high-risk and first-time mothers, many with a history of trauma, which incorporates the reflective functioning, or mentalization, component of certain infant-parent psychotherapy (IPP) models. Program outcomes have shown increases in maternal reflective functioning (RF), decreases in maternal depression and posttraumatic stress disorder (PTSD) symptoms, and no children exhibiting disorganized attachment.[95]

Cicchetti, Rogosch, and Toth[96] have used a modified version of IPP[80] in an effort to increase infant security of attachment in maltreating families. This intervention emphasizes increasing sensitive maternal responsivity via attention to disturbed maternal attachment representations. Outcomes have revealed increased rates of secure attachment, from 3.1% at baseline to 60.7% at follow-up.

Dozier and colleagues in Delaware have developed an evidence-based intervention for very young children in foster care titled "Attachment and Biobehavioral Catch-Up" (ABC).[97] ABC is a manualized, 10-session training program for foster parents, and in a controlled trial, it has been found to be associated with lowered cortisol values and fewer behavioral problems as reported by foster parents.

In Louisiana, the Tulane-Jefferson Parish Human Services Authority Infant Team has partnered with child welfare and judicial, educational, and health care systems to provide assessment and intervention for abused and neglected infants and toddlers (under 48 months) placed into foster care.[98] Following treatment, very young children's rate of risk for a subsequent incidence of maltreatment was reduced by up to 68%.

Finally, in Romania, Zeanah and colleagues have described interventions that result in significant overall improvement in functioning and developmental markers for children with profound disorders of nonattachment. Children who entered the Budapest Early Intervention Program,[68] a foster care placement program with attachment and development sensitized families, demonstrated substantial reduction or remission of emotionally withdrawn/inhibited symptoms. Children living in institutions but enrolled in an enriched, attachment-oriented "pilot unit"[62] showed significantly reduced signs of both RAD subtypes compared with the institutional, care-as-usual group.

PART II: PERSPECTIVES ON THE CAREGIVER AND THE ROLE OF PARENTAL PSYCHOPATHOLOGY
The Role of the Caregiver in Mutual Regulation/Attachment

Hofer[99] first described what he called "hidden regulators," that is, multiple microsystems that subserve the larger macrosystem of what Bowlby had termed "attachment." Hofer discovered that in rodents a bidirectional process of regulation, a mechanism for relational feedback, would help the infant maintain basic physiologic homeostasis with regard to body temperature, arterial blood pressure, as well as sleep, feeding, and elimination patterns. In humans, Stern[100] has referred to "affective attunement" and Tronick and Gianino[101] to "mutual emotion regulation" as psychological extrapolations of hidden physiologic regulation.

In a laboratory paradigm known as the "Still-Face" procedure, infants within the first half of the first year of life are seen to express a range of positive affects that are perceived, mirrored, and modulated by the caregiver under normal circumstances.[101] In the procedure, after a prescribed period of typical interaction, the caregiver is instructed to now maintain a poker face and, therefore, fails to mirror and modulate the infant's affect. The infant initially responds by trying desperately to elicit the caregiver's feedback. When these bids for engagement are unsuccessful, the infant becomes frustrated, agitated, and finally turns away in resignation with visibly flattened affect. In normative dyads, when the caregiver is then instructed to resume interaction, the infant is seen to reengage as well—some infants more eagerly than others.

The Still-Face paradigm has thus become an exquisite measure of maintenance, rupture, and repair of mutual emotion regulation. Although the child-parent attachment, and the many hidden regulators that subserve it, clearly operate within a bidirectional system, the Still-Face paradigm demonstrates the overall *asymmetry* of this system. By definition, the adult caregiver has emotional, cognitive, and physical capacities that permit psychological availability to, understanding of, and communication with the infant or toddler that cannot be reciprocated due to the developmental limitations of the young child. Thus, the caregiver's capacity to self-regulate her own emotion, attention, and behavior is essential to her ability to assist her baby with the regulation of his emotion, arousal, attention, and bodily control.

Indeed, the critical role of the caregiver in determining infant attachment classification was empirically established following the development of the Adult Attachment Interview (AAI) by Main and colleagues.[6] (George C, Kaplan N, Main M. The attachment interview for adults: unpublished manuscript, University of California, Berkeley; 1984.) Main's group found that the degree of coherence and integration characterizing caregiver narratives about their past attachment relationships, on the AAI, could be reliably coded into attachment categories. These adult categories were subsequently found to be highly correlated with infant attachment.[17] "Secure/Autonomous" attachment in the parent was associated with secure attachment in the infant, "Dismissive" with avoidant, "Preoccupied" with resistant, and "Unresolved," with respect to trauma and loss, with disorganized. Attachment theorists suggested that the mechanism responsible for this intergenerational transmission was the caregiver's quality of mental representation of others and self in relation to others.[102,103] In the language of attachment, the infant's "IWM" of self and other is influenced by the quality of the caregiver's internalized attachment representations via interactions with the infant that arise from those representations.

Fonagy and colleagues[104,105] went beyond the content and associated affects involved in caregivers' internalized attachment representations to examine an aspect of metacognitive monitoring of the self and social cognitive awareness of the other. This awareness of self and others is implicit in the more coherent and emotionally rich narrative responses among those adults characterized as "Secure/Autonomous" on the AAI. Fonagy and colleagues[104] defined this aspect that he called "mentalization" (or alternatively, in an operationalized form for research measurement, "reflective functioning") as the awareness of a meaningful relationship between underlying mental states (feelings, thoughts, motivations, intentions) and behavior in and between both self and others. Using the narrative content of the AAI, Fonagy's group found that caregiver RF was significantly predictive of infant attachment classification, even beyond that of AAI classifications. High RF was found to be strongly associated with secure infant attachment and low RF with insecure infant attachment. The caregiver's capacity to read infant mental states accurately, and with inference of meaning, allows for sensitively attuned responses that create a subjective experience of security/safety and support the infant's developing capacity for self-regulation.[93,106]

Slade and colleagues[95] have since moved from considering the caregiver's RF as elicited by inquiring about the caregiver's mental representations of her own caregivers and her relationships with them (ie, in the past) to considering the caregiver's RF as elicited by inquiring about the caregiver's mental representations of her child and her relationship with her child (ie, in the present). Slade and colleagues have developed a developmentally specific interview for parents of infants and toddlers from which transcripts of narrative are coded. A mother's high RF in this context has been associated with more balanced and coherent mental representations of her child[107] and less atypical maternal behavior with her child.[108] Since the work of Slade and colleagues, others have developed alternative coding schemes that can be usefully applied "in vivo" to examine parental mentalizing capacity or "insightfulness" during clinical observations of parent-child interaction as well as during interventions to address disturbances in the attachment.[109]

Disturbances in Caregiver Self-Regulation and Disturbances of Attachment

In her writings on the intergenerational transmission of trauma, Fraiberg[80] long ago noted that disturbed internal attachment representations held by the parent ("Ghosts in the Nursery") give rise to disturbed patterns of caregiving, which then result in disturbed attachment behaviors in the child. Fonagy and colleagues[110] suggested that when engagement in RF leads to highly negative affect, certain aspects of mental functioning may be defensively inhibited to protect against overwhelming affect. A caregiver in a state of defensive inhibition will be incapable of accurately responding to and reflecting the child's mental state, leaving the child to manage states of arousal and anxiety on his or her own.

Within a standard attachment research paradigm during the second year of life, Main and Hesse[12] and later Lyons-Ruth and colleagues[111] identified *dysregulated* and therefore *dysregulating* caregiving behavior(s). Main and Hesse's original conceptualization was one of maternal behaviors that were "frightening" or fight-like, aggressive, and intrusive, and "frightened" or flight-like, withdrawing, and distancing. These behaviors were expanded upon by Lyons-Ruth and colleagues to also include "affective communication errors" (incongruence of affect between child and caregiver response), "disorientation" (freezing, depersonalizing behavior, and dissociative discontinuity), and role reversal (parentified or otherwise adultomorphic behavior). These behaviors, termed "atypical maternal behavior" or "disrupted communication," have been reliably measured using the coding system known as the "Atypical Maternal Behavior Instrument" or "AMBIANCE."[111]

Across multiple studies, dysregulated maternal behaviors have been associated with unresolved trauma and loss in the caregiver's attachment history as well as with insecure, disorganized attachment in the toddler.[112,113] In a 20-year-long prospective study of toddlers originally seen in the Strange Situation Paradigm, atypical maternal behaviors at the time of the SSP were associated with later adolescent dissociation, borderline personality characteristics, and conduct disturbances.[114] Moreover, this type of caregiving behavior is not explained so far by genetic polymorphisms of the dopamine receptor gene *DRD4*—although this marker, when measured in infants, has been shown to render those infants vulnerable to attachment disorganization when interacting with atypical caregiving behaviors.[115]

Parental Psychopathology: Attachment Implications from the Study of Caregiver Posttraumatic Stress Disorder

Any form of psychopathology, be it schizophrenia, bipolar disorder, obsessive-compulsive disorder, or substance abuse, can adversely impact the caregiver's capacity to engage in mutual regulation. The nature of the interference with mutual regulation may be particular to the diagnosis and/or to the individual, but, certainly, it leads to a distinct effect on that individual caregiver's relationship with her child. Maternal Major Depression, as noted in the Still-Face paradigm literature,[116] is a clear example of a disorder that has been demonstrated to disrupt mutual emotion regulation with distinct and enduring biobehavioral effects on the infant.[117]

Recent studies such as STAR*D[118] have underscored how pharmacologic treatment of the depressed mother (only) can improve parent and child outcomes in terms of reduction of child psychiatric symptoms. This is an important point for communities lacking in early childhood mental health resources; however, attachment and interactive behavior have not yet been examined in these studies. One would think that maladaptive patterns of attachment and disruptions of mutual regulation related to maternal depression would need to be addressed, as well as maternal psychopathology, to make a deep and sustained change within the parent-child relationship. It has also been empirically demonstrated that comorbidity as much as, or more than, any particular form of caregiver psychopathology is strongly associated with disturbances in attachment such that treatment for a specific disorder in 1 partner of the dyad may not suffice.[119]

Parental PTSD, a frequently comorbid disorder itself, is one important example of caregiver psychopathology that can disrupt mutual emotion regulation and lead to disturbances of attachment meriting clinical attention. PTSD is of particular interest, because the nature of the disorder is marked by significant affect dysregulation. The individual with PTSD, particularly interpersonal violence-related PTSD, enters a defensive, hypervigilant, self-preservative position relative to other individuals. This defended position prohibits an affiliative stance that would permit psychological availability to another, such as an infant or toddler, and this availability is essential to mutual emotion regulation.[120]

Lyons-Ruth and Block[121] were the first to empirically explore the associations between violence-related PTSD, atypical caregiving behavior, and attachment disorganization in low-income, high-risk mothers and toddlers. They identified a moderate correlation ($r = .35$) between maternal hostile-intrusive (atypical) behavior and self-reported severity of PTSD. Simple exposure to violent trauma in the absence of related psychopathology (ie, PTSD) appears to be a necessary but insufficient predictor of atypical caregiving behavior. Significantly, among insecurely attached toddlers, 88% of those with mothers who have a history of violent trauma and PTSD symptoms exhibited disorganized attachment. In comparison, only 33% of insecure toddlers with mothers *without* such a history exhibited disorganized attachment.

Schechter and colleagues[122,123] explored the possibility that clinically referred mothers with a history of interpersonal violence-related PTSD would display psychobiological dysregulation and that such physiologic dysregulation would also be associated with disturbances in mental representations of the child as well as caregiving behavior. The study indeed found that greater severity of maternal PTSD was associated with lower maternal baseline salivary cortisol and greater likelihood of distorted, inflexible, and negative mental representations of the child. The latter variables were in turn associated with greater atypical maternal behavior.

However, why should a history of interpersonal violence-related PTSD cause such problems for caregivers in the parenting of their very young children? Since very young children cannot regulate their emotional or behavioral responses very well, a toddler or preschooler's tantrums may appear quite violent and frightening to traumatized parents. Additionally, helpless or frightened states of the toddler's mind, such as those that often occur upon separation, may prove intolerable to traumatized parents. Help-lessness, fear, or rage in the toddler may trigger traumatic memories of the caregiver's own (a) past experiences of helplessness and (b) curtailed rage at their abuser. Fright-ened or rageful states in the mind of the caregiver may be so intolerable that they are projected onto the distressed child.[80] Such projections are observable in the motiva-tional misattributions commonly voiced by traumatized parents (eg, "He's just trying to control me"). Alternatively, as Schechter and Willheim have described clinically,[124] the caregiver may defensively inhibit any reflective awareness of the child's mental state, either via dissociation or by physically removing herself from proximity to the child. In either case, the traumatized parent is unavailable to provide a secure base or to support affective regulation for the distressed child.

Posttraumatic Stress Disorder and Secure-Base Distortions

The first author[125] most recently replicated and expanded his 2008 studies of violently traumatized mothers with the goal of examining whether or not secure-base distor-tions[53] would be significantly associated with severity of maternal violence-related PTSD and atypical maternal behavior. More specifically, the operant hypothesis was that atypical maternal behavior would function as a mediator between maternal PTSD and secure-base distortions. As noted in Part I, there has been little, if any, research conducted to establish the validity of secure-base distortion criteria either in isolation or relative to other variables.[53]

In clinical and control samples of 76 mothers and their 12- to 48-month-old children who were recruited from community pediatrics clinics in Northern Manhattan, mothers were assessed for PTSD using the Clinician Administered PTSD Scale[126] and Post-traumatic Symptom Checklist—Short Version.[127] Secure-base distortions of children were measured using the Disturbances of Attachment Interview (DAI),[55,128] a 12-item semistructured interview of the parent that permits observations to be made simulta-neously if the child is present. The DAI consists of 3 sections with 4 items each: DSM-IV-TR RAD-Inhibited Type; DSM-IV-TR RAD-Disinhibited Type; and Secure-Base Distortions. The 4 items in the latter category are separation anxiety, hypervigilance, self-endangering and otherwise risky behavior, and role reversal. Atypical maternal behavior was rated using the coding scheme from the AMBIANCE[111] as applied to a videotaped, laboratory mother-child interaction sequence known as the Modified Crowell Procedure.[129]

Not surprisingly, few children met criteria for RAD, neither the inhibited type (1.3%) nor the disinhibited type (2.6%). However, 27.3% of the sample children met criteria for secure-base distortions. One of the most interesting findings was that the four factors of the secure-base distortions *together* had a Crohnbach's alpha of .75, sug-gesting strong intercorrelations between the four component items of this particular attachment disturbance. All of the children meeting criteria for any of the three attach-ment disturbances had mothers with a diagnosis of PTSD. **Table 1** illustrates the rela-tionship of secure-base distortions to the severity of maternal violence-related PTSD and atypical maternal behavior. The severity of maternal PTSD was significantly asso-ciated with the number of secure-base distortion criteria met on the DAI, with roughly one-third of the variance of secure-base behavior accounted for by the severity of maternal PTSD. Atypical maternal behavior was only weakly related to secure-base distortions in this study, at a trend level of significance. Adjusting the effect of maternal PTSD severity on secure base distortions by entering atypical maternal behavior

Table 1				
Relationship of maternal PTSD and atypical maternal behavior to secure-base distortions (N = 76)				
Unadjusted model				
Dependent Variable	**Predictors**	**F (1,75)**	**R^2**	**β**
Secure base distortion (Number of criterion behaviors on DAI)	Maternal PTSD	32.81[d]	.30	.55[d]
	AMBIANCE	3.20[a]	.04	.20[a]
Adjusted model				
Dependent Variable	**Predictors**	**F (2,74)**	**R^2**	**β**
Secure base distortion (Number of criterion behaviors on DAI)	Maternal	17.32[d]	.32	.53[d]
	AMBIANCE			.12

[a] $\leq .1$
[b] $\leq .05$
[c] $\leq .01$
[d] $\leq .001$

(AMBIANCE) into the regression, did not significantly alter the model. This suggests that further research is needed to understand what other factors may mediate the robust relationship of maternal PTSD to this type of attachment disturbance.

Research Conclusions

Past research has shown PTSD to be related to atypical caregiving behavior, atypical maternal behavior has been related to disorganized attachment, and disorganized attachment has been identified as a risk factor for later pathology. However, the recent data detailed above serve as an example of research investigating the relationship between particular types of maternal psychopathology and particular forms of attachment disturbance. In this case, a parental pathology associated with significant affect dysregulation, namely interpersonal violence-related PTSD, has been found to be associated with secure-base distortion behaviors. The fact that atypical maternal behavior was not found to be a mediator of the effects of maternal PTSD in this study alerts us to the need for further examination of the complex interaction between caregiver pathology and disturbances of attachment.

Research into RAD and the effects of severely deprived or institutional care has made enormous progress over the past decade; however, questions remain regarding secure-base distortions. The category speaks loudly to clinicians who daily encounter children from trauma-ridden, multiproblem families. As noted above, the four subtypes appear to be highly intercorrelated and as a whole are associated with the severity of maternal PTSD. Are the four subtypes really discrete entities or do the behaviors exist on a continuum? Are secure-base distortions relationship-specific or markers for disturbances that may be linked to child traumatization and PTSD? Are there caregiver pathologies that correlate more highly with some secure-base distortion behaviors than with others? In addition, what is the relationship between disorganized attachment classification and secure-base distortions? Such questions await future investigation.

SUMMARY AND CLINICAL IMPLICATIONS

The clinical implications of this review are summarized by the following recommendations concerning the diagnosis and treatment of attachment disturbances. First, there is a need for careful psychiatric evaluation, diagnosis, and active treatment of three patients: the parent, the child-parent relationship, and the child—with attention to the accumulated effects of attachment disturbance on social and emotional development.[130] Interventions that address the child's and parents' individual needs and that directly focus on the child-parent relationship are most likely to interrupt intergenerational transmission of trauma and impairing disturbances of attachment.[131] Second, as has now been demonstrated across multiple studies,[91,104,108] interventions that bolster parental capacities to mentalize, that is, to think about what is going on in their own mind and the mind of their child, are likely to improve child-parent attachment. A mentalizing stance by the caregiver allows for improved caregiver self-regulation and thereby positively influences child-parent mutual regulation, which ultimately supports the child's successful attainment of self-regulation.

Third, treating clinicians should always keep in mind the foundational concepts of attachment; the centrality of fear and distress, the need for safety and comfort, the IWMs that guide expectations and behavior, and the balance between attachment and exploratory systems. Exploration, moreover, can be understood to encompass both that of the external and internal worlds of the child. Fourth, an additional target of intervention, especially in clinical situations in which a caregiver's mental health is significantly and chronically compromised, is that of augmentation of social support. The clinician supports the alliance between the caregiver and child but additionally maximizes the child's social-emotional development via thoughtful recruitment of familial, community, and therapeutic social supports to provide alternative models of attachment that foster the development of mentalization and broader social cognition.[130]

This review has addressed diagnostic categories of child attachment disorder, proposed classifications for disturbances in child-parent attachment, and the manner in which certain forms of caregiver psychopathology serve to severely disrupt child-parent mutual regulation of emotion and arousal. It is clear that, in the context of early development especially, a great deal of plasticity helps the young child to adapt to new relationships, to embrace new models of complex human interaction and individual differences, and to thereby alter his or her IWM of attachment relationships. We have seen, for example, that institutionalized children placed into enlightened foster care, or internationally adopted by a new set of caregivers, can make substantive gains in developmental and relational domains. At the same time, plasticity has its limits such that so-called "indiscriminate sociability" or "glomming on to strangers" does not improve or change substantially in the majority of cases.[55]

Finally, the authors hope that by now readers will have realized that any attempt to "impose" secure attachment on a child, as has been professed by so-called "holding therapies," flies in the face of what attachment theory and related research hold dear,[53] namely, that the process of attachment evolves. It grows and consolidates within a relationship with a caregiver who is able to provide repeated experiences of safety and protection, consistent and sensitive response in times of distress, and the capacity to mentalize the experience of the child. It is therefore essential to model for caregivers, and to provide for our patient families, emotional constancy and availability while continuously striving to understand, follow, and communicate with the child, as an individual with his or her own mind, feelings, thoughts, intentions, desires, and beliefs.[132]

ACKNOWLEDGMENTS

The authors gratefully acknowledge the indispensable help of Ms. Jaime McCaw in the preparation of this manuscript.

REFERENCES

1. Bowlby J. Attachment and loss, vol. I: attachment. New York: Basic Books; 1969/ 1982.
2. Bowlby J. Attachment and loss: retrospect and prospect. Am J Orthop 1982; 52(4):664–78.
3. Marvin R, O'Connor T. The formation of the parent-child attachment following privation. Paper presented at: Biennial meeting of the Society for Research in Child Development; April, 1999; Albuquerque, NM.
4. Mahler MS, Pine F, Bergman A. The psychological birth of the human infant: symbiosis and individuation. New York: Basic Books; 1975.
5. Bowlby J. A secure base: parent-child attachment and healthy human development. New York: Basic Books Inc; 1988.
6. Main M, Kaplan N, Cassidy JC. Security in infancy, childhood, and adulthood: a move to the level of representation. Monogr Soc Res Child Dev 1985; 50(1–2):66–104.
7. Ainsworth MDS, Blehar MC, Waters E, et al. Patterns of attachment: a psychological study of the strange situation. Hillsdale, NJ: Erlbaum; 1978.
8. Crittenden PM. Relationships at risk. In: Belsky J, Nezworski T, editors. Clinical implications of attachment. Hillside, NJ: Erlbaum; 1988. p. 136–74.
9. Lyons-Ruth K, Connell DB, Zoll D, et al. Infants at social risk: Relations among infant maltreatment, maternal behavior, and infant attachment behavior. Dev Psychol 1987;23(2):223–32.
10. Main M, Solomon J. Discovery of an insecure-disorganized/disoriented pattern. In: Brazelton TB, Yogman M, editors. Affective development in infancy. Norwood, NJ: Ablex Publishing; 1986.
11. Main M, Solomon J. Procedures for identifying infants as disorganized/disoriented during the Ainsworth strange situation. In: Greenberg MT, Cicchetti D, Cummings EM, editors. Attachment in the preschool years: theory, research, and intervention. Chicago: University of Chicago Press; 1990. p. 121–60.
12. Main M, Hesse E. Parents' unresolved traumatic experiences are related to infant disorganized attachment status: Is frightened and/or frightening parental behavior the linking mechanism? In: Greenberg MT, Cicchetti D, Cummings EM, editors. Attachment in the preschool years. Chicago: University of Chicago Press; 1990. p. 161–82.
13. Main M, Hesse E. Coding system for identifying frightened, frightening, dissociated, and disorganized parental behavior. Berkeley, CA: University of California at Berkeley; 1992.
14. Main M. Recent studies in attachment: overview, with selected implications for clinical work. In: Goldberg S, Muir R, Kerr J, editors. Attachment theory: Social, developmental and clinical perspectives. Hillsdale, NJ: The Analytic Press; 1995.
15. Campos JJ, Barret KC, Lamb ME, et al. Socioemotional development. In: Haith MM, Campos JJ, editors. Handbook of child psychology: vol. 2. Infancy and developmental psychobiology. New York: Wiley & Sons; 1983. p. 783–815.
16. van IJzendoorn M, Kroonenberg P. Cross-cultural patterns of attachment: a meta-analysis of the strange situation. Child Dev 1988;59:147–56.
17. van IJzendoorn MH. Adult attachment representations, parental responsiveness, and infant attachment: a meta-analysis on the predictive validity of the adult attachment interview. Psychol Bull 1995;117(3):387–403.

18. Cicchetti D. Developmental psychopathology in infancy: Illustration from the study of maltreated youngsters. J Consult Clin Psychol 1987;55(6):837–45.

19. Carlson V, Cicchetti D, Barnett D, et al. Finding order in disorganization: lessons from research on maltreated infants' attachments to their caregivers. In: Cicchetti D, Carlson V, editors. Child maltreatment: theory and research on the causes and consequences of child abuse and neglect. New York: Cambridge University Press; 1989. p. 494–528.

20. Matas L, Arend RA, Sroufe LA. Continuity of adaptation in the second year: the relationship between quality of attachment and later competence. Child Dev 1978;49:547–56.

21. Sroufe LA. The coherence of individual development: early care, attachment, and subsequent developmental issues. Am Psychol 1979;34:834–41.

22. Waters E, Wippman J, Sroufe LA. Attachment, positive affect, and competence in the peer group: two studies in construct validation. Child Dev 1979;50(3):821–9.

23. Main M, Cassidy J. Categories of response to reunion with parent at age 6: predictable from infant attachment classifications and stable over a 1-month period. Dev Psychol 1988;24:415–26.

24. Urban J, Carlson E, Egeland B, et al. Patterns of individual adaptation across childhood. Dev Psychopathol 1991;3:445–60.

25. Elicker J, Englund M, Sroufe LA. Predicting peer competence and peer relationships in childhood from early parent-child relationships. In: Parke RD, Ladd G, editors. Family-peer relationships: modes of linkage. Hillsdale, NJ: Erlbaum; 1992. p. 77–106.

26. Beeghly M, Cicchetti D. Child maltreatment, attachment and the self system: emergence of an internal state lexicon in toddlers at high social risk. Dev Psychopathol 1994;6:5–30.

27. Browne A, Finkelhor D. Impact of child sexual abuse: a review of the research. Psychol Bull 1986;99(1):66–77.

28. George C, Main M. Social interactions of young abused children: approach, avoidance, and aggression. Child Dev 1979;50(2):306–18.

29. Howes C, Segal J. Children's relationships with alternative caregivers: the special case of maltreated children removed from their homes. J Appl Dev Psychol 1993;14(1):71–81.

30. Schneider-Rosen K, Cicchetti D. Early self-knowledge and emotional development: visual self-recognition and affective reactions to mirror self-images in maltreated and non-maltreated toddlers. Dev Psychol 1991;27(3):471–8.

31. Toth SL, Cicchetti D. Patterns of relatedness, depressive symptomatology, and perceived competence in maltreated children. J Consult Clin Psychol 1996;64(1):32–41.

32. Toth SL, Manly JT, Cicchetti D. Child maltreatment and vulnerability to depression. Dev Psychopathol 1992;4:97–112.

33. Zeanah CH, Boris NW. Disturbances and disorders of attachment in early childhood. In: Zeanah CH, editor. Handbook of infant mental health. 2nd edition. New York: Guilford Press; 2000. p. 353–68.

34. Zeanah CH, Smyke AT. Attachment disorders in family and social context. Infant Ment Health J 2008;29(3):219–33.

35. Sroufe LA. The role of infant-caregiver attachment in development. In: Belsky J, Nezworski T, editors. Clinical implications of attachment. Hillsdale, NJ: Erlbaum; 1988. p. 18–38.

36. Carlson EA. A prospective longitudinal study of attachment disorganization/disorientation. Child Dev 1998;69(4):1107–28.

37. DeKlyen M. Disruptive behavior disorder and intergenerational attachment patterns: a comparison of clinic-referred and normally functioning preschoolers and their mothers. J Consult Clin Psychol 1996;64(2):357–65.
38. Green J, Goldwyn R. Attachment disorganisation and psychopathology: new findings in attachment research and their potential implications for developmental psychopathology in childhood. J Child Psychol Psychiatry 2002;43(7): 835–46.
39. Greenberg MT. Attachment and psychopathology in childhood. In: Cassidy J, Shaver P, editors. Handbook of attachment. New York: Guilford Press; 1999. p. 469–96.
40. Lyons-Ruth K, Jacobvitz D. Attachment disorganization: Unresolved loss, relational violence, and lapses in behavioral and attentional strategies. In: Cassidy J, Shaver PR, editors. Handbook of attachment: Theory, research, and clinical implications. New York: Guilford Press; 1999. p. 520–55.
41. van IJzendoorn MH, Schuengel C, Bakermans-Kranenburg MJ. Disorganized attachment in early childhood: Meta-analyses of precursors, concomitants, and sequelae. Dev Psychopathol 1999;11:225–49.
42. Warren SL, Huston L, Egeland B, et al. Child and adolescent anxiety disorders and early attachment. J Am Acad Child Adolesc Psychiatry 1997;36(5):637–44.
43. Bowlby J. Forty-four juvenile thieves: Their characters and their home life. Int J Psychoanal 1944;25:19–52.
44. Robertson J. Some responses of young children to loss of maternal care. Nurs Times 1953;18:382–6.
45. Spitz RA. Hospitalism: an inquiry into the genesis of psychiatric conditions in early childhood. Psychoanal Study Child 1945;1:53–73.
46. Zeanah CH, Boris NW, Scheeringa MS. Psychopathology in infancy. J Child Psychol Psychiatry 1997;38(1):81–99.
47. APA. Diagnostic and statistical manual of mental disorders (DSM-III). 3rd edition. Washington, DC: American Psychiatric Association; 1980.
48. Tizard B, Rees J. The effect of early institutional rearing on the behaviour problems and affectional relationships of four-year-old children. J Child Psychol Psychiatry 1975;16(1):61–73.
49. APA. Diagnostic and statistical manual of mental disorders (DSM-III-R). revised 3rd edition. Washington, DC: American Psychiatric Association; 1987.
50. APA. Diagnostic and statistical manual of mental disorders (DSM-IV). 4th edition. Washington, DC: American Psychiatric Association; 1994.
51. International classifications of diseases, 10th revision (ICD-10). Geneva, Switzerland: World Health Organization; 1992.
52. APA. Diagnostic and statistical manual of mental disorders, 4th edition, text revision (DSM-IV-TR). Washington, DC: American Psychiatric Association; 2000.
53. Boris NW, Zeanah CH. The work group on quality issues. Practice parameter for the assessment and treatment of children and adolescents with reactive attachment disorder of infancy and early childhood. J Am Acad Child Adolesc Psychiatry 2005;44(11):1206–19.
54. Zeanah CH, Mammen OK, Lieberman AL. Disorders of attachment. In: Zeanah CH, editor. Handbook of infant mental health. New York: Guilford Press; 1993. p. 332–49.
55. Zeanah CH, Smyke AT, Koga SF, et al. The BEIP Core Group. Attachment in institutionalized and community children in Romania. Child Dev 2005;76(5):1015–28.
56. Zero To Three/National Center for Clinical Infant Programs. DC:0-3. Diagnostic classification of mental health and developmental disorders of infancy and early

childhood. Arlington, VA: Zero to Three/National Center for Clinical Infant Programs; 1994.

57. Zero To Three/National Center for Clinical Infant Programs. DC:0-3. Diagnostic classification of mental health and developmental disorders of infancy and early childhood. Rev. edition. Washington, DC: Zero to Three Press; 2005.

58. Lieberman A, Zeanah CH. Disorders of attachment in infancy. In: Minde K, editor. Infant psychiatry, child psychiatric clinics of North America. Philadelphia: W.B. Saunders; 1995. p. 571–88.

59. Lieberman AF, Pawl JH. Disorders of attachment and secure-base behavior in the second year of life. In: Greenberg ET, Cicchetti D, Cummings EM, editors. Attachment in the preschool years: Theory, research, and interventions. Chicago: University of Chicago Press; 1990. p. 375–97.

60. Boris NW, Zeanah CH, Larrieu JA, et al. Attachment disorders in infancy and early childhood: a preliminary investigation of diagnostic criteria. Am J Psychiatry 1998;155(2):295–7.

61. Boris NW, Hinshaw-Fuselier SS, Smyke AT, et al. Comparing criteria for attachment disorders: establishing reliability and validity in high-risk samples. J Am Acad Child Adolesc Psychiatry 2004;43(5):568–77.

62. Smyke AT, Dumitrescu A, Zeanah CH. Disturbances of Attachment in young children: I. The continuum of caretaking casualty. J Am Acad Child Adolesc Psychiatry 2002;41(8):972–82.

63. Tizard B, Rees J. A comparison of the effects of adoption, restoration to the natural mother, and continued institutionalization on the cognitive development of four-year-old children. Child Dev 1974;45(1):92–9.

64. Hinshaw-Fuselier S, Boris NW, Zeanah CH. Reactive attachment disorder in maltreated twins. Infant Ment Health J 1999;20(1):42–59.

65. O'Connor TG. Attachment disorders in infancy and childhood. In: Rutter M, Taylor E, editors. Child and adolescent psychiatry: modern approaches. 4th edition. Boston: Blackwell; 2002. p. 776–92.

66. Rutter M, Anderson-Wood L, Beckett C, et al. Quasi-autistic patterns following severe early global privation. J Child Psychol Psychiatry 1999;40: 537–49.

67. Rutter M, Kreppner J, Croft C, et al. Early adolescent outcomes of institutionally deprived and non-deprived adoptees. III. Quasi-autism. Journal of Child Psychology and Psychiatry 2007;48(12):1200–7.

68. Zeanah CH, Smyke AT, Koga S. The Bucharest Early Intervention Project: attachment and disorders of attachment. Paper presented at: the Biennial meeting of the Society for Research in Child Development 2005; Atlanta, GA.

69. Zeanah CH, Boris NW, Bakshi S, et al. Attachment disorders in infancy. In: Osofsky JD, Fitzgerald HE, editors, WAIMH handbook of infant mental health, Volume Four: Infant mental health in groups at high risk. New York: Wiley & Sons; 2000. p. 93–122.

70. O'Connor TG, Bredenkamp D, Rutter M. Attachment disturbances and disorders in children exposed to early severe deprivation. Infant Mental Health Journal 1999;20:10–29.

71. O'Connor TG, Rutter M. Attachment disorder behavior following severe deprivation: Extension and longitudinal follow-up. J Am Acad Child Adolesc Psychiatry 2000;39:703–12.

72. Chisholm K. A three year follow-up of attachment and indiscriminate friendliness in children adopted from Romanian orphanages. Child Dev 1998;69(4): 1092–106.

73. O'Connor TG, Marvin RS, Rutter M, et al. Child-parent attachment following early institutional deprivation. Dev Psychopathol 2003;15:19–38.
74. Stovall KC, Dozier M. The development of attachment in new relationships: Single subject analyses for ten foster infants. Dev Psychopathol 2000;12:133–56.
75. Hodges J, Tizard B. Social and family relationships of ex-institutional adolescents. J Child Psychol Psychiatry 1989;30(1):77–97.
76. Chisholm K, Carter MC, Ames EW, et al. Attachment security and indiscriminately friendly behavior in children adopted from Romanian orphanages. Dev Psychopathol 1995;7:283–94.
77. Richters MM, Volkmar F. Reactive attachment disorder of infancy or early childhood. J Am Acad Child Adolesc Psychiatry 1994;33:328–32.
78. Zeanah CH, Scheeringa MS, Boris NW, et al. Reactive attachment disorder in maltreated toddlers. Child Abuse Negl 2004;28:877–88.
79. Zeanah CH, Smyke AT, Dumitrescu A. Attachment disturbances in young children: II. Indiscriminate behavior and institutional care. J Am Acad Child Adolesc Psychiatry 2002;41(8):983–9.
80. Fraiberg S, Adelson E, Shapiro V. Ghosts in the nursery. A psychoanalytic approach to the problems of impaired infant-mother relationships. J Am Acad Child Psychiatry 1975;14(3):387–421.
81. Ichise M, Vines DC, Gura T, et al. Effects of early life stress on [11C]DASB positron emission tomography imaging of serotonin transporters in adolescent peer- and mother-reared rhesus monkeys. J Neurosci 2006;26(17):4638–43.
82. Schechter DS, Zygmunt A, Davies M, et al. Caregiver traumatization adversely impacts young children's mental representations on the MacArthur Story Stem Battery. Attach Hum Dev 2007;9(3):187–205.
83. Steele B. Psychological effects of child abuse and neglect. In: Call JD, Galenson E, Tyson RL, editors. Frontiers of infant psychiatry. New York: Basic Books; 1983. p. 235–44.
84. Solomon J, George C, DeJong A. Children classified as controlling at age 6: evidence of disorganized representational strategies and aggression at home and at school. Dev Psychopathol 1995;7:447–64.
85. Lieberman AF, Zeanah CH. Disorders of attachment in infancy. Child and Adolescent Clinics of North America 1995;4:571–687.
86. Robertson J, Robertson J. Separations and the very young. London: Free Association Books; 1989.
87. Lieberman AF, Compton NC, van Horn P, et al. Losing a parent to death in the early years. Washington, DC: Zero To Three; 2003.
88. Gaensbauer T, Chatoor I, Drell M, et al. Traumatic loss in a one-year-old girl. J Am Acad Child Adolesc Psychiatry 1995;34(4):520–8.
89. Lieberman AF, Van Horn P, Gosh Ippen C. Toward evidence-based treatment: child-parent psychotherapy with preschoolers exposed to marital violence. J Am Acad Child Adolesc Psychiatry 2005;44(12):1241–8.
90. McDonough SC. Promoting positive early parent-infant relationships through interaction guidance. Child Adolesc Clin N Am 1995;4:661–72.
91. Schechter DS, Myers MM, Brunelli SA, et al. Traumatized mothers can change their minds about their toddlers: understanding how a novel use of videofeedback supports positive change of maternal attributions. Infant Mental Health Journal 2006;27(5):429–47.
92. Cooper G, Hoffman K, Powell B, et al. The circle of security intervention: differential diagnosis and differential treatment. In: Berlin LJ, Ziv Y, Amaya-Jackson L, et al, editors. Enhancing early attachments. New York: The Guilford Press; 2005. p. 127–51.

93. Slade A. Maternal reflective functioning: attachment and caregiving. Paper presented at: meetings of the World Association of Infant Mental Health. 2002; Amsterdam, The Netherlands.

94. Slade A. Keeping the baby in mind: a critical factor in perinatal mental health. Bulletin of ZERO TO THREE: National Center for Infants, Toddlers and Families 2002;22(6):10–6.

95. Slade A, Grienenberger J, Bernbach E, et al. Maternal reflective functioning, attachment, and the transmission gap: a preliminary study. Attach Hum Dev 2005;7(3):283–98.

96. Cicchetti D, Rogosch FA, Toth SL. Fostering secure attachment in infants in maltreating families through preventive interventions. Dev Psychopathol 2006;18(3): 623–49.

97. Dozier M, Lindhiem O, Ackerman JP. Attachment and biobehavioral catch up: an intervention targeting empirically identified needs of foster care infants. In: Berlin LJ, Ziv Y, Amaya-Jackson L, Greenberg MT, editors. Enhancing early attachments. New York: The Guilford Press; 2005. p. 178–94.

98. Zeanah CH, Larrieu JA, Heller SS, et al. Evaluation of a preventive intervention for maltreated infants and toddlers in foster care. J Am Acad Child Adolesc Psychiatry 2001;40(2):214–21.

99. Hofer MA. Relationships as regulators: a psychobiological perspective on bereavement. Psychosom Med 1984;46:183–7.

100. Stern DN. The interpersonal world of the infant. New York: Basic Books; 1985.

101. Tronick EZ, Gianino AF. The transmission of maternal disturbance to the infant. Winter. New Dir Child Dev 1986;34(1):5–11.

102. Bretherton I. Communication patterns, internal working models, and the intergenerational transmission of attachment relationships. Infant Mental Health Journal 1990;11(3):237–52.

103. Crittenden PM. Internal representational models of attachment relationships. Infant Mental Health Journal 1990;11:259–77.

104. Fonagy P, Steele M, Steele H, et al. The capacity for understanding mental states: the reflective self in parent and child and its significance for security of attachment. Infant Mental Health Journal 1991;12(3):201–18.

105. Fonagy P, Steele M, Moran G, et al. Measuring the ghost in the nursery: an empirical study of the relation between parents' mental representations of childhood experiences and their infants' security of attachment. J Am Psychoanal Assoc 1993;41(4):957–89.

106. Bretherton I, Munholland KA. Internal working models in attachment relationships: a construct revisited. In: Cassidy J, Shaver PR, editors. Handbook of attachment. New York: The Guilford Press; 1999. p. 89–114.

107. Schechter DS, Coots T, Zeanah CH, et al. Maternal mental representations of the child in an inner-city clinical sample: violence-related posttraumatic stress and reflective functioning. Attach Hum Dev 2005;7(3):313–31.

108. Grienenberger JF, Kelly K, Slade A. Maternal reflective functioning, mother-infant affective communication, and infant attachment: exploring the link between mental states and observed caregiving behavior in the intergenerational transmission of attachment. Attach Hum Dev 2005;7(3):299–311.

109. Oppenheim D, Koren-Karie N, Sagi-Schwartz A. Emotion dialogues between mothers and children at 4.5 and 7.5 years: relations with children's attachment at 1 year. Child Dev 2007;78(1):38–52.

110. Fonagy P, Steele M, Steele H, et al. The theory and practice of resilience. J Child Psychol Psychiatry 1994;35(2):231–57.

111. Lyons-Ruth K, Bronfman E, Parsons E. Atypical attachment in infancy and early childhood among children at developmental risk. IV. Maternal frightened, frightening, or atypical behavior and disorganized infant attachment patterns. Monogr Soc Res Child Dev 1999;64(3):67–96.

112. Schuengel C, Bakermans-Kranenburg MJ, Van Ijzendoorn MH. Frightening maternal behavior linking unresolved loss and disorganized infant attachment. J Consult Clin Psychol 1999;67(1):54–63.

113. Madigan S, Moran G, Pederson DR. Unresolved states of mind, disorganized attachment relationships, and disrupted interactions of adolescent mothers and their infants. Dev Psychol 2006;42(2):293–304.

114. Lyons-Ruth K, Dutra L, Schuder MR, et al. From infant attachment disorganization to adult dissociation: relational adaptations or traumatic experiences? Psychiatr Clin North Am 2006;29(1):63–86, viii.

115. Gervai J, Novak A, Lakatos K, et al. Infant genotype may moderate sensitivity to maternal affective communications: attachment disorganization, quality of care, and the DRD4 polymorphism. Soc Neurosci 2007;2(3–4):307–19.

116. Weinberg MK, Olson KL, Beeghly M, et al. Making up is hard to do, especially for mothers with high levels of depressive symptoms and their infant sons. J Child Psychol Psychiatry 2006;47(7):670–83.

117. Dawson G, Frey K, Panagiotides H, et al. Infants of depressed mothers exhibit atypical frontal brain activity: a replication and extension of previous findings. J Child Psychol Psychiatry 1997;38(2):179–86.

118. Weissman MM, Pilowsky DJ, Wickramaratne PJ, et al. Remissions in maternal depression and child psychopathology: a STAR*D-child report. JAMA 2006; 295(12):1389–98.

119. Carter AS, Garrity-Rokous FE, Chazan-Cohen R, et al. Maternal depression and comorbidity: predicting early parenting, attachment security, and toddler social-emotional problems and competencies. J Am Acad Child Adolesc Psychiatry 2001;40(1):18–26.

120. Porges SW. The Polyvagal Theory: phylogenetic contributions to social behavior. Physiol Behav 2003;79(3):503–13.

121. Lyons-Ruth K, Block D. The disturbed caregiving system: relations among childhood trauma, maternal caregiving, and infant affect and attachment. Infant Mental Health Journal 1996;17:257–75.

122. Schechter DS, Zeanah CH, Myers MM, et al. Psychobiological dysregulation in violence-exposed mothers: salivary cortisol of mothers with very young children pre- and post-separation stress. Bull Menninger Clin 2004;68(4):319–37.

123. Schechter DS, Coates SW, Kaminer T, et al. Distorted maternal mental representations and atypical behavior in a clinical sample of violence-exposed mothers and their toddlers. J Trauma Dissociation 2008;9(2):123–47.

124. Schechter DS, Willheim E. When parenting becomes unthinkable: interviewing with traumatized parents and their toddlers. J Am Acad Child Adolesc Psychiatry 2009;48:249–54.

125. Schechter DS, Hinojosa C, Kleinman K, Turner J, McCaw JE, Trabka KA. Maternal PTSD, atypical behavior, and joint attention with preschoolers. Paper presented at: American Academy of Child & Adolescent Psychiatry-54th Annual Meeting 2007; Boston, MA.

126. Blake DD, Weathers FW, Nagy LM, et al. The development of a clinician-administered PTSD scale. J Trauma Stress 1995;8(1):75–90.

127. Weathers FW, Litz BT, Keane TM, et al. The utility of the SCL-90-R for the diagnosis of war-zone related posttraumatic stress disorder. J Trauma Stress 1996;9(1):111–28.

128. Smyke A, Zeanah CH. Disturbances of attachment interview. New Orleans, LA: Tulane University School of Medicine, Department of Psychiatry; 1999.
129. Zeanah CH, Larrieu JA, Heller SS, et al. Infant-parent relationship assessment. In: Zeanah CH, editor. Handbook of infant mental health. New York: Guilford Press; 2000. p. 222–35.
130. Wachs C, Jacobs L. Parent-focused child therapy: attachment, identification and reflective function. New York: Jason Aronson Inc; 2006. p. 12–4.
131. Berlin LJ. Interventions to enhance early attachments: the state of the field today. In: Berlin LJ, Ziv Y, Amaya-Jackson L, et al, editors. Enhancing early attachments: theory, research, intervention, and policy. New York: The Guilford Press; 2005. p. 2–5.
132. Cohen NJ, Muir E, Lojkasek M, et al. Watch, Wait, and Wonder. Testing the effectiveness of a new approach to mother-infant psychotherapy. Infant Mental Health Journal 1999;20:429–51.

Preventive Intervention for Early Childhood Behavioral Problems: An Ecological Perspective

Stephanie A. Shepard, PhD[a,b,*], Susan Dickstein, PhD[a,b]

KEYWORDS

- Early childhood • Behavioral problems
- Preventive interventions • Parent training
- Mental health consultation

The early childhood period is associated with profound development across cognitive, social, emotional, behavioral, and physical domains.[1,2] Early childhood mental health is characterized by social-emotional competence and behavior regulation within healthy and supportive relationship contexts.[3] However, children may demonstrate significant disruptions in social, emotional and behavioral functioning from early on, with approximately 12% of preschoolers in the general population and up to 30% in high-risk, low income samples identified as having serious behavioral difficulties.[4–6] These challenges are associated with an elevated risk of future emotional, academic, and relationship problems.[7] Specifically, children exhibiting early-onset behavioral problems are at especially high risk for life-course delinquency, substance use, violent behavior, academic failure, and depression.[8,9] Although conduct problems are the most frequent reason children are referred for mental health services,[10] young children's mental health problems remain underrecognized and undertreated.[11–13] When not addressed early, conduct problems that emerge in early childhood are the most resistant to treatment later in childhood and adolescence.[14]

The purpose of this article is to highlight the importance of parenting-focused early preventive interventions to address early childhood behavior problems. We briefly review evidence-based parenting programs, focusing on one particular program, the Incredible Years Series (IY). We discuss the barriers to embedding evidence-based practice such as IY in community contexts and demonstrate how early

This work was supported by Grant No. K01MH77097 from the National Institute of Mental Health to the first author.

[a] Bradley/Hasbro Children's Research Center, Bradley Early Childhood Clinical Research Center, 1011 Veterans Memorial Parkway, Providence, RI, USA

[b] The Warren Alpert Medical School of Brown University, Providence, RI, USA

E-mail address: stephanie_shepard@brown.edu (S. A. Shepard).

childhood mental health consultation can be used to enhance community capacity to adopt evidence-based practice and improve outcomes for the large number of young children and their families in need.

THE IMPORTANCE OF PARENTING-FOCUSED EARLY PREVENTIVE INTERVENTIONS

Early childhood mental health problems are associated with a host of family factors, including poor parent-child relationship quality and negative/harsh parenting practices.[15–17] Often, families experience co-occurring risks such as parental depression, substance use, unhealthy adult relationships, parenting stress, and sociodemographic challenges such as poverty, lack of access to community resources, and social isolation. Accumulation of family risk has serious consequences for parenting and parent-child relationships and, in turn, for the child's early functioning across multiple domains.[18–22] We know that in high-risk families, the capacity to provide an environment conducive to promoting behavior regulation and social-emotional competence may be seriously limited. In particular, children developing in high-risk family contexts are more likely to have core deficits in forming and engaging in interpersonal relationships, regulating affect, and developing positive sense of self, the very deficits that may set the stage for life-course juvenile delinquency, substance use, violent behavior, academic failure, and depression.[8,23,24]

Early-onset, persistent antisocial trajectories can be identified as young as 18 months of age, typically for children raised within the context of multiple family stressors, disrupted parent-child attachments, parental maladjustment (eg, maternal depressive symptoms, antisocial behavior), and nonresponsive, rejecting, or abusive caregiving.[9,15,17] One proposed mechanism to explain the poor mental health outcomes for these young children is that child behavior challenges combine with parenting risk factors to set the stage for coercive cycles that maintain and exacerbate chronic conduct problems.[25] In the context of child behavior challenges, poor parent-child relationships and parent family-management practices may unintentionally reinforce early disruptive behaviors. The coercive interaction cycles that result are more prognostic of problem behavior trajectories than children's behavior problems alone.[20] This "early starter" model of antisocial behavior underscores the importance of providing family-based interventions focused on parenting in the early childhood years to disrupt these negative developmental trajectories before parent-child interaction cycles become entrenched and behavior problems difficult to treat.[26,27]

Unfortunately, families do not always receive effective or sufficient support that would promote healthy development in their children. The community-based standard of care often falls short of effectively supporting parents to provide the foundations children require for positive developmental outcomes. For example, although families may be offered parenting classes, these programs are rarely evidence based, and estimates are that less than half the families complete the training.[28] Further, families may be offered case management services, but a number of factors limit the effectiveness of these services in promoting positive parenting skills, including (1) delays in accessing services (eg, due to long wait lists); (2) services focused only on immediate crises (such as lack of food or shelter); (3) lack of expertise to address unique factors related to parenting in early childhood; and (4) services are not integrated.

PARENT-MANAGEMENT TRAINING

Parent-management training (PMT) programs in particular are the most well-established treatments available for reducing child disruptive behaviors in families.[29] The primary goals of PMT programs are to change the child's behavior and adaptive functioning by increasing parental involvement and responsivity as well as promoting positive caregiver practices and effective discipline. Indeed, 2/3 of families that participate in PMT experience clinically significant improvements in their child's behavior directly following intervention, with levels of problem behaviors falling into the normal range following intervention and with significant effects lasting up to 4 years.[27,30]

Routed in learning theory (ie, operant conditioning), PMT emphasizes specific behavioral principles and teaches associated techniques including reinforcement techniques to increase desired behaviors and reduce undesired behaviors, and nonpunitive punishment (eg, loss of privileges or time out) and extinction (eg, ignoring) to also reduce undesired behaviors. In addition to these specific techniques, PMT content also typically addresses the parent-child relationship with an emphasis on enhancing parents' skill at engaging in child-directed play as well as strategies to support and encourage children's socioemotional and cognitive development in the context of the play.[27,29] For further details on the conceptual foundations and distinguishing features of PMT, as well as a review of its strong empirical support, Kazdin's book[29] reviewing PMT is highly recommended.

In PMT, parents are considered the change agents and therefore are the focus of the intervention. In sessions, parents are taught techniques to modify their child's behavior such that most of the "treatment" of the child is conducted indirectly through the parents outside of sessions in the family's daily life.[29] In each PMT session, child-management principles and techniques are introduced (eg, through written materials as well as direct instruction and/or modeling) and practiced via experiential methods (ie, role play or live practice and feedback with the child present in session). This active training with parents occurs within the context of a collaborative relationship with a skilled, supportive therapist who facilitates and guides parents' experiential learning. Parents are given practice activities to conduct at home with their child, which are reviewed in session and during telephone contacts between sessions.

Most PMT is delivered in individual sessions in clinic settings. Two well-known, widely adopted examples of evidence-based PMT programs specifically targeting early childhood that are delivered in an individual format are Parent-Child Interaction Therapy (PCIT) and the Positive Parenting Program (Triple P). In addition to targeting parent behavior management skills, one notable feature of PCIT in particular is that parent-child attachments and communication are direct targets of intervention. The defining feature of PCIT is that therapists deliver direct coaching and reinforcement during live parent-child interactions through a communication device placed in the parent's ear (ie, the "bug in the ear" system). This weekly observation of parent-child interactions also allows for ongoing assessment of progress and performance-based treatment planning.[31] Triple P is notable for the provision of a continuum of services in which variations of PMT can be delivered based on problem severity. Parent training variations range from universal, community-based prevention to brief advice (one to two sessions) for a discrete child behavior to individual, clinical intervention with families facing more serious child behavior problems. Ongoing assessment and individualized feedback on parenting skills, along with parent support and stress coping skills, also are core features of Triple P individual, therapist-assisted interventions with parents.[32]

Although PMT is an effective treatment for reducing child disruptive behaviors, current prevalence rates of conduct problems and the vast number of families identified as high risk have created a need that taxes available resources for standard, individual service delivery in clinical settings. One alternative to individual, clinic-based PMT is delivery in a group format, which is a cost-effective approach that can serve large numbers of families and therefore has potential for decreasing the overall prevalence and incidence of behavior problems in the community at large.[27,29,30]

Low-income families facing multiple stressors have been served in this group format,[33] and some evidence suggests that minority families in particular are more likely to participate in services delivered in groups than in individual treatment.[34] One such example is the Community Parent Education (COPE) Program, a large group-based PMT intervention (on average, groups include 18 families or 27 adults) delivered in community settings (eg, schools). Parent training content in COPE is similar to that covered in other, individually administered PMT programs in clinics. A coping problem-solving model is applied, in which parents meet in groups to view video models of parents making less optimal, ineffective parenting choices for addressing child behavior problems and then work together to generate and practice more optimal solutions based on the parenting principles taught.[34] Another outstanding example of a group-based program for parents that reduces early child behavioral problems and increases social-emotional competence, the IY Series,[35] is reviewed in depth below.

The Incredible Years Parent and Children Series

IY has been identified as an exemplary best practice program by the Office of Juvenile Justice and Delinquency Prevention's Family Strengthening Project [35] and has met criteria as a well-established mental health intervention for children with conduct problems by the American Psychological Association Task Force on the Promotion and Dissemination of Psychological Procedures.[36] The IY program is effective with parents of varied economic and education levels and is available in several languages. IY is now implemented in over 40 states and at least 15 countries worldwide.[35] It is delivered as an indicated intervention for parents of children demonstrating early-onset conduct problems and oppositionality and also as a selected prevention program for high-risk samples. Although there are a number of components within the IY series that target children, teachers, and parents, we focus on the IY group-based PMT program designed for parents of young children.

The main goals of the IY Parents and Children Series are to strengthen parenting competencies and confidence and in turn to promote children's social, emotional, and academic competence to reduce or prevent socioemotional and behavioral problems in children.[35] Several IY programs are relevant in the early childhood years. The recently updated IY Basic Preschool/Early Childhood program is designed for children between ages 3 and 6 years[37] and is also available as a manualized home-visiting program for parents who are not able to attend groups or for parents who wish to supplement their group participation with guided practice with a parenting coach in their home.[38] In addition, two new IY parent group programs have recently been developed for younger children, the Parents and Babies Program (birth–12 months) and the Parents and Toddlers Program for ages 1 to 3 years.[39]

The Parents and Babies Program is a six-part program in which parents learn to read their child's cues and to provide nurturance and responsive care. Parents develop skill at observing their babies and understanding their developmental needs. They learn to provide physical, tactile, and visual stimulation, verbal communication, and establish predictable routines. The Parents and Toddlers Program and the updated Basic Preschool/Early Childhood Program extend parents' development of positive parenting skills, including components to develop child-directed play and coaching to promote language, social and emotional competence, and school readiness. This content is significantly expanded in this update of the original Basic Parent and Children Series, with a number of sessions devoted to academic, persistence, social, and emotional coaching. Both the Toddler and Basic Preschool/Early Childhood programs also cover how to encourage cooperative behavior through praise, encouragement and incentives, and positive discipline (rules, routines, and effective limit setting) as well as handling misbehavior. The Toddler program has an additional component in which parents learn about handling separations and reunions. In the updated Basic Preschool program, parents also learn a number of strategies for handling misbehavior, including ignoring, timeouts, natural and logical consequences, and teaching their children problem solving and self-regulation. All programs also promote parents' abilities to maintain self-control and to calm down, and encourage parents to develop and access support networks.[37,39]

The Parents and Babies Program is covered in approximately 8 sessions, and the Parents and Toddlers Program requires an additional 13 sessions.[39] The updated Basic Preschool/Early Childhood Preschool program extends the original Basic program from 12 sessions to 14 sessions (prevention samples) or 18 to 20 sessions for parents with children with behavioral diagnoses and in high-risk populations.[37] Sessions typically occur once per week for 2 to 2.5 hours. In general, the programs rely on collaborative group discussion, video modeling, and rehearsal as the primary teaching methods.[40] Sessions always include a detailed review of home activities, approximately 25 to 30 minutes of video review (see below), and at least four or five guided role plays or "practices." Role plays allow participants to practice strategies generated through the group collaborative process and to anticipate and overcome barriers to successful implementation at home. Additional rehearsal takes place during home activities assigned weekly, and group leaders make regular telephone contact with each member to support learning and application of skills to their home environments.

A key component to training is the use of video vignettes portraying parents and children interacting in typical family situations. The updated Basic Preschool/Early Childhood program contains the same vignettes from the original Basic program, supplemented with a number of new vignettes representing greater diversity, including families of African American, Asian, Caucasian, and Hispanic backgrounds. By using video models, parents observe ways to encourage their children's positive behaviors and discourage their inappropriate behaviors across a wide range of situations. Parents also view less successful interactions and witness the outcomes of less optimal choices, thereby fostering problem-solving discussions of alternative solutions and opportunities to rehearse alternative responses. Watching the videos of parent-child interactions also promotes parents' ability to observe their child's behavior, analyze situations, and to determine when and how best to intervene. As parents practice observing child behavior, they begin to identify problems when they are small and to be proactive to prevent larger disruptions that are more difficult to address. Through watching and discussing video vignettes, parents also have opportunities to become more aware of their child's positive behaviors and to identify opportunities to deliver praise and positive attention. Using the videos as the primary training method also standardizes group content to ensure coverage of specific content, increasing the feasibility of disseminating widely and delivering with fidelity.[29,35]

The program is designed to include 10 to 14 parents in a group. The collaborative group process is intended to build parents' confidence in their own ideas and their ability to solve problems and handle difficult situations that arise with their child. The group format encourages parents to give and get support from peers, fosters supportive connections, and reduces parents' feelings of isolation.[35] Participants are asked to make a "buddy call" each week to check in with another participant to further encourage the development of social connections and sources of support for participants.[35]

Detailed manuals for leaders prescribe the sequence of topics. General group process strategies are discussed in the manual, and each video vignette is reviewed, including provision of specific questions to encourage parents to draw out relevant parenting principles. Background content on parenting principles and information on normative child development also are provided for leaders, as well as specific guidelines and recommendations for group discussion topics and rehearsal activities. Additional materials provided include digital versatile discs (DVDs) of approximately 280 vignettes of parent-child interactions, homework assignments, and handouts.

A Review of the Evidence: IY Efficacy and Effectiveness

Webster-Stratton and colleagues conducted six randomized control trials of the original Basic Parenting series for families with children ages 3 to 8 years referred for oppositionality and early-onset conduct problems, and three randomized control prevention trials for families with children enrolled in Head Start.[35] To date, there have been no randomized trials of the new Babies and Toddler programs. However, preliminary evidence derived from an application of the original preschool curriculum for parents with children ages 2 and 3 years enrolled in daycare centers serving low-income urban families supports its adoption.[41] The efficacy of the updated Basic Preschool/Early Childhood program is currently under investigation.

In both treatment and prevention samples, parent participation in the original IY Basic parenting program resulted in sustained improvement in parents' self-reports and independent observations of their behavior management skills compared with control groups, replacing the use of harsh, ineffective parenting strategies with positive parenting, and improving observations of parent-child interactions and self-reports of parent involvement. In turn, program participation led to reductions in observed and reported child conduct problems at home and school and increased compliance with parental commands among children ages 3 to 8 years referred for treatment due to high levels of noncompliance, aggression, and/or oppositionality. Children in Head Start whose parents participated in the IY Parent groups, particularly those with initially elevated behavior problems, demonstrated enhanced social competence and reductions in negative affect, noncompliance, and disruptive behaviors.[42–44] Children with comorbid attentional problems, including inattention, impulsivity, and hyperactivity, were especially responsive to their parents' participation in the IY Basic parenting program, as demonstrated by declines in observed and parent-reported, but not teacher-reported, conduct problems.[45] Finally, studies show that the IY Basic parenting program delivered in a group format is as effective, if not more effective, than individual, personalized parent therapy applying IY practices and principles in individual sessions with parent-child dyads; it is considerably more cost effective, and parents report higher satisfaction ratings with the IY Basic parenting group program relative to the individual treatment.[46,47]

A number of independent replications of the original IY Basic parenting program with both treatment and prevention samples report similar positive outcomes for parents and children's behavior at home and in daycare settings, improvements that were maintained up to 2 years following participation.[41,46,48–50] These replications demonstrate the feasibility and effectiveness of implementing the IY program in applied community settings serving high-risk, low-income inner city families from ethnic minority backgrounds [41,46,49,50] and extend its applicability to parents with children as young as 2 years of age.[41,49] In addition, results of one study demonstrate the power of this parenting program for altering one proposed biologic underpinning of children's conduct problems, cortisol levels during social challenges; Relative to controls, high-risk children who demonstrated atypical (low) cortisol responses in anticipation of social challenges at baseline demonstrated more typical responses of normally developing, low-risk children (ie, normal increases in cortisol levels) following their parents' participation in the parenting program.[51] Finally, results of two replication studies demonstrate positive changes in families that generalize beyond the target child; both found that improved parenting behaviors were accompanied by reductions in problem behavior for siblings who were not the direct target of the intervention.[49,52]

Studies consistently demonstrate that families facing multiple stressors, including poverty, single parent status, social isolation, family conflict, substance use, and psychological distress, can be served in this group format and make measurable gains.[33] For example, IY program effects are robust among parents who experience depression, anger problems, or antisocial behavior and among parents with a prior history of child maltreatment.[33,48,49,53] Even when parents' adjustment (ie, depression) does not change with the intervention, depressed parents are still able to make positive changes to their parenting behaviors following IY, which in turn are associated with reductions in child negative behavior.[49] However, children whose parents continue to report high levels of depression following the IY parent groups are less likely to maintain treatment gains over time.[54]

Parent Engagement and Treatment Responsiveness

Group-based PMT is typically delivered in fairly fixed doses, but the number of sessions required to make meaningful change is not well understood.[55] Examining the dosage question with respect to the original IY Basic parenting program in particular, some researchers report that parents begin to demonstrate parenting skill improvements after attending three sessions,[33] whereas others found that attendance at 50% of IY sessions discriminated parents who benefit.[56] Although IY program developers find that parents who agree to participate attend, on average, as many as 87% of sessions in treatment samples, the rate is much lower in prevention samples (participants attend, on average, 58% of sessions) and in replication studies conducted in community settings, where the average is closer to approximately 60% of sessions. Further, the level of engagement as defined by number of sessions attended, homework completion, and participation in group discussion is related to the amount of progress made in a dose-response fashion, with the strongest outcomes found for parents who attended at least two-thirds of the sessions.[33,41]

The impact of expanding the original IY Basic parenting program to 20 sessions on initial enrollment, attendance and adherence, and outcomes remains to be determined. However, one adaptation of IY that expands the program to 22 sessions reports that families, on average, attend only 55% of sessions; results were strongest for those families who attended more than 50% of sessions.[48] Preliminary data on the updated, extended version of the Basic program suggests that parents who participated in the 20-week group report feeling more confident in handling their children's behavior and report fewer, and less intense, child behavior problems and better child-emotion regulation than did families who participated in a shorter (10 week) version.[57]

Indeed, inconsistent attendance, poor treatment adherence, and premature termination remain major obstacles to fully realizing the benefits of PMT. Several strategies are consistently recommended to support attendance given our current understanding of the stressors families face (for review, see[58]). These include running groups in convenient community locations on a variety of days and times that best fit parents' schedules. Providing transportation and childcare may also make it more feasible for parents to attend. Making meals available reduces another burden to participants, particularly when group schedules overlap with mealtimes.

Even when families are helped to overcome these pragmatic barriers, the high demands placed on parents in PMT relative to other forms of treatment must also be appreciated. For example, there can be a mismatch between parents' expectations of therapy for their child's behavior problems and the realities of PMT. A number of treatment supplements have been developed to enhance attendance and adherence by addressing parents' expectations for treatment and incorporating motivation-enhancing strategies.[55,59] Motivational strategies have been incorporated into intake procedures, including initial phone contacts with parents and initial sessions, to increase the likelihood of attendance and promote stronger treatment adherence.[60,61] Typically, this involves engaging parents in problem solving regarding identified barriers to treatment, such as lack of familial support for attending. Parents' perceptions of treatment demands and beliefs about treatment relevance or efficacy are also addressed. Clarifying the helping process, including a focus on parents as the agents of change, is also an important element of engagement-enhancing procedures. Using brief, motivation-enhancing strategies (ie, 5–15 minutes in length incorporated in up to three of the first few treatment sessions) enhances parents' desire to participate in the treatment to change their parenting behaviors, which in turn leads to higher attendance and adherence to individually administered PMT.[61] The extent to which these approaches engage parents in group-based PMT, particularly when encouraged on a preventive basis, has not been examined.

Given that parent, family, and contextual risk factors associated with early-onset conduct problems also influence treatment responsiveness and maintenance of gains, some parents may require additional services beyond parent training to address these undermining factors.[29] Parent stress, psychopathology, and family conflict all have the potential to compromise parents' adherence and responsiveness to treatment.[62] Supplementing traditional programs with strategies to address these issues may reduce attrition and increase adherence and treatment responsiveness. For example, incorporating focus on non–parenting-specific, family, and adult concerns (eg, marital discord, family conflict, job stress, health problems) throughout parenting programs helps families cope with life stress while remaining in treatment, which in turn leads to reductions in dropout rates.[28] IY in particular includes a supplemental series of 10 to 14 weeks to address the family stressors that tend to diminish effective parenting and treatment responsiveness. The ADVANCE program, which can be offered following completion of the Basic program, is designed to directly target parental stress and communication, problem solving, and collaboration among parents.[63]

Building Capacity to Meet the Need

The need for service for young children with conduct problems far exceeds the current capacity to provide high-quality, evidence-based service. Meeting this need requires innovative approaches to service delivery, particularly for families otherwise not willing or able to engage in group-based treatment. This includes making available self-administered programming and capitalizing on technology to identify new service delivery formats (ie, television programming, distribution of video vignettes and instructional content on DVD, Internet delivery). Such strategies are more cost effective, reduce the need for highly trained therapists, and build capacity for a greater number of families to access the treatment.[64–65] Several efforts to develop self-administered programs for parents yield clinically significant parent and child behavior changes, including parents' independent review of IY video vignettes.[64,66] In addition, the provision of self-help workbooks adapted from empirically supported programs (eg, Triple P) combined with professional telephone consultation and, more recently, delivering parenting program content via primetime television coverage coupled with the self-help workbooks and web-based support, both led to improved parenting skills and reductions in children's disruptive behaviors.[67,68] Another innovative approach, delivering IY curriculum via the Internet combined with opportunities for parents to gain social support through Internet blogs and a home visiting program to provide direct coaching and practice to parents, is currently under investigation.[69]

However, reaching those families with children at highest risk for conduct problem trajectories who require more intensive services than these self-administered options remains a formidable task. To meet the need, service delivery must be expanded beyond traditional mental health clinics. One approach may be for empirically supported programs to be embedded within other existing service structures that serve the largest proportion of families.[70] For example, providing PMT in community daycares and Head Start, schools, and other community settings may considerably increase the number of families who can be served, particularly those families who otherwise might not have access to good quality mental health services. Recent attempts to embed IY parent groups in medical homes also have been successful in reaching families and provide an opportunity to identify eligible families not enrolled in daycare or school.[71,72] Recruiting for parenting interventions through the Women, Infant, and Children Nutritional Supplement Program is another way to identify, recruit, and engage families at high risk who are not yet known to educational or social service programs and who may not attend regular primary care wellness visits.[73] Offering services in these settings increases access and reduces barriers to participation, such as concern regarding stigmatization, transportation, and mistrust of mental health providers. Another innovative approach to wide dissemination of PMT that currently is under investigation is to incorporate behavior management training into training programs for pediatric residents so that pediatric providers may integrate relevant content and principles in primary care visits when behavioral or parenting issues are raised.[74]

PARENT-MANAGEMENT TRAINING IN REAL-WORLD SETTINGS

Despite the abundance of evidence supporting PMT programs such as IY, the ways in which these manualized curricula are implemented in the community require local adaptation not necessarily addressed in the context of strictly controlled university-based research trials. Real-world barriers in community settings have the potential to undermine successful implementation of evidence-based treatments and diminish their efficacy.[75,76] Program effectiveness may be diluted because of a lack of resources (ie, funding, time, administrative support), infrastructure, and personnel with "buy-in" to program principles and processes and the need to adhere to a manualized curriculum. In addition, personnel in community settings often lack the training and background in early childhood mental health principles needed to deliver the programs with fidelity and to support what may be significant mental health needs of parents and children that co-occur with presenting behavioral problems in young children.

Early childhood mental health consultation can address some of these barriers. Mental health consultation specifically includes relationship building between consultants and programs; enhancing staff capacity through training and ongoing support; identifying and addressing program needs; and incorporating family, caregiver, and contextual factors to provide a comprehensive perspective that supports social-emotional competence and behavior regulation of young children.[77] When community-based programs serving young children have access to high-quality mental health consultation, children do better. For example, lower rates of expulsion from prekindergarten are found when programs have access to mental health consultation.[78] Although specific mechanisms have not been adequately studied, mental health consultation may improve early childhood outcomes by increasing developmentally appropriate practices and expectations; enhancing early identification of problem behaviors; reducing staff stress and turnover; addressing programmatic issues that affect service delivery; and otherwise supporting the child care community, families, and children who are manifesting (or are at risk for) problematic behaviors.[77] In our program, we augment PMT with mental health consultation to address barriers typically associated with the implementation of evidence-based practice in the community.

Example of Parent Management Training Implementation with Local Adaptation

The Bradley/Hasbro Early Childhood Clinical Research Center (BECCRC), affiliated with Brown Medical School, has worked in the community for 20 years developing an ecologically-based consultation model integrating early childhood mental health principles and evidence-based practice into a continuum of mental health consultation services. All service delivery is embedded in research focused on high-risk children, emotion regulation, social competence, parenting, and family process. We illustrate below how we provide mental health consultation in conjunction with evidence-based PMT to enhance service delivery and achieve optimal outcomes for young children and their families in community settings. For ease of narrative, we have synthesized and integrated our collective experiences with numerous community partners, including community family support agencies, Head Start programs, and other child-care settings. We use the factitious name "Child Care Academy" (CCA) to refer to this collection of experiences.

CCA is a community-based support service for families with children, birth to age 5 years, growing up in contexts that put them at significant risk of behavior problems and maladjustment. Their mission is to (1) promote healthy parent-child relationships including sensitivity to children's developmental needs; (2) facilitate healthy family environments that promote effective childcare routines and family-management practices; and (3) decrease family isolation. Their program director was eager to move beyond provision of general support services to deliver evidence-based programs to help accomplish their goals. Establishing a relationship with the BECCRC was motivated by their intrinsic desire to expand their capacity to meet the needs of the children and families they serve and an awareness that they lacked the necessary knowledge base, training, and infrastructure to select and provide such services.

BECCRC worked with the CCA program director to select a program that best fit the agency culture, goals, and practices. The director's goal was to identify a program to promote effective family-management strategies in enormously high-risk families who have children with high rates of behavioral difficulties. She was looking for a program that was culturally relevant, could service their large caseloads, and that had empirical support. Through discussions with staff at various levels of the agency and structured observations, we identified IY Basic and ADVANCE parenting programs as the best fit. However, in the face of limited resources, overburdened staff lacking requisite mental health training, and high turnover, it was deemed neither cost effective nor feasible to train CCA staff to be able to independently maintain a high standard of IY delivery.

The partnership between BECCRC consultants and CCA staff was necessary to enhance CCA's emergent capacity to offer high-quality services to their families.

Community settings such as CCA typically do not employ mental health professionals with advanced degrees who can lead IY groups with fidelity, and they often lack sustainable funding to support leaders' training and ongoing supervision. The IY program developer recommends that group leaders, who have at least a masters-level degree, participate in a 3-day, standardized training provided by IY certified trainers and mentors. Ongoing consultation and tape review by IY trainers and mentors and attendance at consultation workshops at least every 2 years are also strongly encouraged to maintain program fidelity.[32,41] High staff turnover rates that plague agencies such as CCA diminish the cost effectiveness of such training, further undermining sustainable delivery.

Instead, CCA case managers are experts in family engagement and support, and have longstanding relationships with families through their home visiting program. CCA provides individualized home visiting services ranging from daily to monthly to help stabilize families, meet their basic needs, and improve parent-child interactions. They also provide educational and social programming for families and have a state-of-the-art playroom that is staffed by trained CCA personnel and available for daily use by families. Their program therefore was well suited for adopting the IY parenting programs and supporting successful, sustainable outcomes, although expertise to do so was limited. The partnership determined that BECCRC consultants, who already deliver IY programs in a number of community agencies across our state, were better poised for direct IY delivery. At the same time, much of the 8 to 10 h/wk required to run IY groups involves support activities that could be more cost efficiently, and effectively, implemented by CCA case managers and staff who were well connected with families. Their IY delivery responsibilities are described below.

BECCRC consultants are formally trained to deliver IY programs and receive ongoing consultation by the IY program developer as part of a longer-term academic and service agenda. All BECCRC consultants are clinical psychologists, offering expertise in early childhood development in high-risk contexts and an understanding of the influence of multiple levels of context and organizational structures and processes. BECCRC therefore was uniquely suited to help CCA embed IY into their current service delivery model and to integrate IY principles into existing program elements, which would support its efficacy and sustainability. At the same time, BECCRC was afforded the opportunity to disseminate evidence-based practice on a larger scale in community settings, extending our clinical-research agenda.

Local incredible years series delivery

All CCA case managers participated in IY groups as coleaders to train them on IY principles. Involving case managers in group delivery also established continuity in follow-up supporting activities. That is, CCA case managers serving as group coleaders reviewed and provided feedback on weekly home activities with families. They made planned phone contacts with each family between sessions to follow up on homework completion and addressed barriers to implementing strategies at home. They made a second reminder phone contact the night before or morning of each session. In this way, families experienced the continuity of a relationship with their case managers inside and outside of the group. CCA case managers previously trained in IY principles and strategies then provided childcare while parents attend groups, enhancing the quality and continuity of care that all family members received.

Similar to others who have extended the IY curriculum for especially high-risk families,[48] we supplemented delivery of the IY Basic parent program with guided parent-child interactions during family meals and family play time before and after each session. Parents were supported in practicing skills learned in the group during this family time in the CCA playroom. BECCRC and CCA coleaders provided coaching, guidance, and modeling of skills. In addition, observation during this time allowed for ongoing assessment of progress and needs with respect to the group. CCA staff also sponsored additional family "play dates" in their playroom both during and after completion of the IY group. Parents attended these "play dates" primarily to maintain the social connections formed in the group, but the guidance and support provided by trained case managers and staff provided booster IY training.

In CCA, already established home visits also provided opportunities to reinforce parents' learning of the IY program content. CCA caseworkers' involvement in the IY groups prepared them to help families integrate IY content to meet their specific family needs and values. They worked intensively with families between sessions to individualize learning and generalize skills, and then shared with the group examples of each family's successes observed during home visits. By bridging home and IY group experiences in this way, CCA caseworkers provided further reinforcement for participation and built parents' sense of self-efficacy and confidence. Following parents' completion of the group, ongoing CCA home visits served as booster training to support continued learning and practice.

Indeed, successful IY program delivery relied heavily on caseworkers' trusting relationships with families; caseworkers became the linchpin to ongoing attendance and engagement. The core CCA components of family-driven case management and regular home visits further supported IY delivery by addressing factors that may undermine attendance and the likelihood that parents would engage in learning and adapt new strategies. For example, they worked with families on problem solving and prioritizing to avoid allowing other obligations and crises that inevitably emerge during groups to impede attendance and engagement.

Augmenting incredible years series with early childhood mental health consultation

BECCRC provided early childhood consultation on a variety of levels to address issues that emerged with children and families, staff needs, and programmatic or systems concerns as related to delivery of evidence-based programs. We describe these consultation services and illustrate how embedding IY within a continuum of mental health consultation supports positive outcomes for families and sustainable agency practice.

Enhancing IY delivery: mental health consultation with families The following three vignettes illustrate how mental health consultation augmented implementation of the IY program in CCA to meet individual family needs.

Example 1 Mother 1 was a teenage mother with a significant trauma history who had been living in foster care for much of her life; she was participating in IY as one of many requirements imposed by Child Protective Services to help her regain custody of her own son, who was also living in foster care. She requested private consultation with the IY leader following the first session to discuss additional steps she might take to increase the likelihood of reunification. Mother 1 also expressed concern about her visits with her son; a lack of consistent, predictable visits in a setting conducive to positive, developmentally appropriate interactions could undermine her efforts to build their relationship and inhibit her ability to practice what she was learning in the IY program. The consultant leading her IY parent group advocated for Mother 1 and her son to have regular, weekly visits in the safety of the CCA playroom during which the consultant provided parent-child dyadic coaching. The focus of their work was relationship building: helping Mother 1 read her son's cues and develop positive attributions regarding his behaviors in order that she provide nurturing, responsive care. The consultant guided Mother 1's practice of IY skills and helped her understand her son's developmental needs and make sense of his behaviors within the context of attachment disruptions. The consultant also helped Mother 1 learn coping strategies and positive self-talk to remain calm in response to her son's distress. Facilitating intensive dyadic treatment in the context of the IY group was critical for helping this young mother adopt effective skills and reestablish a healthy relationship with her son.

Example 2 During the course of an IY group, it became clear that a number of family context issues were interfering with Mother 2's ability to make progress toward her explicit goal of reducing sibling conflict in her family. Consultation sessions were scheduled to help Mother 2, in her third trimester of pregnancy, address the significant marital conflict and stressors (ie, their impending eviction) that were undermining her efforts to address her sons' aggressive behaviors. Mother 2's partner did not support her participation in the group and was not willing to attend IY sessions. Consultation sessions helped Mother 2's partner gain trust and "buy-in" to allow her continued participation in the IY group and helped the couple establish clear communication around IY principles and problem-solving strategies to establish consistency. Additional consultation meetings involved both parents practicing IY principles with their sons and helping Mother 2 develop the confidence she needed to implement consistent, effective limit-setting strategies.

Example 3 Mother 3 shared in her IY parent program that her daughter was at risk of expulsion from preschool due to severe behavioral disruptions in the classroom, and that her own level of distress about the situation had led to a number of volatile exchanges with the teacher and school personnel. The BECCRC consultant attended meetings between Mother 3 and school personnel to improve communication and establish a constructive working relationship; Describing Mother 3's efforts in the IY group improved the view the school personnel held of this mother and increased their willingness to work together to support her daughter. School-based consultation was then provided to build consistency between the home and school environment. The consultant worked with Mother 3 and the teacher to develop a behavior plan to support progress across contexts, including educating the teacher on IY principles and strategies to facilitate a "common language" and common approach to implementing the behavior plan. Finally, the consultant attended the celebration planned by the mother at the end of the year when her daughter was named Student of the Year.

These examples illustrate how early childhood mental health consultation to community partners can augment IY delivery by helping families apply program principles to the specifics of their daily lives and their individual goals, thereby increasing its relevance for parents. By addressing non–parenting-specific parent, family, and contextual issues beyond what CCA case managers can address with families, consultation services can also address factors that otherwise risk undermining program engagement and treatment responsiveness.

Enhancing IY delivery: mental health consultation with staff Initial buy-in of agency frontline staff for IY was low, despite provision of an extensive description of the IY series and its objectives and a thorough review of its research efficacy by BECCRC consultants before adopting the program. CCA staff enthusiasm for new services was tempered by their concern regarding additional job responsibilities, distress over the amount of change introduced, and their guard for whether IY would be respectful of their families and applicable for meeting their needs. We quickly learned that garnering their full support required tangible experience; enthusiasm developed organically through their own participation in the group as coleaders and in observing firsthand the progress families were making in the context of their home visits.

"When I went for my visit this week, the television was off for the very first time! Maria was on the floor playing with her son, talking with her son. I saw him smile for the very first time that day. I have noticed since that time he has been talking a lot more; he has a lot more words now that his mom has been trying so hard. This group made a huge difference for this mother and her son."

Notably, as case managers gained an appreciation for the group through their own participation, retention rates increased. Once they saw its cultural relevance and the extent to which parents were respected and empowered, case workers were more willing to do the work required to recruit families and support their ongoing participation, and retention rates improved from 75% to as many as 90% of parents attending enough sessions to be considered "meaningful attenders" (ie, enough to be able to make measurable gains[79]). The passion for the program they then exuded had a contagion effect on the families, and this enthusiasm was critical for embedding IY programs.

Additional staff consultation focused on training caseworkers and childcare workers on IY principles and strategies to increase consistency across all service providers within CCA. Following initial training, the consultant met weekly with childcare providers to support their individual work with families. Consultants also attended regular family case-management reviews to provide reflective supervision and psychoeducation on early childhood mental health principles, thereby increasing understanding of families' mental health needs and enhancing their capacity to address concerns beyond the delivery of the parenting group (as well as understanding when best to refer a family to the mental health consultant).

Enhancing IY delivery: mental health consultation with program management A variety of constraints may lead an agency to alter a program they plan to adopt in order that the program fit within its existing service structure and available resources. For example, by shortening the length of sessions or changing the duration of the group, reorganizing the order of topics or omitting specific content, or omitting components such as buddy calls or mid-week phone calls. Because making such adaptations runs the risk of diluting its effects and undermining the delivery of empirically supported practice, a critical consultation component was helping CCA identify their unique needs and generating viable solutions with the least likelihood of undermining fidelity to the IY curriculum. However, some flexibility for local adaptation and choice is also important to "make it their own" and ensure a good fit with their agency culture and therapeutic style.[80] At the inception of our partnership, a Collaborative Working Group (CWG) was formed of key agency leaders representing agency, staff, and parent perspectives and the BECCRC consultant. The CWG met to establish coordinated plans for IY delivery. This included the consultant advising the careful balance between adapting IY to meet local needs and adhering to the curriculum.

Program-management consultation also was used to improve CCA organizational functioning to advance their capacity to provide evidence-based services. CCA lacked experience needed to adhere to a prescribed curriculum, and the CWG required significant support to prioritize requirements for effective delivery given competing demands on staff time and agency resources. Critical work involved revising their program mission and staff job descriptions to integrate IY delivery and supporting activities. This included evaluating the "fit" between IY and other program practices to reduce duplication of efforts. Responsibilities had to be reorganized such that new IY support activities were an integrated, rather than additional, part of their job. Carving out the time to offer the support services detailed here and finding the time for regular case-management reviews and group supervision required significant shifts in personnel responsibilities.

The BECCRC consultant also provided weekly reflective supervision to the program director to enhance her leadership abilities and help her recognize and address aspects of the organizational climate and structure that undermine successful implementation. For example, the consultant worked with the director on time-management skills to help her prioritize her own regular attendance at IY group sessions over other demands. Through reflective supervision, she became aware of her own ambivalence about implementing evidence-based practice and how her ambivalence negatively influenced staff efforts. She became aware of how staff motivation to do the work improved as her own appreciation for the process grew. She also learned to identify communication patterns and practices that led to deteriorations in staff engagement and morale. One outcome of this work was the initiation of individual supervision with staff to provide the support needed to feel comfortable with their new job responsibilities; ongoing supervision advanced her capacity to provide that support to her staff.

Conclusions
The partnership we describe has a number of important advantages to combat the challenges agencies face in adopting evidence-based practice. First, this arrangement profits from community expertise in engaging and supporting families and increases cost efficiency. Second, contracting with trained mental health consultants for direct delivery of the manualized curriculum allows underresourced agencies with high turnover rates, which typically employ staff who lack advanced backgrounds in mental health fields, to be able to offer high-quality, evidence-based practice. Third, provision of consultation services to support delivery can help agencies integrate program principles into all service delivery and build capacity for coordinated services. Finally, building on agency expertise and resources for providing families with ongoing support in turn builds mental health consultants' capacity to simultaneously meet the service delivery needs of multiple agencies.

The model we describe also has the potential to build capacity for delivering evidence-based practice in a variety of settings beyond the one described. For example, we are about to begin a project integrating IY parent programs into family's medical homes. Mental health consultants will provide consultation services and IY training to practitioners to integrate principles into primary care visits and will offer IY Basic and ADVANCED parenting programs on site. We also adopted a similar model for implementation in early childcare settings. Taken together, this model therefore has great potential for increasing community capacity to provide high-quality, sustainable, evidence-based PMT such as IY.

SUMMARY

PMT is the treatment of choice for families with children who have early-onset behavior problems, and programs such as IY that are delivered in group format in community settings have the potential for providing highly effective prevention and intervention services to the large number of families in need. IY is now being offered in diverse settings to further expand service capacity, including medical homes, childcare settings, schools, and social service/support agencies in addition to traditional mental health clinics. However, overcoming the barriers to reaching and serving the large number of families in need remains a formidable task. We believe that a key to successful transfer of evidence-based PMT practice into community-based PMT requires unique service delivery models and partnerships between applied delivery settings and mental health consultants that capitalize on the expertise and resources each provides.

REFERENCES

1. Nelson CA, Bosquet M. Neurobiology of fetal and infant development: implications for infant mental health. In: Zeanah CH, editor. Handbook of Infant mental health. New York: Guilford; 2000. p. 37–59.
2. Thompson RA, Easterbrooks MA, Padilla-Walker LM. Social and emotional development in infancy. In: Lerner RM, Easterbrooks MA, Mistry J, editors. Handbook of psychology: developmental psychology. Hoboken (NJ): John Wiley and Sons; 2003. p. 91–112.
3. Zeanah CH. Handbook of infant mental health. 2nd edition. New York: Guilford; 2000.
4. Egger HL, Angold A. Common emotional and behavioral disorders in preschool children: presentation, nosology, and epidemiology. J Child Psychol Psychiatry 2006;47(3–4):313–37.
5. Qi CH, Kaiser AP. Behavior problems of preschool children from low income families: review of the literature. Topics in Early Childhood Special Education 2003; 23(4):188–216.
6. Snyder H. Epidemiology of official offending. In: Loeber R, Farrington D, editors. Child delinquents: development, intervention and service needs. Thousand Oaks (CA): Sage; 2001. p. 25–46.
7. Shonkoff JP, Phillips DA. From neurons to neighborhoods: the science of early childhood development committee on integrating the science of early childhood development. Washington, DC: National Academy Press; 2000.
8. Moffitt TE. Life-course-persistent and adolescence-limited antisocial behavior: a developmental taxonomy. Psychol Rev 1993;100:674–701.
9. Shaw DS, Gilliom M, Ingoldsby EM, et al. Trajectories leading to school-age conduct problems. Dev Psychol 2003;39(2):189–200.
10. Kazdin AE. Evidence-based psychotherapies for children and adolescents. New York: Guilford Press; 2003.
11. Costello EJ, Burns BJ, Costello AJ, et al. Service utilization and psychiatric diagnosis in pediatric primary care: the role of the gatekeeper. Pediatrics 1988;82(3): 435–41.
12. Horwitz SM, Gary LC, Briggs-Gowan MJ, et al. Do needs drive services use in young children? Pediatrics 2003;112(6):1373–8.
13. Horwitz SM, Kelleher KJ, Stein REK, et al. Barriers to the identification and management of psychosocial issues in children and maternal depression. Pediatrics 2007;119(1):208–18.
14. Loeber R, Dishion T. Early predictors of male delinquency: a review. Psychol Bull 1983;94(1):68–99.
15. Aguilar B, Sroufe LA, Egeland B, et al. Distinguishing the early-onset/persistent and adolescence-onset antisocial behavior types: from birth to 16 years. Dev Psychopathol 2000;12:109–32.
16. Campbell SB, Shaw DS, Gilliom M. Early externalizing behavior problems: toddlers and preschoolers at risk for later maladjustment. Dev Psychopathol 2000;12:467–88.

17. Shaw DS, Bell RQ, Gilliom M. A truly early starter model of antisocial behavior revisited. Clin Child Fam Psychol Rev 2000;3:155–72.
18. Planos R, Zayas LH, Busch-Rossnagel NA. Mental health factors and teaching behavior among low-income Hispanic mothers. Fam Soc 1997;78(1):4–12.
19. Sameroff AJ, Seifer R, Bartko WT, et al. Environmental perspectives on adaptation during childhood and adolescence. New York. In: Luthar SS, Burack JA, Cicchetti D, editors. Developmental psychopathology: perspectives on adjustment, risk, and disorder. Cambridge [England]: Cambridge University Press; 1997. p. 507–26.
20. Shaw DS, Gross H. Early childhood and the development of delinquency: what have we learned from recent longitudinal research. In: Lieberman A, editor. The yield of recent longitudinal studies of crime and delinquency. New York: Springer; 2008. p. 79–127.
21. Yoshikawa H. Prevention as cumulative protection: effects of early family support and education on chronic delinquency and its risks. Psychol Bull 1994;115: 28–54.
22. Seifer R, Dickstein S. Parental mental illness and infant development. In: Zeanah C, editor. Handbook of infant mental health. New York: Guilford; 2000. p. 145–60.
23. Cicchetti D, Toth S. Developmental perspectives on trauma: theory, research, and intervention. Rochester (NY): University of Rochester Press; 1997.
24. Kaufman J, Henrich C. Exposure to violence and early childhood trauma. In: Zeanah CH, editor. Handbook of infant mental health. New York: The Guilford Press; 2002. p. 195–207.
25. Patterson GR, Reid JB, Dishion TJ. Antisocial boys. Eugene (OR): Castalia; 1992.
26. Mrazek PJ, Haggerty RJ. Reducing Risks for Mental Disorders: Frontiers for Preventive Intervention Research. Washington, DC: National Academy Press; 1994.
27. Webster-Stratton C, Taylor T. Nipping early risk factors in the bud: preventing substance abuse, delinquency, and violence in adolescence through interventions targeted at young children (0–8 years). Prev Sci 2001;2(3): 165–92.
28. Prinz RJ, Miller GE. Family-based treatment for childhood antisocial behavior: experimental influences on dropout and engagement. J Consult Clin Psychol 1994;62(3):645–50.
29. Kazdin AE. Parent management training: treatment for oppositional, aggressive, and antisocial behavior in children and adolescents. New York: Oxford University Press; 2005.
30. Taylor TK, Biglan A. Behavioral family interventions for improving child-rearing: a review of the literature for clinicians and policy makers. Clin Child Fam Psychol Rev 1998;1(1):41–60.
31. Eyberg SM, Funderburk BW, Hembree-Kigin TL, et al. Parent-Child Interaction Therapy with behavior problem children: one and two year maintenance of treatment effects in the family. Child Fam Behav Ther 2001;23:1–20.
32. Sanders MR. The Triple P-Positive Parenting Program: towards an empirically validated multilevel parenting and family support strategy for the prevention of behavior and emotional problems in children. Clin Child Fam Psychol Rev 1999;2:71–90.
33. Baydar N, Reid JM, Webster-Stratton C. The role of mental health factors and program engagement in the effectiveness of a preventive parenting program for Head Start mothers. Child Dev 2003;74(5):1433–53.

34. Cunningham CE, Bremner R, Boyle M. Large group community-based parenting programs for families of preschoolers at risk for disruptive behavior disorders: utilization, cost effectiveness, and outcome. J Child Psychol Psychiatry 1995; 36:1141–59.

35. Webster-Stratton C. The Incredible years training series. OJJDP Juvenile Justice Bulletin 2000;1–23.

36. Brestan EV, Eyberg SM. Effective psychosocial treatments of conduct-disordered children and adolescents: 29 years, 82 studies, and 5272 kids. J Clin Child Psychol 1998;27:180–9.

37. Webster-Stratton C. Incredible years parents and children series: basic preschool/early childhood program curriculum. Seattle (WA): Carolyn Webster-Stratton; 2008.

38. Webster-Stratton C. Basic preschool home visiting-coaches and parents manual. Seattle (WA): Carolyn Webster-Stratton; 2008.

39. Webster-Stratton C. Incredible years parents and children series: baby and toddlers program curriculum. Seattle (WA): Carolyn Webster-Stratton; 2008.

40. Webster-Stratton C, Hancock L. Training for parents of young children with conduct problems: content, methods, and therapeutic processes. In: Schaefer CE, Briesmeister JM, editors. Handbook of parent training. New York: John Wiley & Sons; 1998. p. 98–152.

41. Gross D, Fogg L, Webster-Stratton C, et al. Parent training of toddlers in day care in low-income urban communities. J Consult Clin Psychol 2003;71:261–78.

42. Webster-Stratton C, Hammond M. Treating children with early-onset conduct problems: a comparison of child and parent training interventions. J Consult Clin Psychol 1997;65(1):93–109.

43. Webster-Stratton C, Reid J, Hammond M. Preventing conduct problems, promoting social competence: a parent and teacher training partnership in head start. J Clin Child Psychol 2001;30(3):283–302.

44. Webster-Stratton C, Reid J, Hammond M. Treating children with early-onset conduct problems: intervention outcomes for parent, child, and teacher training. J Clin Child Adolesc Psychol 2004;33(1):105–24.

45. Hartman RR, Stage SA, Webster-Stratton C. A growth curve analysis of parent training outcomes: examining the influence of child risk factors (inattention, impulsivity, and hyperactivity problems), parental and family risk factors. J Clin Child Psychol 2003;44(3):388–98.

46. Taylor TK, Schmidt F, Pepler D, et al. A comparison of eclectic treatment with Webster-Stratton's Parents and Children Series in a children's mental health center: a randomized controlled trial. Behav Ther 1998;29(2):221–40.

47. Webster-Stratton C. A randomized trial of two parent-training programs for families with conduct-disordered children. J Consult Clin Psychol 1984;52(4):666–78.

48. Brotman LM, Gouley KK, Huang K, et al. Preventive intervention for preschoolers at high risk for antisocial behavior: long term effects on child physical aggression and parenting practices. J Clin Child Adolesc Psychol 2008;37(2):386–96.

49. Gardner F, Burton J, Klimes I. Randomised controlled trial of a parenting intervention in the voluntary sector for reducing child conduct problems: outcomes and mechanisms of change. J Child Psychol Psychiatry 2006;47(11):1123–32.

50. Scott S, Quentin S, Doolan M, et al. Multicentre controlled trial of parenting groups for childhood antisocial behavior in clinical practice. BMJ 2001;323:1–6.

51. Brotman LM, Gouley KK, Huang K, et al. Effects of a psychosocial family-based preventive intervention on cortisol response to a social challenge in preschoolers at high risk for antisocial behavior. Arch Gen Psychiatry 2007;64:1172–9.

52. Brotman LM, Dawson-McClure S, Gouley KK, et al. Older siblings benefit from a family-based preventive intervention for preschoolers at risk for conduct problems. J Fam Psychol 2005;19(4):581–91.
53. Hurlburt MS, Nguyen K, Reid J, et al. Efficacy of the Incredible Years group parent program with families in Head Start with a child maltreatment history. Child Abuse Negl, in press.
54. Reid JM, Webster-Stratton C, Hammond M. Follow-up of children who received the Incredible Years intervention for oppositional defiant disorder: maintenance and prediction of 2-year outcome. Behav Ther 2003;34:471–91.
55. Nock MK, Ferriter C. Parent management of attendance and adherence in child and adolescent therapy: a conceptual and empirical review. Clin Child Fam Psychol Rev 2005;8(2):149–66.
56. Linares LO, Montalto D, Li M, et al. A promising parenting intervention in foster care. J Consult Clin Psychol 2006;74(1):32–41.
57. Webster-Stratton C, Herman KC. Incredible Years early intervention programs: integrating services across school, home, and community settings. Psychology in the Schools, In press.
58. Gross D. What motivates participation and dropout among low-income urban families of color in a prevention intervention? Fam Relat 2001;50(3):246–54.
59. Staudt MM. Helping children access and use services: a review. J Child Fam Stud 2003;12(1):49–60.
60. McKay MM, Stoewe J, McCadam K, et al. Increasing access to child mental health services for urban children and their caregivers. Health Soc Work 1998; 23(1):9–15.
61. Nock MK, Kazdin AE. Randomized trial of a brief intervention for increasing participation in parent management training. J Consult Clin Psychol 2005;73: 872–9.
62. Kazdin AE, Holland L, Crowley M. Family experiences of barriers to treatment and premature termination from child therapy. J Consult Clin Psychol 1997;65: 453–63.
63. Webster-Stratton C. Advancing videotape parent training: a comparison study. J Consult Clin Psychol 1994;62(3):583–93.
64. Webster-Stratton C, Kolpacoff M, Hollinsworth T. Self-administered videotape therapy for families with conduct-problem children: comparison with two cost-effective treatments and a control group. J Consult Clin Psychol 1988;56(4): 558–66.
65. Webster-Stratton C. Enhancing the effectiveness of self-administered videotape parent training for families with conduct-problem children. J Abnorm Child Psychol 2000;18(5):479–92.
66. Webster-Stratton C. Individually administered videotape parent training program: who benefits? Cognit Ther Res 1992;16(1):31–5.
67. Morawska A, Sanders MR. Self-administered behavioral family intervention for parents of toddlers: effectiveness and dissemination. Behav Res Ther 2006;44: 1839–48.
68. Sanders M, Calam R, Durand M, et al. Does self directed and web-based support for parents enhance the effects of viewing a reality television series based on the Triple P-Positive Parenting Programme? J Child Psychol Psychiatry 2008;49(9): 924–32.
69. Taylor TK, Webster-Stratton C, Feil EG, et al. Computer-based intervention with coaching: an example using the incredible years program. Cogn Behav Ther 2008;37(4):233–46.

70. Spoth RL, Kavanagh K, Dishion TJ. Family-centered preventive intervention science: toward benefits to larger populations of children, youth, and families. Prev Sci 2002;3:145–52.

71. Lavigne JV, LeBailly SA, Gouze KR, et al. Treating oppositional defiant disorder in primary care: a comparison of three models. J Pediatr Psychol 2008;33(5): 449–61.

72. Sheldrick RC, McMenamy J, Kavanaugh K, et al. A preventive intervention for ADHD in pediatric settings. Paper presented at: Annual Convention of the Pediatric Academic Societies; May 14–17, 2005; Washington, DC.

73. Shaw DS, Dishion TJ, Supplee L, et al. Randomized trial of a family-centered approach to the prevention of early conduct problems: 2-year effects of the Family Check-Up in early childhood. J Consult Clin Psychol 2006;74(1):1–9.

74. Bauer NS, Sullivan P. Parenting prescriptions: an educational outpatient behavior pediatrics initiative. Paper presented at: Society for Developmental and Behavioral Pediatrics Educational Workshop; September 29, 2007; Providence, RI.

75. Saul J, Wandersman A, Flaspohler P, et al. Research and action for bridging science and practice in prevention. Am J Community Psychol 2008;41(3–4): 165–70.

76. Webster-Stratton C, Taylor TK. Adopting and implementing empirically supported interventions: a recipe for success. In: Buchanan A, Hudson BL, editors. Parenting, schooling and children's behavior: interdisciplinary approaches. Hampshire [England]: Ashgate Publishing; 1998. p. 1–24.

77. Early childhood mental health consultation. In: Cohen E, Kaufmann RK, editors. Promotion of mental health: prevention of mental and behavioral disorders. Rockville (MD): Center for Mental Health Services, Substance Abuse and Mental Health Services Administration; 2005. p. 3–20.

78. Gilliam WS, Shahar G. Prekindergarten expulsion and suspension: rates and predictors in one state. Infants Young Child 2006;19:228–45.

79. Reid MJ, Webster-Stratton C, Baydar N. Halting the development of conduct problems in head start: the effects of parent training. J Clin Child Adolesc Psychol 2004;33(2):279–91.

80. Schmidt F, Taylor TK. Putting empirically supported treatments into practice: lessons learned in a children's mental health center. Prof Psychol Res Pr 2002; 33(5):483–9.

Giving Voice to the Unsayable: Repairing the Effects of Trauma in Infancy and Early Childhood

Alicia F. Lieberman, PhD[a],*, Patricia Van Horn, PhD, JD[b]

KEYWORDS

- Infancy and early childhood trauma
- Child-parent psychotherapy • Traumatic stress
- Intergenerational transmission • Evidence-based treatment

The impact of traumatic events on infants, toddlers, and preschoolers is a well-documented phenomenon, which, in spite of its gravity, has failed to galvanize the actions demanded by the scope of the problem, either in terms of clinical attention or in the form of broad and sustained public policy initiatives. In spite of pervasive evidence to the contrary, there is a widespread misconception among mental health professionals and the public at large that young children are immune to trauma, because they are too cognitively immature to understand, remember, and be affected in other than transitory ways by acts of violence, accidents, intrusive medical procedures, witnessing accidental injury or death, and other traumatic events. The research on early trauma establishes conclusively that, although there are marked individual differences in how children in the first 5 years of life respond to and recover from trauma, they consistently show negative biologic, emotional, social, and cognitive sequelae after enduring traumatic events (see[1] for a review). This evidence lends particular urgency to the development, evaluation, and implementation of approaches to prevention and treatment, which are both empirically supported and can be effectively adapted to

Support: The writing of this manuscript was made possible by the generous support of the SAMHSA National Child Traumatic Stress Network and the Irving B. Harris Foundation.

[a] Irving B. Harris Endowed Chair in Infant Mental Health, Department of Psychiatry, University of California San Francisco, 305 Cape Court, Mill Valley, CA 94941, USA

[b] Associate Professor, Department of Psychiatry, University of California San Francisco, Child Trauma Research Program, San Francisco General Hospital, 1001 Potrero Avenue, Suite 2100, San Francisco, CA 94110, USA

* Corresponding author. Department of Psychiatry, University of California San Francisco, Child Trauma Research Program, San Francisco General Hospital, 1001 Potrero Avenue, Suite 2100, San Francisco, CA 94110.

E-mail address: alicia.lieberman@ucsf.edu (A.F. Lieberman).

Child Adolesc Psychiatric Clin N Am 18 (2009) 707–720
doi:10.1016/j.chc.2009.02.007
1056-4993/09/$ – see front matter

mental health community programs and other service systems that serve traumatized children and their families. This article describes the clinical applications and community dissemination of child-parent psychotherapy (CPP), a relationship-based trauma treatment for young children and their families, which has substantial empiric evidence of efficacy in decreasing symptoms of traumatic stress and restoring young children's normative developmental trajectories (see Lieberman and colleagues[2] for a review).

EARLY EXPOSURE TO TRAUMATIC EVENTS: A CONTEXTUAL FRAME FOR INTERVENTION

The statistics about the prevalence of traumatic events in early childhood are staggering, yet mental health professionals do not, as a rule, receive training in age-appropriate assessment and treatment for children in the birth–5 years age range. There is a profound gap between the prevalence of early trauma and the recognition of this phenomenon in the field of mental health. Among abused children, 40% are younger than 6 years of age.[3] Children in the first year of life account for 44% of abuse-related fatalities, and 78% of the fatalities are children younger than 3 years of age.[4,5] Children younger than 5 years of age are at greater risk of hospitalization and death than older children as the result of drowning, burns, falls, chocking, and poisoning.[6] The immediate postpartum period is particularly vulnerable: one-third of maltreated infants younger than 1 year are injured in the first week of life.[7] Contextual violence is also prevalent in young children's environments. Children younger than 5 years of age are disproportionately represented in homes with domestic violence, and exposure to domestic violence in the first 6 months of life is a significant predictor of child neglect through 5 years of age.[8,9] Some subgroups are at greater risk than others as a result of the cumulative effect of numerous risk factors.[10] A nationally representative sample of children aged 2 to 9 years showed that those at highest risk for victimization were in families exposed to multiple stresses, including single-parent and step-parent households as well as ethnic minority and low-income groups.[11]

These figures provide a frame for designing assessment and treatment models, because exposure to traumatic events has grave mental health repercussions for infants and young children. Clinicians must be prepared to ask specific questions about trauma exposure to provide appropriate intervention. For example, in a pediatric sample of 305 children aged 2 to 5 years, 42% of the 2-year-olds and 52.5% of the entire sample had experienced at least one severe traumatic stressor, and there was a strong association between the number of traumatic events and the likelihood of an emotional or behavioral disorder according to the Diagnostic and Statistical Manual of Mental Disorders, fourth edition (DSM-IV), which was documented in 17.4% of the children.[12]

The importance of adopting diagnostic criteria specifically geared to the developmental characteristics of infants and toddlers is highlighted by findings that using the standard DSM-IV criteria yielded a posttraumatic stress disorder (PTSD) diagnosis in only 13% of severely traumatized infants and toddlers, whereas using developmentally appropriate alternative criteria led to the diagnosis of PTSD in 69% of the sample.[13] Using the same alternative criteria with preschoolers referred to treatment as the result of exposure to domestic violence and physical maltreatment, Lieberman and colleagues[14] found that the diagnosis was met by 45% of the sample. It is important of point out, however, that children exposed to traumatic stressors may be in need of treatment even in the absence of a formal diagnosis, because the psychological impact of traumatic events often derails the child's normative acquisition of developmental capacities, with long-term consequences for emotional, social, and cognitive competence.[15,16]

Assessment and treatment of traumatic stress in young children must be geared to identifying and addressing environmental risk factors. It is now widely accepted that child development is best understood using an ecological-transactional model that encompasses the biologic characteristics of the child in the context of family, community, and cultural protective and risk factors.[17,18] For children exposed to chronic sources of adversity and cumulative traumatic stressors, the combined effect of multiple risk factors and scarcity of protective resources has far-ranging effects on mental health and overall functioning.[16,19] Contextual factors were identified in the DSM-IV field trials as having a major effect on the extent of psychological damage. Primary predictors of the child's functioning are the child's age at first traumatization, the frequency of traumatic experiences, and the extent to which caregivers were implicated in the traumatic event.[20] The parents' psychological status and responsiveness to the child significantly influence the child's functioning and ability to recover from the impact of traumatic events.[17,21–23] Unless clinicians are alert to these findings, they might focus narrowly on the traumatized child's symptoms and miss the ecological context that triggers and sustains these symptoms. These findings highlight both the need for prompt clinical attention to early trauma and the importance of incorporating the child's primary caregivers into the treatment.

IDENTIFYING TRAUMATIC STRESS IN INFANCY AND EARLY CHILDHOOD

Assessment and treatment must also attend to how the child's developmental capacities influence her response to trauma.[16,24] The expression of traumatic stress in infants, toddlers, and preschoolers is shaped by the rapid pace of development in the first 5 years of life, including the acquisition and consolidation of patterns of attachment, affect regulation, discrete emotions, independent locomotion, and language. Students of trauma going back to Freud[25] pointed out that early trauma involves a shattering of the young child's "protective shield" represented by the parents' care and nurturance. The young child's developmentally appropriate expectation that the parent will be available as an effective protector is violated by the experience of trauma, with possible long-term ramifications for the capacity to place trust in intimate relationships. Fraiberg[26] observed that preverbal infants use fighting, freezing, and avoidance to defend against the overwhelming emotions elicited by perceived danger. Toddlers in the second year of life may also show aggression against the parents as perceived aggressors or failed protectors. They may also turn aggression against the self in an effort to deflect their anger away from the all-important attachment figure who failed to protect them, as shown for example in biting or hitting themselves, banging their head, pulling their hair, holding their breath, and engaging in reckless and self-endangering behavior. These behaviors can be misinterpreted as expressions of the child's constitutional regulatory problems in the absence of a clinical lens that incorporates systematic assessment for the possibility of trauma.

Careful clinical observations of very young children have not yet yielded a widely accepted diagnostic classification relevant to them. In planning assessment and treatment, clinicians should be aware of the finding that the DSM-IV category of PTSD resulted in a high number of false negatives when applied to young children.[13] In an effort to develop a more useful diagnostic instrument for infancy and early childhood, the DC: 0-3 classification[27] maintained the three PTSD symptom clusters defined in the DSM IV (reexperiencing, withdrawal, and hyperarousal) but made the category more relevant to the first 5 years of life by adopting the following changes: (1) calling the condition traumatic stress disorder to highlight the role of ongoing traumatic events in the child's life, such as recurrent physical abuse, sexual abuse, and domestic violence; (2) including threat to the *psychological* (not only physical) integrity of the child or others in the definition of a traumatic event; (3) giving specific examples of age-appropriate behavior, such as posttraumatic play, loss of previously acquired developmental skills, play constriction, and sleeping problems; (4) adding a fourth cluster comprising symptoms not present before the traumatic event, such as new fears, somatic symptoms, separation anxiety, aggression, or sexualized behavior; and (5) requiring that the child display only one symptom in each of the symptom clusters. In its recent revision, DC: 0-3R[28] adopted the DSM-IV nomenclature of PTSD to make the diagnostic language consistent across the age spectrum and opted to categorize new symptoms as an associated feature of the disorder rather than as a fourth cluster. Although DC: 0-3R offers clinicians the best available instrument for diagnosis in infancy and early childhood, the diagnostic criteria will undoubtedly continue to change as new research data emerge. An example is the current interest in developmental trauma disorder as a distinct diagnostic category to conceptualize the pervasive disorganization of core competencies that characterizes the psychiatric effects of chronic, cumulative trauma.

THE RELATIONAL IMPACT OF TRAUMATIC STRESS

Traumatic events occurring in infancy and early childhood tend to affect every member of the family regardless of the nature of the event. Accidents such as car collisions, dog bites, falls, burns, and near-drownings occur frequently in the first years of life and may leave both the child and the parents with enduring fears and anticipatory anxiety. Adult caregivers may blame themselves or each other for their failure to protect the child. These emotions may trigger a cascade of changes in the parent-child relationship, with mutually reinforcing negative feelings and difficulty repairing lapses in empathy.

Most children and parents recover from these challenges and use the experience to become more consciously alert to realistic danger. For those who are unable to do so, the traumatic event can mark a turning point for the worse in their ability to trust themselves and each other. The security of attachment may be affected in the aftermath of trauma, particularly when there is chronic exposure to danger. From this perspective, patterns of disorganized attachment may be an overlooked expression of the child's traumatic stress response, which denotes fear of the parent as the source of maltreatment or uncertainty about the parent's capacity to protect from danger.[29] For example, when there is family violence, there is a significant relationship between the child's traumatic experiences and the mother's symptoms of PTSD.[30] This finding complements the findings by Scheeringa and Zeanah[31] that young children show higher symptoms of PTSD when they witness their mother being the victim of domestic violence than when the child himself or herself was the victim of abuse. Taken together, these two sets of findings suggest that the mother and the young child are each deeply traumatized by the trauma of the other. This relational impact of child trauma is the foundation for focusing on the child-parent relationship as the most expedient vehicle toward the child's recovery. For traumatized young children, a simultaneous clinical focus on attachment issues and on traumatic responses holds the greatest promise for improvement.

CPP AS A RELATIONSHIP-BASED APPROACH TO EARLY TRAUMA TREATMENT

CPP is based on the premise that the most effective and long-lasting means of supporting and restoring the mental health of traumatized young children is to enable the child and the parents to accomplish the following goals:

(1) Create a common language to describe what happened; (2) regulate the overwhelming affects associated with the experience; (3) enhance the parents' capacity

to respond in developmentally appropriate ways to the child's basic needs for protection, nurturance, and socialization; and (4) restore trust in the parent's ability to protect the child from external and internal danger.[32]

Clinical focus on the parent-child relationship as the quintessential mutative factor in treatment for infants and toddlers dates back to the pioneering work of Fraiberg,[33] whose careful clinical studies illustrated the intergenerational transmission of psychopathology when the baby becomes the representative of figures from the parent's past who were associated with now unrecognized fear, anger, and unfulfilled longings. Fraiberg created a treatment approach called *infant-parent psychotherapy* to guide parents of children aged birth–3 years to the early sources of their conflicted feelings toward the child, and she stated that as a result of this process, the "baby is liberated, as it were, from the distortions and displaced affects which have engulfed him in the parental neurosis."[33] Intimate relationships are particularly colored by the metaphorical "angels in the nursery" of having felt unconditionally loved and protected while growing up[34] and the "ghosts in the nursery" of early experiences of loneliness, rejection, and terror.[35,36] The past lives on in a multiplicity of guises, including perceptions of the present and expectations of the future that carry the imprint of what was already experienced in the formative stages of one's life.

The concept of the baby as a transference object who evokes unresolved parental conflicts is also a core element of trauma-focused CPP. Parental negative attributions to the child are often the manifestation of a process of projective identification in which the child becomes the recipient of unconscious wishes, fears, and fantasies that were rooted in early traumatic experiences but that the parents cannot acknowledge as a part of their own self. These unconscious processes lead the parent to become selectively attuned to child behaviors that can be interpreted as confirming the parent's attributions. The meanings that the parent attributes to the child become the substrate for childrearing attitudes and behaviors that bring pressure on the child to align his or her behavior in conformity to the parent's attributions.[35] Harsh physical maltreatment and abuse can result when the parent's negative perceptions are enacted in outbursts of rage, which may be justified by the parent as efforts to discipline the child.

Clinical Example

A child-mother dyad was referred for treatment after the childcare provider found bruises on the 15 month-old's bottom. The child protection worker who investigated the possibility of abuse described the child as "out of control," "impossible to stop," and "recklessly throwing himself on the floor and running off" when frustrated. She made a referral for treatment after accepting the mother's explanation that he was bruised when he fell while trying to climb on the dining room table to reach his bottle. During the initial assessment, the mother described her 15-month-old son as "diabolical," "impossible to control," "reckless," and "suicidal." As she spoke, the child hit the cat and tried to climb on the windowsill of the family's fourth-floor apartment. The mother did nothing to stop the child's behavior but pointed to it as an example of the accuracy of her perceptions. As treatment unfolded, this mother described horrific episodes of maltreatment by her psychotic mother as she was growing up. In her mind, her son had become the representative both of her "diabolical" mother and of the repressed self-destructive aspects of herself that were shaped by her mother's abuse. The son, in turn, dutifully enacted his mother's expectations in an effort to please his mother by becoming the uncontrollable, aggressive, suicidal child that she was pressuring him to be.

During a session 1 month into the treatment, the clinician asked the mother whether she ever found herself doing to her son the same things that her mother had done to her. The mother at first denied this possibility. The clinician gently persisted, explaining that her query was prompted by the intense frustration that the mother often showed in her interactions with the child. Very slowly and hesitantly, the mother disclosed that she sometimes lost control of herself and could not stop hitting the child, although she always managed to hit him over his clothes in order not to leave marks. The bruises that prompted the referral to Child Protective Services occurred when the child was in the bathtub and started splashing water on the mother's new cashmere sweater. The mother had interpreted this behavior as a purposeful effort to ruin her beautiful new garment and was flooded by a feeling that she was trapped in a relationship with this "monster" who gave her "no peace." As she spoke, the mother started crying, and the clinician asked her what the tears meant. The mother said, "I want to be a good mother. I don't want to be a monster like my mother." The equation linking her own mother, herself, and her child to the identity of the "monster" became clear and would become a key motif in the treatment that ensued. While the mother described this event, her son stood at a distance, looking at her with wide eyes and a sober expression. The clinician said to the mother, "He is listening very seriously. What you are saying is very important to him." There was a silence. The clinician turned to the child and said, "Your mommy is telling me that she hit you. That is very scary." The child nodded solemnly, staying firmly in his place. The clinician added, "Your mommy doesn't want to scare you. She is sorry that she hurt you." The child stood still. Turning to the mother, the clinician said, "Can you tell him that yourself?." In a shaky voice, the mother told the child that she was sorry that she hit him and would not do that again. It was notable that the mother and child continued to keep their distance from each other. The promise of safety was too incipient to be trusted–either by the mother or by the child.

Child trauma at the hands of the parent, as in this case, often emerges only after careful observation of the child-parent interactions and exploration of the parent's attributions to the child. One of the consequences of uncovering child abuse is that the clinician is legally mandated to make a referral to Child Protective Services. The clinician explained this obligation to the mother, who became both angry at the clinician and terrified that the child would be placed in foster care. The clinician told the mother that, although she could not predict what measures the agency would take, she would recommend against foster care placement, because the mother had voluntarily disclosed that she hit the child and was participating in treatment. The clinician also suggested that the mother herself make the call to Child Protective Services in the clinician's presence and coached the mother in what to say. This approach had a productive outcome. The mother felt some sense of control by making the call herself. The child protective worker accepted the clinician's recommendation against foster care and instead maintained the case open under a "family preservation" category that would enable the worker to visit the family monthly and monitor for abuse during a period of at least 6 months. Although the mother expressed anger at the clinician for making the referral, she also acknowledged that she felt as if a burden had been taken off her shoulders as a result of not having to keep secret this deeply shameful part of herself.

In the treatment of this mother-son dyad, the clinician made extensive use of clinical strategies that linked the mother's relentlessly punitive and derogatory treatment of her child in the present with her own past as a terrified young girl who both internalized a profound sense of inner badness and was enraged by her mother's abuse. Her son's defiance triggered within her psyche memories of her early helplessness and provoked aggression as a desperate effort at self-protection. The child had become, in the mother's mind, a new version of this persecutory figure that continued to hound her and would give her no peace.

Simultaneous attention to the influence of the past and the immediate demands of the present is one of the hallmarks of psychoanalytic relationship-based interventions as developed by Fraiberg and colleagues.[33,36,37,39] Insight-oriented interventions need to be supplemented with unstructured developmental guidance when the parent lacks age-appropriate childrearing information. The clinician helped the mother to understand the developmental meaning of her son's moment-to-moment behavior by explaining the normative motivations and anxieties of the first 2 years of life and helping her to learn protective responses to the child's aggression and self-injurious behavior. The core mutative factor, however, is seen as enabling the parents to correct their distorted perceptions of the child and to redirect the associated negative affects to their legitimate original recipients in the parents' childhood. In this sense, psychoanalytically oriented CPP is emblematic of Faulkner's dictum that "the past is never dead. It's not even past."[38]

Therapeutic focus on how the parent's past affects the child's trauma experience is most feasible during the child's preverbal period, when language, independent locomotion, and self-assertion are still incipient and the parents and clinician are not distracted by the verbal and mobile child's motivation for individual attention and active participation.[34,40] When the child has acquired language and symbolic skills, trauma treatment must incorporate the creation of a shared trauma narrative between child and parent, as described below.

CREATING A SHARED TRAUMA NARRATIVE BETWEEN CHILD AND PARENT

Present trauma and the child's age are two factors that call for significant clinical modifications that extend beyond attention to the parental reenactment with the child of experiences and conflicts from the past. When the child is the victim of traumatic events in the present, the claims of the parents' past must give space to accommodate the urgent demands of the present circumstances. This is particularly important after the first year of life, when toddlers and preschoolers can participate actively in the treatment by verbalizing and playing out their emotional distress. At present, CPP is an umbrella term that encompasses the age ranges covered by the terms *infant-parent psychotherapy*,[37,38] *toddler-parent psychotherapy*,[40–43] and *preschooler-parent psychotherapy*.[44] Trauma treatment for older toddlers and preschoolers involves a major clinical challenge, because the therapist must attend simultaneously to the child's individual experience of the trauma, to the parents' individual experiences and how their past is connected to the child's trauma, and to parental responses to the child that may alleviate or exacerbate the child's traumatic response.

As a general rule, trauma-focused CPP with verbal children shifts clinical priorities away from linking the parent's past with the child's present experience of trauma and becomes more focused on giving the child a safe emotional space to name and process the traumatic experience. The clinician attends to the moment-to-moment interactions between parent and child to address the specific emotional meanings that parent and child have for each other around issues of trust and protection from danger.

As is the case with preverbal young children, therapeutic sessions are jointly attended by the parent and the child. When more than one parent needs clinical attention and is willing to participate in treatment, the format is expanded to include the child and both parents. Similarly, when siblings are close in age and have clinical needs that can be addressed simultaneously, two or more children may attend sessions jointly. Treatment traditionally involves weekly 1-hour sessions lasting approximately 1 year, but these parameters can vary depending on clinical needs and program resources. Treatment can be conducted in the home, office, or community settings convenient for the family, such as childcare center or family resource center. Individual sessions with the parent are introduced when attention to the parent's individual experience is necessary to promote improvement in the child. Individual sessions for parent and/or child may also be used as adjuncts or substitutes to the joint child-parent sessions when the joint sessions are not conducive to improvement in the child's mental health or the parent's capacity to provide appropriate caregiving.[33]

The urge to avoid thinking, feeling, and speaking about the trauma compounds the clinical challenge of treating traumatized young children who are capable of verbalizing the traumatic event or enacting it in play. When the parent gives the child the implicit or explicit message that the traumatic event must remain a secret—not only to outsiders but also within the family and within the self—the trauma as an *unsayable* event puts the child in the untenable position of "knowing what you are not supposed to know and feeling what you are not supposed to feel."[45] CPP has the goal of making the trauma *knowable* and *sayable* as a shared child-parent experience in which the parent becomes capable of acknowledging the reality of the events and the legitimacy of the child's resulting terror, anger, and broken trust. The emotional connection made possible by this recognition enables the clinical process to place the trauma in perspective and to move on to build protection, nurturance, and pleasure in everyday life. The clinician acts as an emotional translator between child and parent, communicating to the parent the developmental or symbolic meaning of the child's behavior and trying to establish bridges between the often discordant developmental agendas and affective needs of traumatized children and their parents.[33] Treatment manuals are used to organize and clarify the premises of intervention and provide clinical examples for the use of specific therapeutic modalities.[46,47]

Treatment begins with an initial assessment that may comprise four or five sessions and includes individual sessions with the parent(s) to learn about the nature of the traumatic event(s), the family circumstances, the psychological functioning of the parents, and the child's functioning before the traumatic events and in their aftermath. It is very useful to administer a trauma-screening inventory, because parents tend to consciously or unconsciously omit or minimize the traumatic experiences endured by the child. The sessions with the parent also provide an opportunity to plan how the parent will explain to the child the reasons for the treatment. In this process, the clinician models for the parent a way of talking about the trauma directly but tactfully, using words that the child can understand. The child usually joins the assessment process in the third session. When there is reason for concern about the child's cognitive functioning, a structured cognitive assessment is conducted. Alternatively, the session involves unstructured play with a combination of toys that are evocative of the specific traumatic event (eg, ambulance, police car, doctor's kit, a family of dolls matching the family's composition and ethnicity), wild and farm animals, and toys associated with nurturing (eg, kitchen set). Early in the session, the clinician asks the child whether the parent explained the reason for the session and corroborates the parent's explanation. For example, the clinician might say, "Your mom told me that you got very scared when you saw your dad hitting her, and now you are sad and angry because he does not live with you any more." This description of the traumatic circumstances is followed by an explanation that the mother is bringing the child to treatment as a way of helping with the feelings and behaviors that are troubling the child. From the beginning, the clinician normalizes the negative feelings created by the traumatic events and instills hope that the child and the parent will together find ways to feel better.

CPP intervention modalities include the following: (1) using play, physical contact, and language to help regulate the expression of affects associated with stress and trauma and promote developmental progress; (2) unstructured, reflective developmental guidance; (3) modeling protective behavior; (4) insight-oriented interpretation; (5) addressing traumatic reminders; (6) retrieving and creating benevolent memories; (7) emotional support; and (8) attention to reality through crisis intervention, case management, and concrete assistance. Through the use of these modalities, the therapist cultivates during the sessions an emotional climate in which frightening memories can be retrieved safely and painful affect can be tolerated, because there is understanding and support.

Clinical Example

A father and his 4-year-old daughter were referred for treatment by Family Court after the child witnessed the father hitting his wife, who was also the child's stepmother. The child had become sad and withdrawn, started wetting the bed at night, and woke up crying several times every night. The preschool teacher reported that she seemed preoccupied and listless and had started calling her peers by abusive names. The father had acknowledged the incident, which he justified as the result of excessive drinking. He agreed to the Court's stipulation that he participate in treatment for alcohol abuse, anger management, and CPP. During the initial assessment, the father and clinician planned how he would explain to the child the reason for the treatment. The father spontaneously came up with the idea that he would tell the child that he had made a bad mistake when he hit his wife, that he was drinking too much, and that he was trying hard to learn not to hit, because he wanted everybody in the family to be safe.

In the initial session following the assessment, the father started out by saying that they had had a very nice week and everything was going fine. The clinician turned to the child and said, "Daddy told me the other day that a lot of things happened in your family." The child nodded and said, "Daddy went to jail on Saturday." Surprised, the clinician asked, "How come?" The child answered, "He was beating up my brother." (This brother was the 14-year-old son of the stepmother). The clinician responded, "That is very scary!" The child nodded in agreement and added, "I was scared. My stomach hurt. And daddy was mean because my cousin was crying and daddy yelled at him and told him he was a crybaby." The clinician looked questioningly at the father, who turned to the child and said, "I am sorry I did that." The clinician asked what happened. There was a silence, which was interrupted by the child saying, "Daddy was drinking." The clinician replied, "It sounds like daddy becomes mean when he drinks. How do you feel when that happens?" The child answered, "I feel sad." The therapist answered, "Yes, I can understand that. It is sad that you have to worry so much because daddy drinks and gets angry. It makes you cry even at night when you are sleeping." The father told the child, "I am very sorry I made you sad. Your brother and I were texting each other and I apologized to him. I am sorry I was mean. Will you accept my apology?" The child nodded and asked to play with the jail toys. She found a doll to represent the father and set up the jail while the father spoke to the therapist, giving her the business card for the social worker who had been assigned to the case. He then turned to the child and said, "The social worker told me that drinking is a sickness. I have to get well, and I am going to a class to help me get better." The child nodded and started playing with the jail. She took the father doll, put its arms behind its back, and said, "This is what the policeman did to daddy." The father took the doll and put it in the jail cell, saying, "And then this is what happened. They put me in a little room like this and I stayed there all night." The therapist asked, "How were you feeling then?" The father looked at the child and said, "I was thinking that I really missed my kids. I missed your brother, I missed you, and I missed mommy." The child said, "Daddy told the policemen that they smelled like pigs." The therapist asked the child if she knew what that meant. The child answered, "No, but I don't think that it's very nice." The father looked sheepish. The child added, "And then daddy got in trouble at church. He grabbed the pastor's shirt." The father explained that he had gotten angry when the pastor told him not to drink and grabbed his shirt; the pastor asked him to leave and not come back until he could talk without becoming aggressive. The therapist asked what happened then. The father said that his wife and the children were very upset about what happened in church, and he had called the pastor and apologized. Turning to the child, the therapist said, "It sounds like everyone gets sad and upset when daddy drinks and gets mean. What can we do to get rid of mean daddy?" The child said, "No, we can't get rid of daddy." The therapist answered, "No, we won't get rid of the nice daddy. That is the daddy who is sitting here. But there is also a mean daddy who scares you and makes everybody sad." The child answered, "There is only one daddy." The therapist, realizing that the child was right, answered, "Yes, you are right. There is only one daddy. He sometimes is nice and sometimes is mean." The child nodded. The father looked very embarrassed. The therapist added, "It sounds like daddy gets very mean and scary when he drinks." The child nodded. She then asked to play with the play dough, and father and child spent the rest of the session making play dough figures that represented the family members. At the end of the session, the therapist said, "You talked about really important things today." The father said, "I have a lot of homework to do." The clinician agreed and turned to the child saying, "Your dad is telling us that he really heard what you were saying." The child gave a little smile and took the father's hand as they left the room.

This session illustrates the extraordinary ability of young children to describe in detail frightening events when they are given permission to do so. One strength of this father was his ability to listen to his child and to show remorse, although he was somewhat facile in his contrition. The session also illustrates a potential pitfall of treatment when the therapist wants to offer simplistic solutions, as when she talked about "getting rid" of the "mean daddy." The child's refusal to go along with this untenable plan led the therapist to a more accurate (if sadder) acknowledgment that the same father held two mutually incompatible facets and needed to be accountable for the frighteningly aggressive parts of himself. This initial session laid the foundation for a clear-eyed focus on the challenges that he faced in living up to the promise of recovery that he made to his daughter.

EMPIRICAL EVIDENCE OF EFFICACY

CPP efficacy has been documented in five separate randomized, control trials with high-risk infants, toddlers, and preschoolers. The samples include anxiously attached toddlers of newly immigrated Latina mothers with histories of exposure to violence,[48] toddlers of middle-class depressed mothers,[42] maltreated infants in the child welfare system,[49] maltreated preschoolers in the child welfare system,[44] and preschoolers who witnessed domestic violence against the mother in addition to other violence-related traumatic stressors.[14] Outcome findings include reductions in child and maternal psychiatric symptoms; more positive child attributions of parents, themselves, and relationships; improvement in quality of child-mother relationship and measures of security of attachment; and improvements in child cognitive functioning. CPP is currently under review by the Substance Abuse and Mental Health Services Administration for inclusion in the National Registry of Evidence-based Practices.

SUMMARY

The treatment of traumatic stress in infants and young children calls for careful evaluation of the individual manifestations of the child's traumatic response and the family and environmental factors involved. Acknowledging the concrete reality and emotional sequelae of the trauma is the primary building block of treatment. The capacity of children and parents to tolerate talking and playing about the trauma varies widely. Some children are confidently ready to speak about what happened; others take a long time to do so. Similarly, parents vary widely in their ability to open themselves to their child's emotional experience. Although clinical timing and tone are always important in therapeutic interventions, therapists working with traumatized young children should cultivate a readiness to speak about the trauma using manageable words that address the concrete characteristics of the traumatic event in ways that the child can understand. The therapist's courage in giving voice to previously unspeakable experiences enables the child and the parent to give themselves and each other permission to know what must be known and to feel what is legitimate to feel.

REFERENCES

1. Van Horn P, Lieberman AF. Psychological impact and treatment of children exposed to domestic violence. In: Jenny C, editor. Medical evidence in child maltreatment. New York: Elsevier; 2009.
2. Lieberman AF, Ghosh Ippen C, Marans S. Psychodynamic treatment of child trauma. In: Foa EB, Matthews Friedman JA, Cohen A, et al, editors. Effective treatments for PTSD: practice guidelines from the international society for traumatic stress studies. 2nd edition. New York: Guilford Press; 2008. p. 370–87.
3. Administration for Children and Families, U.S. Department of Health and Human Services. Child maltreatment 2004. Available at: http://www.acf.hhs.gov/programs/cb/pubs/cm04/chapterthree.htm#ten. Accessed January 28, 2009.
4. National Clearinghouse on Child Abuse Neglect Information. Child abuse and neglect fatalities: statistics and interventions, 2006. Available at: http://www.childwelfare.gov/pubs/factsheets/fatality.cfm. Accessed January 15, 2009.
5. Administration for Childen and Families, U.S. Department of Health and Human Services. Child welfare information gateway, child abuse and neglect fatalities: statistics and interventions. Available at: http://www.childwelfare.gov/pubs/factsheets/fatality.cfm. Accessed January 28, 2009.
6. Grossman DC. The history of injury control and the epidemiology of child and adolescent injuries. In: Behrman RE, editor. The future of children. Los Altos, CA: David and Lucile Packard Foundation; 2000. p. 4–22.
7. Centers for Disease Control and Prevention. Nonfatal maltreatment of infants – United States, October 2005–September 2006. Morb Mortal Wkly Rep 2008;57:336–9.
8. Fantuzzo JW, Fusco RA. Children's direct exposure to types of domestic violence crime: a population-based investigation. J Fam Viol 2007;22:543–52.
9. McGuigan WM, Pratt CL. The predictive impact of domestic violence on three types of child maltreatment. Child Abuse Negl 2001;25:869–83.
10. Sameroff AJ, Fiese BH. Transactional regulation: the developmental ecology of early intervention. In: Shonkoff JP, Meisels SJ, editors. Handbook of early childhood intervention. 2nd edition. New York: Cambridge University Press; 2000. p. 135–59.

11. Turner HA, Finkelhor D, Ormond R. The effect of lifetime victimization on the mental health of children and adolescents. Soc Sci Med 2006;62:13–27.
12. Egger H, Angold A. Stressful life events and PTSD in preschool children. Paper presented at: Annual Meeting of the American Academy of Child and Adolescent Psychiatry; 2004; Washington DC.
13. Scheeringa MS, Zeanah CH, Drell MJ, et al. Two approaches to the diagnosis of posttraumatic stress disorder in infancy and early childhood. J Am Acad Child Adolesc Psychiatry 1995;34:191–200.
14. Lieberman AF, Van Horn P, Ghosh Ippen C. Towards evidence-based treatment: Child-parent psychotherapy with preschoolers exposed to marital violence. J Am Acad Child Adolesc Psychiatry 2005;44:1241–8.
15. Carrion VG, Weems CF, Reiss AL. Stress predicts brain changes in children: A pilot longitudinal study on youth stress, PTSD, and the hippocampus. Pediatrics 2007;119:509–16.
16. Pynoos RS, Steinberg AM, Piacentini JC. A developmental psychopathology model of childhood traumatic stress and intersection with anxiety disorders. Biol Psychiatry 1999;46:1542–54.
17. Cicchetti D, Lynch A. Toward an ecological/transactional model of community violence and child maltreatment: consequences for children's development. Psychiatry 1993;56:96–118.
18. Sameroff AJ. Models of development and developmental risk. In: Zeanah CH Jr, editor. Handbook of infant mental health. New York: Guilford Press; 1995. p. 659–95.
19. Rutter M. Poverty and child mental health: Natural experiments and social causation. JAMA 2003;290(15):2063–4.
20. van Der Kolk B, Pelcovitz D, Rosh S, et al. Dissociation, somatization, and affect dysregulation: The complexity of adaptation to trauma. Am J Psychiatry 1996; 153:83–93.
21. Laor N, Wolmer L, Cohen D. Mothers' functioning and children's symptoms 5 years after a SCUD missile attack. Am J Psychiatry 2001;58:1020–6.
22. Linares LO, Heeren T, Bronfman E, et al. A mediational model for the impact of exposure to community violence on early child behavior problems. Child Dev 2001;72:639–52.
23. Schechter DS, Coates SW, Kaminer T, et al. Distorted maternal mental representations and atypical behavior in a clinical sample of violence-exposed mothers and their toddlers. J Trauma Dissociation 2008;9(2):123–47.
24. Marans S, Adelman A. Experiencing violence in a developmental context. In: Osofsky JD, editor. Children in a violent society. New York: Guilford Press; 1997. p. 202–22.
25. Freud S. Inhibitions, symptoms and anxiety. In: Strachey J, editor. and trans. The standard edition of the complete psychological works of Sigmund Freud. Vol. 4. London: Hogarth Press; 1926;1959:87–156.
26. Fraiberg S. Pathological defenses in infancy. Psychoanal Q 1982;5:612–34.
27. Zero To Three/National Center for Clinical Infant Programs. Diagnostic classification 0-3: diagnostic classification of mental health and developmental disorders of infancy and early childhood. Arlington, VA: Zero to Three/National Center for Clinical Infant Programs; 1994.
28. Zero To Three/National Center for Clinical Infant Programs. Diagnostic classification 0-3: diagnostic classification of mental health and developmental disorders of infancy and early childhood. Rev. ed. Washington, DC: Zero to Three Press; 2005.

29. Lieberman AF, Amaya-Jackson L. Reciprocal influences of attachment and trauma: using a dual lens in the assessment and treatment of infants, toddlers, and preschoolers. In: Berlin LJ, Ziv Y, Amaya-Jackson L, editors. Enhancing early attachments: theory, research, intervention, and policy. New York: Guilford Press; 2005. p. 100–24.

30. Schechter DS, Zygmunt A, Coates SW, et al. Caregiver traumatization adversely impacts young children's mental representations on the MacArthur Story-Stem Battery. Attch Hum Dev 2005;9(3):187–205.

31. Scheeringa MS, Zeanah C. Symptom expression and trauma variables in children under 48 months of age. Infant Ment Health J 1995;16:259–70.

32. Lieberman AF, Van Horn P. Psychotherapy with infants and young children: re-pairing the effects of stress and trauma on early attachment. New York: Guilford Press; 2008.

33. Fraiberg SH. Clinical studies in infant mental health: the first year of life. New York: Basic Books; 1980.

34. Fraiberg S, Adelson E, Shapiro V. Ghosts in the nursery. A psychoanalytic approach to the problems of impaired infant-mother relationships. J Am Acad Child Psychiatry 1975;14(3):387–421.

35. Lieberman AF. Negative maternal attributions: effects on toddlers' sense of self. Psychoanalytic Inquiry 1999;19(5):737–56.

36. Lieberman AF, Silverman R, Pawl JH. Infant-parent psychotherapy: core concepts and current approaches. In: Zeanah ZH Jr, editor. Handbook of infant mental health. 2nd edition. New York: Guilford Press; 2000. p. 472–84.

37. Lieberman AF, Padrón E, Van Horn P, et al. Angels in the nursery: The intergen-erational transmission of benevolent parental influences. Infant Ment Health J 2005;26:211–38.

38. Faulkner W. Requiem for a nun. New York: Random House; 1951.

39. Lieberman AF. Infant-parent psychotherapy with toddlers. Dev Psychopathol 1992;4:559–75.

40. Cicchetti D, Rogosch FA, Toth SL. The efficacy of toddler-parent psychotherapy for fostering cognitive development in offspring of depressed mothers. J Abnorm Child Psychol 2000;28:135–48.

41. Cicchetti D, Toth SL, Rogosch FA. The efficacy of toddler-parent psychotherapy to increase attachment security in offspring of depressed mothers. Attach Hum Dev 1999;1:34–66.

42. Toth SL, Rogosch FA, Manly JT, et al. The efficacy of toddler-parent psycho-therapy to reorganize attachment in the young offspring of mothers with major depressive disorder: A randomized preventive trial. J Consult Clin Psychol 2006;74(6):1006–16.

43. Toth SL, Maughan A, Manly JT, et al. The relative efficacy of two interventions in altering maltreated preschool children's representational models: Implications for attachment theory. Dev Psychopathol 2002;14(4):877–908.

44. Bowlby J. A secure base: parent-child attachment and healthy human develop-ment. New York: Basic Books Inc; 1988.

45. Lieberman AF, Compton N, Van Horn P, et al. Losing a parent to death: guidelines for the treatment of traumatic bereavement in infancy and early childhood. Washington, DC: Zero to Three Press; 2002.

46. Lieberman AF, Van Horn P. Don't hit my mommy! A manual for child-parent psychotherapy with young witnesses of family violence. Washington, DC: Zero to Three Press; 2005.

47. Lieberman AF, Weston D, Pawl JH. Preventive intervention and outcome with anxiously attached dyads. Child Dev 1991;62:199–209.
48. Cicchetti D, Rogosch FA, Toth SL. Fostering secure attachment in infants in maltreating families through preventive interventions. Dev Psychopathol 2006;18(3): 623–49.
49. Lieberman AF, Ghosh Ippen C, Van Horn P. Child-parent psychotherapy: six month follow-up of a randomized control trial. J Am Acad Child Adolesc Psychiatry 2006;45:913–8.

A New Model of Foster Care for Young Children: The Bucharest Early Intervention Project

Anna T. Smyke, PhD[a],*, Charles H. Zeanah, Jr, MD[a],
Nathan A. Fox, PhD[b], Charles A. Nelson III, PhD[c]

KEYWORDS

- Psychosocial intervention • Institutions • Foster care
- Attachment • Infants and toddlers

The Bucharest Early Intervention Project (BEIP) is a randomized, controlled trial of foster care as an intervention for infants and toddlers following institutionalization.[1,2] The feasibility phase of the study, conducted in Bucharest, Romania, began in November 2000, and the study itself began in April 2001. The participants in this unique study were 208 young Romanian children who were assessed at baseline and then at regular intervals during the next 3 years.[1] Of this group, 136 institutionalized children were randomized into conditions of either care as usual (CAU) (ie, institutional care), or transfer into Romanian foster families. Comparison children, recruited from local health centers, had never been institutionalized and lived with their families in Bucharest. On average, children were 21 months old when the study began (range, 5–30 months). The institutionalized children had spent well over half their lives in institutional care.

BEIP personnel were Romanian psychologists and social workers who were recruited in Bucharest. The project manager was a Romanian-born American citizen

The Bucharest Early Intervention Project (BEIP) was funded by the John D. and Catherine T. MacArthur Foundation Research Network on Early Experience and Brain Development (Charles A. Nelson, Network Chair).

[a] Department of Psychiatry and Neurology, Tulane University School of Medicine, 1440 Canal Street (TB-52), New Orleans, LA 70112, USA
[b] Department of Human Development, University of Maryland College Park, MD 20742, USA
[c] Boston Children's Hospital and Harvard Medical School, Harvard Medical School/Children's Hospital Boston, DMC Lab of Cognitive Neuroscience, 1 Autumn Street, Mailbox #713, Office AU621, Boston, MA 02115, USA
* Corresponding author. Department of Psychiatry and Neurology, Tulane University School of Medicine, 1440 Canal Street (TB-52), New Orleans, LA 70112.
E-mail address: asmyke@tulane.edu (A. T. Smyke).

Child Adolesc Psychiatric Clin N Am 18 (2009) 721–734
doi:10.1016/j.chc.2009.03.003
1056-4993/09/$ – see front matter © 2009 Elsevier Inc. All rights reserved.

who was particularly adept at understanding and addressing the cross-cultural issues that were inevitable with such an effort. For a complete description of the study design and the sample, see Zeanah and colleagues, 2003.[1]

The essential question that the project is designed to address is whether a quality foster care program can enhance the development of children who have been abandoned and placed in institutions in early life. The design of the study also allowed us to examine moderators of intervention effects, including timing of placement, gender, and caregiving quality. The comparison group of never-institutionalized Romanian community children allowed the assessment of the degree of recovery of children in foster care.

The purpose of this article is to describe details of the foster care intervention, which we designed to be informed by the latest thinking in infant mental health regarding early intervention. Because of space limitations, we refer the interested reader to other sources in which we have considered the many ethical issues involved in the project in detail.[3,4] Here, we describe the process and content of the intervention before briefly reviewing the results of the project. We conclude with some of the remaining challenges of child protection for abandoned and maltreated infants and toddlers.

THE BUCHAREST EARLY INTERVENTION PROJECT FOSTER CARE NETWORK

We sought to establish child-centered foster care, a model in which foster parents became fully invested in and psychologically committed to the children in their care, loving them as their own. To describe how we implemented this intended model, we begin by describing the context of foster care when we began the project.

Context of Foster Care in Bucharest

Creating a foster care network for BEIP was challenging because of the particulars of the Romanian context at the time the project began. Institutional care, which had been the chief form of care for orphaned and abandoned children for more than 200 years in Romania, became even more widespread during the Communist era there from 1945 to 1989. Following the revolution of 1989, it became clear that tens of thousands of young children were living in institutions, most in appalling conditions. Adoption of thousands of these children into North American and Western European families was common for about 12 years. Foster care was implemented on a small scale by international adoption agencies who placed some young children in foster homes for a few months before they were adopted out of the country. They had used the French model, in which a designated foster parent was paid a salary and benefits for the job of being a foster parent, in contrast to the US system in which generally modest board payments follow the child in care wherever they are placed.

The international adoption process in Romania was widely perceived to be corrupt, and in response to pressure from the European Union, international adoption was ended by the government in April 2001. The international adoption agencies that had previously supported some modest foster care networks in Bucharest had no money to maintain them, and they were eliminated.

We also encountered widespread suspicions about foster care, because it had such a limited tradition in Romania. We heard rumors that foster care was a front for plans to sell children for their organs or for pedophilia. Some government officials believed that institutional settings were more likely to provide children with professional caregiving, including the structure and activities they require to develop optimally.

The Bucharest Early Intervention Project Social Work Team

We believed that the key to success of the foster care intervention was the social work staff who would implement and maintain it. Therefore, hiring social workers who were enthusiastic, eager to learn, and able to innovate was essential.

A major challenge was that the tradition of social work in Romania was limited at the time the project began. During the communist era, there were no social workers, meaning that there were neither traditions nor senior mentors for the new social work graduates who had begun to practice in the decade following the revolution. We hired three recently graduated social workers who had had no previous experience with institutionalized children or foster care. On the other hand, they embodied the characteristics we sought, and they approached the task enthusiastically.

We trained these social workers extensively in basic principles of infant mental health, including building attachment relationships, understanding children's postinstitutional adjustment, and managing common behavior problems. The guiding principle was to develop open relationships with foster parents based on trust and on respect for their important work.

We recognized that the challenges for foster parents of caring for postinstitutionalized infants and toddlers were considerable. The BEIP foster care network would require extensive support, both for the foster parents working directly with the children and the social workers working with the foster parents. Each of the social workers was responsible for a third of the study participants in foster care and their foster parents. They visited with each foster family on a weekly basis and after a year reduced these visits to three per month. Frequent phone contact was maintained with each family throughout the project.

Following in-person training at the outset of the project, experienced US clinicians provided weekly video consultation with the social work team throughout the life of the project.

Foster Parent Recruitment and Training

We recruited foster parents for the BEIP in much the same way that they are recruited in the United States, with newspaper advertisement, posted flyers, and radio interviews of BEIP project personnel. Background checks of foster parents were conducted to verify education, employment, and absence of criminal histories once parents had expressed an interest in the project.

The initial foster parent training was subcontracted to an NGO experienced in providing foster parent training in Romania. This NGO used manuals of foster care that had been developed in the United States and then modified for and by Romanians who had been involved in the international adoption agencies using foster care.

BEIP social workers also organized groups for prospective foster parents, helping them to obtain their licenses. These early efforts helped the social workers to gain a better understanding of the foster parents and to anticipate appropriate matches between foster child and foster parent. We sought foster parents who seemed to understand young children and who seemed to possess the requisite emotional availability for the intensive work of caring for a postinstitutionalized infant or toddler. Demographic characteristics of the 56 foster parents in the BEIP network were similar to those of foster parents in the United States They averaged 46 years of age and most had a gymnasium (34.5%) or high school (52.7%) education. Some had previous experience caring for young children as they transitioned from institutions to international adoption (27%) but most had never fostered before (73%). Most foster mothers were married (54.5%), and the remainder were single (7.3%), divorced (18.2%), or widowed (20%). On average, there were 2.5 other persons in the foster household.

BEIP social workers next attempted to match the children who were randomized to foster care to specific foster parents. The US consultants held frequent discussions with the social workers regarding the needs and problems of young, postinstitutionalized children. This allowed the social workers to orient foster parents to the process of the children's transition from institutional care to family care, using attachment theory and research as the foundation for the work.

Social workers had foster parents spend time with the child with whom they were matched in the institutional setting before the child was placed in their home. The goals were, first, to begin the establishment of a relationship between the foster child and the foster parent and, second, to give the foster parents some appreciation of the child's institutional experience.

As the project continued, BEIP social workers also provided counseling, support, and parenting to biological parents who contacted Child Protection authorities to recover their children. Initially, during the consent process for the project, Romanian Child Protection officials had asked the BEIP social workers to obtain consent from as many biological parents as they could locate for their children to be placed in foster care. The social workers worked hard to locate parents by going to old addresses and asking neighbors and relatives where parents might be. In some cases, parents had not known where their children were located once they entered the Child Protection system, and they were relieved to receive information about them. Some of these parents eventually came forward and sought to be reunited with their children. They were assisted in the establishment of a relationship with their children in several cases in which Child Protection officials decided that reunification was appropriate.

Challenges of Caring for Young, Postinstitutionalized Children

Although most children navigated transitions from institutional care to family care successfully, there were challenges requiring special support. A number of children displayed 1 or more problems, including regulatory problems (eg, sleep, eating, and toileting), developmental problems (eg, cognitive, speech and language delays, and gross motor delays), social interaction problems (eg, extreme withdrawal, indiscriminate behavior, and aggression), as well as problems with agitation and stereotypies. One of the most ubiquitous early challenges for foster parents was the children's "loudness." This was a real problem for many foster parents living in large apartment buildings separated from neighbors by thin walls.

Our approaches to these issues were based on our experiences in a program for maltreated infants and toddlers in foster care in the southern United States.[5] Consultants from the United States visited quarterly and accompanied the social workers on home visits to talk with foster parents. For example, the social workers were working with a quiet, seemingly depressed foster mother who had received a loud, agitated, $2\frac{1}{2}$ -year-old boy from the institution into her home. Her husband and her son liked the child but were irritated by the child's agitation and his inability to sleep at night. The foster mother was desperately worried about her neighbors' reaction to the child's loud screaming. The team had made serious efforts to make good matches between foster children and foster mothers. However, they reported during weekly supervision that the foster mother had decided that the job was too difficult and she did not want the child to remain in her home. This prompted intensified visits from the BEIP social worker.

The social worker had phoned and visited the foster mother many times, and the foster mother, resistant to openly discussing the problems that the child was having and the effect on her family, initially had reported no problems before requesting the child's removal 3 weeks later. The request coincided with the visit of the US consultant, so a visit to the foster mother's home was arranged. We spoke with the foster mother, interpreting back and forth between English and Romanian, and she talked about her many concerns about the young child. She told the social workers and the consultant that her young foster son had ceased to use the toilet, had very delayed language, and showed many stereotypies.

As we talked back and forth, we stressed that it was the child's experience of institutional living that was directly responsible for the behavior that he displayed. This was important, because we wanted to stress that the child was reacting to his experience and was not a "bad child." We also noted an important point: the first 6 weeks of a placement are often the most challenging. In our experience, if a family weathered the first 6 to 8 weeks, the relationship generally becomes more satisfying for both foster parent and child. In addition, we pointed out a number of behaviors that we observed in the home that clearly indicated that the boy was becoming attached to his foster mother. Finally, knowing that there was "nothing to lose" we detailed the profound impact on the child that would come if he were moved from her home. It had taken a great deal for him to learn to trust his foster mother, and we explained forthrightly how difficult it would be for this young toddler to be sent away.

The foster mother related that her family was due to go on vacation and said that they would take the young boy with them, think carefully about what the social workers and the consultant had suggested, and then make a final decision about his placement with them after they returned. The child and his foster parents seemed to relax and to get to know each other better during their time on vacation. In the carefree environment of the sunny beach, the boy recovered his ability to use the toilet. His sleep problems disappeared, and his stereotypies decreased significantly. As the family returned from vacation, their foster son was calmer, more comfortable, and potty trained. He had begun to thrive as he learned to trust his foster mother who had chosen to keep the youngster with her. The family kept the young boy for another 2 ½ years, and eventually, they helped to facilitate his transition back to his biological family. The foster mother later reported that she occasionally visits the little boy who was part of their family for more than 2 years.

Toilet training was also a concern for many of the foster parents, particularly as the children grew older. Children in the institution had been potty trained by placing them simultaneously as a group on plastic potties placed on the floor at the designated "potty time," sometimes for more than an hour, until they "produced." BEIP social workers provided each foster family with a potty seat, but parents were stunned by the absolute refusal of the young children to even sit on the seats. The consultants, based on experiences with children in foster care in the United States, encouraged them to wait at least 6 months after the children had been in the home before attempting toilet training. Of course, many children were willing to resume use of the potty after a shorter period of time, but this plan removed pressure from the foster parents to train the children.

Similarly, during observations of young children in institutions, we had noted that bath time was rarely a time of positive interaction between caregiver and child. Young children seemed terrified of their baths, looking on in grim, fearful anticipation as they watched their unit mates screaming during the bath, knowing that their turn would soon come. Soon after placement, foster parents remarked on the children's abject fear of the bath. With encouragement and a "normalization" of this behavior, foster parents developed a variety of ways in which to make bath time more enjoyable.

As the foster children grew older, it was evident that some of them would benefit from a preschool program. Several of the foster children reacted strongly and in a dysregulated manner to visiting hospitals and clinics, presumably from prior experiences. However, one of the most appropriate preschool programs was located on the grounds of a local hospital. After discussing this dilemma with the consultants, the social workers negotiated with the director of the program to do preliminary home visits, getting to know each child before he came into the preschool. The director was open to working with the children to get them acclimated to the preschool, and the children were able to have a gradual transition into a program that allowed them peer interaction as well as access to special education.

The social workers noted that some foster parents called them very frequently to discuss the adjustment of their young children, whereas other foster parents rarely had any concerns. They noticed as well that although most foster parents had developmental expectations that were appropriate for their foster children, some foster parents expected way too much of their young foster children, and some foster parents placed no demands on their children at all, vastly underestimating the child's abilities. Some foster parents expressed ongoing sadness about children that they had fostered before they were employed in our foster care network. The consultant and the social workers felt that foster parents might feel supported if they met together.

From these concerns, we created what we believe to be the first foster parent support group in Romania. It became clear that issues of loss were prevalent for many of the foster mothers and several of them cried openly in the group. The foster mothers seemed to benefit from talking to one another about their experiences and provided support to one another. Notably, this occurred despite the fact that the foster parents had concerns about sharing private feelings with others. During the Ceaucescu regime, the secret police had actively encouraged people to inform on one another. As a result, no one had felt safe, as even family members had been known to inform on one another. At the support group, the foster parents seemed to appreciate very much the opportunity to discuss their hopes and concerns. This theme of reluctance to share feelings and concern about what might happen as a result was one of the major ones that had to be addressed in our Romanian-American collaboration. The establishment of the foster parent support groups and the foster parent training groups, conducted by the BEIP social workers, helped foster parents to see that the difficulties that they were experiencing were far from unusual and provided them with concrete suggestions regarding methods with which to manage their young foster child's behavior.

Support to Social Workers

Supervision as a professional process was virtually unknown in Romania when we first began our collaboration. The social workers and research assistants had experienced "administrative" supervision in previous settings. For example, they might be questioned regarding the number of children they had placed or quizzed about the amount of paperwork they had prepared. Having a "boss" rather than a "consultant" meant that the focus was on administrative issues rather than on discussion of psychological issues for parents and young children.

The consultation model that we introduced was one of reflective/supportive supervision.[6] We hoped to support our Bucharest team in their very stressful work. The US consultants spent time getting to know the BEIP social workers during the early phases of the study, and we began weekly group supervision.[7] Initially, our hourlong sessions were conducted via telephone and included both the social workers and the research assistants. There was a great desire on their part to learn as much as they could about the various theoretical foundations of the work we were doing. Questions regarding administration of the study measures were soon supplanted by questions regarding the adjustment of infants and toddlers to family life and the reaction of foster mothers to their new charges.

Several key elements were introduced to the team in Romania. First, we wanted them to recognize that there was an art to talking to foster parents if one wanted to gain a clear understanding of how a foster child is doing. Our experience in the United States had shown us that many foster parents had difficulty telling us when problems had developed. General questions about how things are going were usually met with the response that everything was fine. We knew that it was essential to ask specific questions regarding eating, sleeping, toileting, and other areas to learn about the child's actual behavior in the home.[8] In our experience, foster parents are rarely comfortable reporting problems, because they do not want to seem as if they are not successful at their jobs. Persistence and nonjudgmental interest was an important means to put the foster parent at ease and engage her in the task of making the young foster child's life better.

The social workers had some initial worries about the process of consultation/ supervision. They had wondered if supervision was actually ongoing evaluation. Would the consultant go straight to the boss with the information gleaned in supervision, possibly causing them to be fired? Would the consultant understand what the supervisee thought? What if we disagreed? What if the consultant did not really understand how things were in Romania? What if their English was not good enough on the phone?

There were other challenges. All of the social workers were required to be bilingual. Nevertheless, they had varying levels of comfort expressing themselves in English, especially since the topics being discussed were also new to them. Additionally, the consultants were talking to them via telephone, and the absence of visual cues made the consultation experience difficult for both parties.

These concerns diminished after we obtained a simple videoconferencing system that allowed for access to visual cues. In addition, the consultant began to learn Romanian, and the social workers became more comfortable and knowledgeable in English. These developments reduced the technical barriers to communication.

There were also psychological barriers that gradually emerged. Talking about one's feelings and reactions in front of colleagues was unfamiliar and difficult. It took time for their reservations about this to be disclosed because of their uncertainty about the process of reflective supervision. After these problems emerged gradually in the consultation sessions, the social workers later pointed out that this was likely a parallel process with their interactions with foster parents who also felt evaluated and put on the spot when asked to talk about their feelings about young foster children.

Many of the concepts discussed with the team were new to them. Initially, they found it difficult to think about implementing an idea if they had not seen it in practice. However, there were no obvious ways in which they could practice techniques other than actually trying them with the families. When the consultant asked if they thought they could implement a particular plan, a dilemma presented itself. Was the consultant literally asking if the social worker could implement the intervention, or was she giving an "order?" The consultant sensed occasional reticence but attributed this to lack of confidence rather than to confusion about whether a command had been issued. In turn, the social workers were not sure if they were allowed to disagree with the consultant, because open discussions had not been tolerated in their previous job experiences.

Building trust was a gradual process. Consultants traveled quarterly to the study site to meet with the social workers and research assistants. They worked to listen to their experiences and to understand the ways in which American approaches were foreign to them. Although many American and Romanian work sites are based on a hierarchical model of power distribution, the particular model that we were offering for team development was more egalitarian, based on a system that invited all members of the team, regardless of their educational level or experience, to share their experiences and their impressions of a given child or caregiver. The social workers were unfamiliar with such a model and took time to trust that consultants really meant what they said.

At one point, the team reported that a foster mother was having marked difficulty managing the challenging behavior of a 3-year-old foster child. The child was dysregulated at times and frequently "tested the limits" of what behavior would be tolerated. The team had talked to the foster mother about helping the child to develop more appropriate behavior. They visited her in the home and discussed several techniques with the foster mother. Team members noted on subsequent visits that the child's behavior had changed little. There were clearly barriers to implementation of the behavior plan, but they were not immediately clear. The consultant suggested that the social workers carefully begin to discuss the foster mother's own early experiences to determine if there were issues that could be identified as a barrier. The social workers were uneasy about asking the foster mother such personal questions about her early experiences. With encouragement, the social workers practiced role playing the interaction, and they agreed to try.

Later, they reported that their efforts to talk to the foster mother had been richly rewarded. She revealed that she and a sibling had been placed in an institution when she was 9 years old, because her mother could not afford to feed them. She had remained there for 2 years, and she remembered them as the worst years of her life. As she took on the care of her foster daughter, she thought painfully about how difficult the child's experiences had been. The social workers were surprised to see how much the foster mother's early experiences had affected her current behavior. The social workers talked with the foster mother about how important it was to help her foster daughter to learn how to regulate her emotions and shape her behavior so that she could engage with her peers and with other adults. The foster mother eventually mastered this idea and was proud of the progress that her foster daughter had made.

Some topics that are common in US mental health settings were almost taboo in Romania. For example, the team asked for suggestions regarding behavior management for a 42-month-old child after he had been reunited with his biological family at the direction of Child Protection officials. After his return, the child had stabbed his father in the hand with a small knife. The parents called the BEIP social worker and asked for help. The social worker was initially uncertain about what to say, and she asked for help from the consultant.

The consultant wondered immediately if domestic violence were an issue in this child's life. She told the social workers that the level of the child's aggression was quite unusual at his age and that it seemed plausible that this child had witnessed serious violence. She recommended that the social worker inquire about the possibility of domestic violence in the family. At first, the social workers discounted this possibility, but following much further discussion and review of the literature, they agreed to consider domestic violence as a possible way of understanding the boy's behavior. They approached the parents to discuss the child's aggressive behavior. The parents acknowledged that they had been fighting before the child got the knife, but they said that it was only "play fighting." The social workers used their new understanding to talk with parents regarding the effects of witnessing such "play" on a young child, particularly as he was just making the adjustment to their home. They used the literature they had reviewed to inform their discussions with the parents and felt more confidant making recommendations.

This clinical dilemma also led to a discussion among the social workers and the consultant about the experiences they had had with domestic violence involving their own relatives and friends. They indicated that the topic had been largely taboo in Romania and that they found it hard to discuss. Their experience in applying what they had learned to the family of the 3-year-old boy described here increased their comfort in considering contextual influences on the behavior of young children. Additionally, they later had a daylong group discussion about ways in which small children exhibit distress through dysregulated behavior and in their everyday tasks, such as eating, sleeping, and interaction with their family members.[9]

DISSEMINATING THE INTERVENTION WITHIN ROMANIA AND BEYOND

As the project moved toward permanency planning for each child, an agreement with the local Bucharest Child Protection agencies went into effect, and in several of the sectors, the BEIP foster parents were transferred into local government foster care. The team continued to provide some support to foster parents. The transition was difficult for the foster parents and for the social workers, as they recognized that the model that they had implemented was not always continued. As different questions arose regarding rapid changes of placement for foster children, the team reached out to the governmental social workers regarding their thoughts about the best interest of the child. They seemed somewhat disinterested in what the BEIP social workers had to say. About this time, the project organized one of several continuing education events, and one of the US consultants conducted a workshop regarding the importance of attachment in foster care, which was attended by 60 child protection personnel. It was clear from the discussion that followed the presentation that individuals working with institutionalized children often knew that a given arrangement is not in a child's best interest but that they were uncertain of viable alternatives. Broadening the perspective of a variety of professionals charged with protecting children remains a challenge.

A model for training social work students from Bucharest University by BEIP social workers was created and included a team-teaching approach. The social workers explained the developmental and behavioral interventions they performed with foster parents and children. The students alternated their weekly meetings between the BEIP social workers and the research assistants. This enabled them to learn about the effects of institutionalization on child development and to view videotapes of children's behavior in institutions and in foster homes. The social workers explained how attachment theory could be used to understand the needs of home-reared and institutionalized infants and toddlers.

PARALLEL PROCESSES

We hoped that our interactions with the BEIP team would be a positive start in a parallel process supported by supervision. As we treated the team with warmth and respect, we hoped that they would interact similarly with the foster parents with whom they worked. In turn, we hoped that foster parents, treated with respect and warmth, would bestow these same gifts on their young foster children. We approached our interactions with foster children, foster mothers, and the biological families from an attachment perspective, and it is for that reason that there was little movement from one caregiver to another. Interestingly, child protection personnel were surprised that so many of the BEIP foster parents were interested in adopting their foster children, even though it meant losing their foster care salary. They did not understand that the use of an attachment perspective in foster parenting means that the foster parents form an attachment to the young child as well as the child's attachment to the foster parent. One of the most rewarding aspects of our work on this project has been the way in which the Romanian foster care team mastered the concept of attachment and its essential application to work with young children.

Future Collaboration

BEIP social workers developed many ideas about ways in which to effectively use the knowledge that they had gained in the course of their work with the project. They talked about editing and updating the foster parent training manual in a way that emphasized the importance of attachment in our orientation to foster care. They also thought of ways to work toward actively promoting in-country adoption. Additionally, they were concerned that, although they believed institutionalized children should be reunified with their families as a general principle, this should not happen if the families were not ready to receive them. They understood the importance of working with parents to establish a consistent relationship with their young children before the child's return home.

OUTCOMES OF THE INTERVENTION

The BEIP foster care intervention was designed to change the *experience* of young children and thereby to favorably alter their developmental trajectories. For that reason, the children's development and the intervention itself were carefully assessed. Following baseline assessments, 136 institutionalized children were randomly assigned to CAU (continued institutional care) or to removal from institutions and placement with foster families. The 68 children in the foster care group (FCG), the 68 children in the CAU group, and the 72 children in the never-institutionalized community group (NIG) all were seen for follow-up assessments at 30 and 42 months, and for some measures, also at 54 months. To test the effects of the foster care intervention, we contrasted outcomes in the FCG and the CAU. To assess the degree of recovery, we contrasted the FCG with the NIG.

All assessments of effects of the intervention were assessed using intent-to-treat analyses, meaning that whatever group the child was originally assigned to (foster care or CAU), the child continued to be included in that group when evaluating outcomes. In fact, there was movement out of institutions during the course of the study, as many institutionalized children were returned to their biological families, adopted by Romanian families, or placed in government-sponsored foster care that did not exist at the time the study began. Because we used intent-to-treat analyses, the results reported are conservative estimates of intervention effects. Before turning to child outcomes, however, we first report results related to the child protection system that we created.

Child Protection Outcomes

One of the central outcomes to be considered in evaluating foster care from the perspective of child protection is that it provides quality caregiving as well as necessary safety and stability for young children who have already experienced serious adversity. Judged from these perspectives, BEIP was successful. First, we conducted formal assessments of the children's caregiving environment at baseline and again at 30 and 42 months of age using the Observational Record of the Caregiving Environment.[10,11] We demonstrated that the quality of caregiving was significantly better in foster care than that in institutions at both 30 and 42 months of age. Further, the quality of caregiving in foster care was indistinguishable from the quality of caregiving in the families of never-institutionalized children from the community. Second, during the 4 years of the initial phase of the project, there were only two foster care disruptions. The first occurred because 1 foster mother developed signs of a major mental illness and had to be hospitalized. The second was a single foster mother who died suddenly.

After the children turned 54 months of age, we arranged for the foster care network that had been supported by the project to be transferred by the local governmental sectors in Bucharest, as we had negotiated at the outset of the project. Because Romania was undergoing a transition from institutional care to foster care at that time, the local governments hired the foster parents and used governmental social workers to monitor the needs of these families. Thus, we established and supported a high-quality foster care network throughout the life of the project and then transferred it to local government support at the project's conclusion.

Child Outcomes

Developmental outcomes
Cognitive functioning was assessed with the Bayley scales at 30 and 42 months and the Wechsler Preschool and Primary Scale of Intelligence at 54 months. Developmental quotients at 30 and 42 months and intelligence quotients at 54 months were significantly higher in the FCG than those in the CAU, though they remained significantly lower than the NIG at every age assessed.[3] Interestingly, the younger the child was when placed in foster care, the more the cognitive gains. In fact, there was little intervention effect for children older than 24 months of age at the time of placement. Language results were similar.[12] Both expressive and receptive language was significantly higher in the FCG compared with the CAU at 30 and 42 months of age, but the FCG did not attain the language level of the NIG. The one exception was that children placed before 15 months of age had language skills that were indistinguishable from the NIG children.

There was also a powerful intervention effect for emotional responsiveness.[13] In tasks designed to elicit positive emotional responses in young children (puppets and peek-a-boo activities), the FCG demonstrated significantly more positive affect and attention to task than the CAU. In fact, they exhibited more positive affect than the NIG at 54 months of age.

Attachment, measured by Strange Situation classifications, indicated powerful intervention effects.[14] Significantly more FCG children (49%) had secure attachments at 42 months of age compared with those of CAU children (17.5%). Continuous ratings of security showed that all three groups were significantly different from one another, with CAU children having the lowest scores and NIG children having the highest scores. In addition, significantly fewer FCG children had disorganized, controlling, or insecure/other classifications compared with those of the CAU.

Brain functioning outcomes
Brain functioning was assessed by recordings of electroencephalograms (EEGs) and event related potentials (ERPs). The former was used to assess general brain activity and the latter to detect responses to facial expressions of emotion. EEG spectral power and coherence were not greater in the FCG than those in the CAU at 30 or 42 months, but there were correlations between length of time in care and increased

EEG power and decreased coherence for children in the FCG at 42 months. These findings indicate more electrical activity and more hemispheric differentiation for children who had been placed in foster care at younger ages. For ERPs, at three assessments (baseline, 30 months, and 42 months), institutionalized children showed markedly smaller amplitudes (ie, brain activity) and longer latencies (ie, processing speed) for the occipital components compared with noninstitutionalized children. By 42 months, ERP amplitudes and latencies of children placed in foster care were intermediate between the institutionalized and noninstitutionalized children, indicating that foster care was partially effective in ameliorating deficits caused by institutionalization. The age at which children were placed into foster care was unrelated to their ERP outcomes at 42 months. Facial emotion processing was similar in all three groups of children; specifically, fearful faces elicited larger amplitude and longer latency responses than happy faces for frontocentral components. Taken together, these results indicate that foster care was somewhat effective in restoring normal brain functioning.

Clinical outcomes
Psychiatric morbidity was assessed by structured interviews with institutional caregivers, foster parents, and biological parents. Several major areas of functioning were assessed in the clinical domain. First, there was no demonstrated benefit of foster care for reducing externalizing disorders (ie, aggressive behavior disorders, Attention-deficit/hyperactivity disorder) at 54 months of age among the children with a history of institutional rearing. In contrast, there was a significant reduction in internalizing disorders (ie, anxiety and depression) at 54 months for children in foster care compared with children in CAU. Third, there was a significant reduction in signs of the emotionally inhibited type of reactive attachment disorder for children in foster care at 30, 42, and 54 months of age. For the disinhibited type of reactive attachment disorder, the only significant difference was at 42 months, when the group in foster care had fewer signs than the group in CAU. Regarding clinical outcomes, intervention effects were evident, but they were more readily demonstrable in the emotional rather than the behavioral realms.

As Romania moves away from institutional care and into foster care, one of the challenges will be discovering ways in which to ensure the quality of foster care for infants and toddlers who cannot be cared for by their parents. We value the contributions of the BEIP social workers and study personnel to this model of child-centered foster care and look forward to learning other ways in which to ensure that foster care provides young children with the emotional and developmental support that they need. We seek to increase the recognition among Child Protection professionals that, far from being a "place to stay," foster care is actually a proactive, important intervention aimed at supporting young children in their recovery from maltreatment and abandonment.

SUMMARY

An attachment-based, child-centered approach to foster care for young, previously institutionalized children was developed in Bucharest, Romania, as part of the BEIP, a randomized, controlled trial of foster care versus CAU, including institutionalization. Regular, weekly consultation from clinicians in the United States was used to provide support to the social workers who were responsible for the day-to-day implementation of the intervention. Consultation included discussion of specific ways to manage challenging postinstitutionalized behaviors and ways in which to support foster parents so that they could scaffold infants and toddlers in the development of socioemotional, communicative, and problem-solving skills. Ways in which to understand the young child's response to traumatic events such as witnessing domestic violence were also discussed. In turn, the social workers were charged with providing support to foster parents as they assisted children in making the difficult transition to family life and came to understand their own feelings about caring for the needs of these young children. The BEIP examined outcomes for infants and toddlers in developmental areas, such as cognitive development, speech and language, behavior, and brain development. Children placed in foster care, compared with CAU, made significant gains in a variety of spheres of development. The BEIP demonstrates that a child-centered approach to foster care is not only feasible but preferred in supporting the socioemotional development of young children who have experienced deprivation during their early rearing.

ACKNOWLEDGMENT

We gratefully acknowledge the Romanian children and caregivers who have taught us so much. We are indebted to the BEIP Foster Care Team (Veronica Ivascanu, Amelia Greceanu, and Alina Mihai) for their important contributions to the BEIP and to the formulation of this article. Multumesc foarte mult!

REFERENCES

1. Zeanah CH, Nelson CA, Fox NA, et al. Designing research to study the effects of institutionalization on brain and behavioral development: the Bucharest early intervention project. Dev Psychopathol 2003;15:885–907.
2. Smyke AT, Koga SF, Johnson DE, et al. The caregiving context in institution-reared and family-reared infants and toddlers in Romania. J Child Psychol Psychiatry 2007;48:210–8.
3. Nelson CA, Zeanah CH, Fox NA, et al. Cognitive recovery in socially deprived young children: the Bucharest early intervention project. Science 2007;318: 1937–40.
4. Zeanah CH, Koga SF, Simion B, et al. Ethical considerations in international research collaboration: the Bucharest early intervention project. Infant Ment Health J 2006;27(6):559–76.
5. Larrieu JA, Zeanah CH. Treating infant-parent relationships in context of maltreatment: an integrated, systems approach. In: Sameroff A, McDonough S, Rosenblum K, editors. Treatment of infant-parent relationship disturbances. New York: Guilford; 2003. p. 243–64.
6. Gilkerson L, Irving B. Harris distinguished lecture: reflective supervision in infant-family programs: adding clinical process to nonclinical settings. Infant Ment Health J 2004;25(5):424–39.
7. Wajda-Johnston V, Smyke AT, Nagle G, et al. Using technology as a training, supervision, and consultation aid. In: Finello K, editor. The handbook of training and practice in infant and preschool mental health. San Francisco, CA: Jossey-Bass; 2005. p. 357–74.
8. Heller SS, Smyke AT, Boris NW. Very young foster children and foster families: Clinical challenges and interventions. Infant Ment Health J 2002;23(5):555–75.
9. Lieberman A, Van Horn P. Don't hit my mommy: a manual for child-parent psychotherapy with young witnesses of family violence. Washington, DC: Zero to Three; 2004.
10. NICHD Early Child Care Research Network. Characteristics of infant child care: factors contributing to positive caregiving. Early Child Res Q 1996;11:269–306.

11. Early Child Care Research Network. The effects of infant child care on infant-mother attachment security: results of the NICHD study of early child care. Child Dev 1997;68:860–79.
12. Windsor J, Benigno JP, Wing CA, et al. Language recovery in young children. Child Dev (under review).
13. Ghera MM, Marshall PJ, Fox NA, et al. Social deprivation and young institutionalized children's attention and expression of positive affect: effects of a foster care intervention. J Child Psychol Psychiatry 2009;50:246–53.
14. Smyke AT, Zeanah CH, Fox NA, et al. Placement in foster care enhances quality of attachment among young institutionalized children. Child Dev, in press.

Video Feedback in Parent-Infant Treatments

Sandra Rusconi-Serpa, FSP[a], Ana Sancho Rossignol, FSP[a],
Susan C. McDonough, PhD[b]

KEYWORDS

- Video feedback interventions • Parent-infant interactions
- Parent-infant treatments • Infant pre-attachment
- Caregiver sensitivity

Studies focusing on parent-infant interactions have developed considerably since the 1970s and have led to an understanding that disturbances in interactive behavior underlie much of infant psychopathology. This understanding has facilitated the development of interventions that focus on the quality of the infant-parent relationship using video feedback analysis of mother-infant interaction. Video feedback has been used in several therapeutic approaches with families that include young children as a way of engaging parents to focus with the clinician on interactive behavior with their child. Several studies have shown that the thoughtful use of this therapeutic tool can improve the quality of interactions in a short period of time.[1–6] Video feedback interventions that focus on attachment quality have also been shown to result in a notable increase in maternal sensitivity.[7–9]

Video feedback has been used in different therapeutic models. Several adaptations to particular settings have been developed using this therapeutic tool, albeit with different goals and targeting a large variety of outcome variables. This article describes how video feedback techniques are used in parent-infant interventions, with attention to their different treatment goals and their different ways of effecting change. Four clinical approaches representing the most important video feedback–based interventions are presented: (a) the attachment-based approach (ie, interventions that seek to enhance parental sensitivity at a behavioral level); (b) the psychoanalytically oriented approach (ie, interventions designed to develop parental reflective functioning and representations using the parents ability to observe and process nonverbal interactions); (c) the systemic approach (ie, interventions that

[a] Service of Child and Adolescent Psychiatry, Department of Child and Adolescent, University Hospitals of Geneva and University of Geneva, 41, Crêts-de-Champel, CH- 1206 Geneva, Switzerland
[b] School of Social Work, University of Michigan, 1080 S. University, Ann Arbor, MI 48109, USA
E-mail address: sandra.rusconi-serpa@hcuge.ch (S.C. McDonough).

Child Adolesc Psychiatric Clin N Am 18 (2009) 735–751
doi:10.1016/j.chc.2009.02.009
1056-4993/09/$ – see front matter © 2009 Published by Elsevier Inc.

childpsych.theclinics.com

target family relationships through behavioral interactions and bodily communication of the different family members); and (d) the transactional model (ie, interventions designed to target the social environment as the primary source of positive and negative development for the child). A clinical case illustrates the transactional model as used in the Interaction Guidance-Geneva Model.

Video feedback interventions may differ in terms of the infants' age at the start of the intervention, the number of sessions, the principal therapeutic target (ie, parent-infant behavior, parental perceptions or the quality of family alliance, quality of parents-infant communication), and their theoretical basis for psychic change (ie, parental sensitivity, maternal reflective functioning, strengthening of positive, corrective experiences, recognizing patterns of negative reciprocity, and so forth). These interventions may also vary in terms of their duration, from a 15-minute videotaped intervention providing behavioral feedback in a single session to an intensive and weekly individual meeting over several years of the child's life.

ATTACHMENT-BASED INTERVENTIONS

In the last decade, a considerable number of systematic intervention programs driven by attachment theory and research have been developed using video feedback as an important tool to increase parents' sensitivity and responsiveness to their infant's signals.[10,11] The principal goal of these programs is to develop a theory and evidence-based protocol that can be used in a partnership between professionals who are trained in scientifically based attachment procedures, and appropriately trained community-based practitioners.[7] These programs developed rapidly in the field of early intervention because there was an increasing demand by parents and professionals for interventions that are effective in shifting problematic or at-risk attachments toward more adapted developmental pathways.

One of the models developed in this approach is the Video feedback Intervention to promote Positive Parenting (VIPP).[12] This intervention is based on attachment and coercion theories and it focuses on positive parenting defined as the appropriateness of parents' responses to infant's behaviors. To prevent a further increase of externalizing problems in young children screened for externalizing behaviors, the VIPP approach was extended with a focus on parental sensitive discipline (VIPP-SD).[10] The VIPP-SD intervention aims to enhance parental sensitivity and sensitive discipline, that is, the parents' ability to take into account the child's perspective and signals, when discipline is required. This intervention emphasizes the importance of early childhood parenting as an important contributor to socialization processes in the first years of life. In this model, the therapist makes an association between early maladaptive parent-infant interaction patterns, especially inconsistent parental discipline and the failure to provide positive reinforcement for compliant and prosocial behaviors, and the emergence of externalizing problems in infants.

The VIPP-SD is a brief, focused, and standardized program in which parent and child are recorded on videotape during daily situations at home. Video feedback is provided to stimulate the parents' sensitive interactive skills, and targets parenting and information on the development of young children. This model is used by trained interveners during six 1.5-hour sessions with families at home. Each intervention session starts by recording a standardized mother-child interaction (like reading a book together) on videotape. Between home visits, the intervener selects specific video fragments and prepares comments based on the themes of each specific intervention session. The first four sessions have different themes. The first session focuses on teaching parents to recognize the differences between exploratory behavior and contact seeking (sensitivity), and on the importance of distraction and induction as noncoercive responses to conflict situations. The second session is centered on teaching parents to use positive reinforcement by praising the child for positive behavior and ignoring negative attention seeking (discipline). The third session focuses on the importance of adequate and prompt responses to the child's signals by showing interaction chains with three components: the child's signal, the mother's sensitive response, and the child's positive reaction to that response. The central theme of the fourth session is the sharing of positive and negative emotions and the promotion of empathy for the child, using consistent and adequate discipline strategies and clear limit setting (discipline). The last two sessions consolidate intervention effects by integrating all tips and feedback given in the previous sessions, in video feedback and intervention. The video feedback is adjusted to specific mother-infant dyads, depending on their particular needs and the nature of the video-taped interventions.

In studies using the VIPP approach, positive effects have been documented on parental sensitivity or attachment security in nonclinical groups, for example, in adoptive families,[11] and in at-risk and clinical groups, such as mothers with an insecure representation of attachment,[13] mothers screened for low sensitive responsiveness, and mothers with eating disorders and their infants.[14] Bakermans-Kranenburg and van Ijzendoorn[8] also investigated the differential effectiveness of VIPP-SD in changing basal cortisol secretion in infants, examining the role of the DRD4 gene. The exon III DRD4 7-repeat allele has been associated with several forms of externalizing problems across the lifespan, such as aggression and attention-deficit/hyperactivity disorder. The 7-repeat allele has been linked to lower dopamine reception efficiency; and the dopaminergic system is known to be engaged in attentional, motivational, and reward mechanisms. These investigators found that parental insensitivity was associated with externalizing behaviors in preschoolers, but only in the presence of the DRD4 7-repeat polymorphism. The increase in externalizing behaviors in children with the 7-repeat allele exposed to insensitive care compared with children without these combined risks was sixfold. The dopamine system may affect susceptibility to environmental influences, and may thus play an important role in gene-environment interactions.[9,15]

Marvin and colleagues[7] developed a group-based intervention named the Circle Of Security (COS) designed to shift patterns of attachment-caregiving interactions in high-risk toddlers to more appropriate developmental pathway. This model of intervention is based on attachment theory and on current theory and research on child development, in particular the notions of emotion regulation, interactive synchrony, states of mind regarding attachments and intimate relationships, and reflective functioning.

The core construct of this intervention embraces Ainsworth's ideas of a Secure Base and a Haven of Safety.[16] The COS investigators adapted graphic aides for the intervention, which they share with parents to illustrate both sides of this construct: the child's exploratory system and his tendency to venture away from the attachment figure to explore the world if he feels safe to do so, versus the activated child's attachment system and his need to seek proximity and protection, as well as help in organization of his feelings if feeling threatened by internal or external factors, or if feeling that he has gone beyond the safe limits of exploration. A key component of the COS is to help parents understand that smooth interactions between children and their caregivers are often disrupted and need "repair," and that this ability to repair the disruption is the essence of a secure attachment. This "repair" requires clear cues from each partner and clear understanding and responsiveness to each other's signals. The intervention uses video feedback of caregiver-children interactions to increase caregiver sensitivity and appropriate responsiveness to the child's signals, to increase their ability to reflect on their own and the child' behaviors, thoughts, and feelings regarding attachment-caregiving interactions, and to reflect on experiences in their own histories that affect their current caregiving patterns.

The COS intervention involves at-risk mothers of toddlers or preschoolers meeting as a small group with a therapist for 20 weeks. In the context of the group, each parent reviews edited video vignettes of interactions with their infant. These video feedback vignettes of interactions recorded during a pre-intervention assessment, and the related psycho-educational and therapeutic discussions, are individualized to each dyad's specific attachment-caregiving pattern and associated internal working models. An identical assessment is conducted immediately after the 20-week intervention to track changes in patterns of child-caregiver interaction. During the first weeks, video vignettes are used to enhance parents' observational skills and understanding of children's needs. As their observational skills increase, parents are asked to evaluate the interactions and to discuss the child's primary need (exploration versus attachment) presented in the video vignettes. Educational videotapes are then use to clarify the role of defensive process within personal interaction, and parents are invited to begin exploring how their defensive process may impact their particular caregiving strategy. Attention is paid to the flexibility/rigidity of the caregiver's defensive process, to her capacity to regulate her own emotions in the group, to her capacity for reflective functioning, and to her willingness to develop a therapeutic relationship with the group leader. Marvin used the COS with 75 dyads and the results showed a significant shift from disordered to ordered child attachment pattern (from 55% to 20%), an increase in the number of children coded as secure (from 32% to 40%), and a decrease in the number of caregivers classified as disordered (from 60% to 15%).

Brisch[17] developed an early attachment–oriented intervention composed of supportive group psychotherapy, attachment-oriented focal individual psychotherapy, a home visit and video-based sensitivity training with families of preterm infants. These infants are known to be at high risk for poor psychomotor, behavioral, and emotional outcomes, and the quality of attachment and parent-infant interaction can be considered as protective factors. In this intervention model, video feedback is used at 3 months of age (corrected for prematurity); mothers and fathers are invited to the laboratory in the hospital for a 1-day, individualized, video feedback sensitivity training session. A 10-minute video of semi-structured play and diaper-changing situations is recorded using a split screen. The aim of this training is to enhance parental capability to recognize their infants' signaling, to reflect on the possible interpretations, and to give positive feedback on interactions in which parents are sensitive to and have a correct interpretation of their infant's needs. This model of intervention is based on the importance of parental sensitivity for the development of the infant's secure attachment.

Egeland[18] implemented a preventive attachment-based intervention called STEEP, which stands for Steps Toward Effective, Enjoyable Parenting. This intervention involves providing ongoing home visits and group education beginning during the second trimester of pregnancy and continuing through the early years of the child's life. Families are referred to the program by obstetric clinics and health care providers and this intervention was originally developed to serve first-time parents whose personal history and life circumstances present challenges to good parent-child relationships. It was later adapted to special populations, such as families with premature babies, teen parents, or mothers with postpartum depression. The principal goal of this program is to enhance the quality of the parent-child relationship in the early years by bringing support and learning to new mother-infant pairs. During home visits, parent-infant interactions are videotaped regularly in a variety of routine situations. The centrepiece of STEEP is its strategy of videotaping parent-infant interaction (called Seeing is Believing), which is used to engage parents in a process of self-observation as they watch the tape with their home visitor. Video feedback is used to encourage parents to focus on what their baby is telling them and to recognize their own skills in adapting to the baby's needs. Videotaping is considered to help in keeping the parent-child relation at the center of the intervention, to provide a permanent record for monitoring the family's progress, and it is also seen as a valuable aid when seeking supervisors. For the families, the tape is often seen as a treasured keepsake and a powerful incentive for participating in the STEEP program.

Psychoanalytically Oriented Interventions

The applied psychoanalytic approach aims to clarify, confront, and interpret defensive maternal representations that mark relational disturbances. This form of treatment is focused on declarative and verbalized modes of exchange,[19,20] whereas the interactional approaches tend to intervene on specific behavioral transactions and focus on the procedural mode of exchange. However, outcome studies using different types of interventions[21] have shown that representational and behavioral approaches are both effective and that the dichotomy between these two approaches overestimated.[22]

Changes in maternal representations can be achieved equally by way of behaviourally focused or representationally focused interventions.

Beebe[2] developed a video-based intervention by adapting microanalytic methods of infant observation used previously in parent-infant research. Affective exchange among other indices of communication became the observational focus by which patterns of interactive regulation could be clarified and verbalized. This brief treatment model includes face-to-face split-screen videotaping and a therapeutic observation of the videotape with the parents. It uses the video feedback within a psychoanalytic framework, often as a consultation to an ongoing psychoanalytically oriented nonvideo treatment of the parent. This consultation model includes positive reinforcement, modeling, information giving, and interpretation while watching the videotape with the parent and her analyst/therapist, focusing especially on the areas of attention, arousal, affect, and timing regulation. This intervention aims to link the history of the presenting "complaints" with the patterns of interactive regulation seen in the videotape and the story of the parent's own upbringing. This model also tries to identify the specific representations of the baby that may interfere with the parents' capacity to observe and process the nonverbal interaction. It argues that the mother's experience of watching herself and her baby interact, and the joint attempts of the therapist and the parent to translate the sequences of behaviors into words, facilitates the mother's ability to "see" and to "remember," stimulating the integration of procedural and declarative modes of processing. The concepts of self-regulation (the capacity of the partners to regulate their respective states) and interactive regulation (the continuous process in which each partner makes moment-to-moment adjustments to the behavior of the other) are important in this model because one of its aims is to identify the relative contributions of self and interactive regulation of the partners in the disordered interactions. Beebe prefers to see infants as young as possible and the typical age is 5 to 9 months. The treatment, which can consist of one or more video feedback consultation visits is generally concluded before the infant's second birthday.

Beebe[2] concluded that observed interactive sequences are the critical ingredients in the process of translating the procedurally encoded action sequences into language and thus into declarative knowledge. For this author, the video feedback method has the advantage of being simultaneously visually concrete and "distant" because it is not happening right now. It also allows concentration on a particular modality and slowing it down, whereas in the live interaction all modalities and words flood the senses. The visual information of videotaped interactions speaks on its own and helps the clinician to emphasize certain aspects, to underscore the positive elements as well as identify derailments. This video microanalysis method allows the interactive organization of the mother-infant disturbance to be identified but the success of that method depends on the clinician's capacity to "hold" the mother: staying with the parent as the video is shown, the therapist is alert to any signs of distress and uses these empathically to understand the parent's experience with the infant and her inner world.

Zelenko and Benham[3] use an infant-parent psychodynamic therapy that involves the videotaping of sessions, with subsequent reviewing and discussion with the mother. In this therapeutic technique, past and current maternal experiences and associated representations are considered central aspects to understand the relational pathology. Videotape replay is seen as a tool accelerating the access to early maternal memories and to promote enlightening awareness of the links between maternal past experience and present behaviors with her child. Video feedback is considered to facilitate therapeutic alliance, especially if maternal ability to develop a trusting relationship with a therapist is of particular concern. Videotaping is seen as a unique vehicle for discussion, providing a distancing effect and permitting observations impossible with the human eye during the session.

Videotape replay can facilitate the therapeutic process in three ways: (a) it provides a unique opportunity to observe the mother's own nonverbal behaviors during interactions with the child, behaviors considered as enacted mental representations; (b) watching herself in the maternal role may promote identification with the child and access to her own childhood memories; (c) identification with the child may also lead to a better understanding of her child's immediate experiences with her as a mother.

Schechter and colleagues[23] developed a brief experimental intervention called CAVES (Clinician-Assisted Video feedback Exposure Sessions) that integrates the principles of infant-parent psychotherapy, video feedback, controlled exposure to child distress in the context of parental posttraumatic stress disorders (PTSD), and stimulation of parental reflective functioning. This clinician-assisted video feedback intervention was initially developed to study the process by which change in maternal mental representations can be effected using video feedback in the presence of a mentalizing therapist. The intervention was designed to support emotional self-regulation of mothers with violence-related PTSD. Unlike other video feedback interventions discussed thus far, CAVES, after establishing a positive, supportive frame by showing "the most joyful, contingent, and mutually responsive" moment during mother-child play, focuses the parent and therapist's attention on a video excerpt of child separation, a situation that exposes traumatized mothers to avoided mental states of helplessness, distress, and perceived loss of protection. Schechter and colleagues[23] posited that negative maternal attributions are an aspect of violent trauma-associated emotion dysregulation and projected self-representations of the maltreated mother.

Schechter and colleagues[23] were especially interested in the question of whether a mothers' perception of her child could be changed in a single session of video feedback, given that the traditional target of parent-infant video feedback interventions has been mother-infant interactions and not maternal perceptions. In mothers with violence-associated PTSD, Schechter and colleagues[4] found that distorted, negative, and poorly integrated maternal representations of her child were associated with the severity of PTSD; these mothers had a tendency to view their own children as significant life stressors rather than as sources of joy.

This intervention aims to model and stimulate a mother's reflective functioning (ie, associated with balanced, integrated mental representations). It encourages joint attention with the therapist to the video feedback excerpts. However, because this intervention was developed as an experimental condition designed to test the hypothesis that PTSD interferes with maternal capacity to engage in mentalization and mutual emotion regulation in the "heat" of distressing interactions, Schechter and colleagues[4] state that further research with this manualized approach is needed to replicate the findings and to determine how many sessions helping mothers "to step out of the heat of the moment" would be needed to sustain the observed changes in mental representations.

Cummings and Wittenberg[24] proposed a brief psychodynamic parent-infant psychotherapy called Supportive Expressive Therapy – Parent-Child version (SET-PC) to address the emotional and behavioral problems of toddlers and preschoolers influenced by the parent-infant relationship. SET-PC addresses the parent's internal representations, negative affects, and attributions about the child, and recurrent behavioral responses underlying and maintaining coercive cycles. This intervention applies a social learning approach to the treatment of parent-child coercive transactions. This approach supports the notion that oppositional and aggressive behavior is learned and maintained within the parent-infant relationship, and that children's disruptive behavior is inadvertently reinforced by their parents.

SET-PC is a brief, manualized intervention that includes a structured assessment phase, a socialization interview, and 16 therapy sessions. The parent's Core Conflictual Relationship Theme (CCRT) is formulated in the assessment phase of therapy (two to three sessions), during which the parent is seen without the child. During the socialization interview with the parent, the CCRT is shared and agreement is reached that the CCRT does in fact match the child's presenting problem and that it provides some explanation for it. The therapeutic process is reviewed with the parents and dates are set for 16 subsequent sessions.

Each dyadic therapy session begins with a 20-minute parent-child play session recorded on videotape, followed by a 50-minute therapist-parent session. The first 10 minutes are spent watching a portion of the videotape chosen by the therapist. The therapist uses supportive interventions to help the parent recognize the recurring and maladaptive nature of the CCRT and the therapeutic change through the therapy. After termination, a 3-month follow-up appointment is scheduled. Videotaped interactions are used: (1) to enhance the parent's ability to observe and reflect on their own states of mind, their children's states of mind, and the influence of the interaction on both; (2) to help the parent to recognize recurring attributions, affects, and behavioral responses in themselves (CCRT in action), and to understand how these influence the child's symptomatic behavior; (3) to help the parents recognize developmental capacities in the child. This intervention is considered as a powerful experiential learning, and it allows the development of the parent's observational capacities and reflective functioning. Reflective functioning capacity is associated with better parental functioning because the parent more accurately perceives, accepts, and attunes to the child's mental state.

SYSTEMIC INTERVENTIONS

Video feedback techniques are also used in interventions focusing on family relationships. Fivaz-Depeursinge and Corboz-Warnery[25] developed a method of "systems consultations" for therapists caring for high-risk families with infants and young children that involves parental psychopathology, conflict between spouses/parents, or functional problems in the case of the child. In systems consultations, the therapist asks the consultant for assistance to identify or clarify a situation and consider different options for intervention. The goal of consultation for the parents is to receive feedback on their child's resources or possible deficits, and to help them in parenting their child. This model of intervention was later applied to extended therapeutic work with families to complement the assessment of the triad or of the larger family system, with separate assessments of the family's dyadic subsystems.[6] The model has been used in training professionals to work with families in infant mental health in several countries, in particular in a nationwide, early childhood psychiatry program in Israel.[26]

This model of intervention is based on the Lausanne Triadic Play (LTP) paradigm, which is a clinical research paradigm developed to systematically observe family interactions in a three-way relationship between the father, the mother, and the infant. As the goal of triadic play is to share playful moments of affective communication, the LTP assessment targets the family's intersubjective communication. Three-way communication is attained by means of complex coordination between the three partners' (mostly nonverbal) signals. The infant's active participation in affect sharing by means of his/her triangular capacity is observable from early on. In good-enough family alliances, the three partners are included in the interaction; no one is excluded; they keep to their roles (active versus third party); the parents support each other in front of the child. In problematic alliances, exclusion, or interferences or withdrawal from roles are the main patterns; the parents undermine or fail to support each other and the infant is not engaged. Thus, each type of family alliance has specific strong and weak points that point to the exact target of intervention. For example, if there is a family pattern of exclusion of one of the members, the intervention will be directed at this exclusion. If a parent self-excludes himself, micro-episodes of triangular family play of the LTP previously selected by the consultant may be reviewed during the video feedback with the therapist and the parents, and the context of exclusion identified. The consultant might then reframe the parent's disengagement from the child following the techniques elaborated by family therapists, such as the exclusion being the result of his "invisible loyalty" to his family of origin. Assuming the therapist and family return later for a consultation to check on the progress of the therapy, this context of exclusion may be contrasted with micro-episodes in which all family members share triangular positive affect.

There are four parts in the triadic play: (1) one parent plays and the other is a third party; (2) the two parents reverse roles; (3) all three play together, and (4) the two parents interact with one another and the infant is a third party. These four episodes are recorded on videotape and later used by the consultant for video feedback. The paradigm can be adapted for older children, namely toddlerhood, childhood, and adolescence. A prenatal version (with a doll representing the future infant) has also been developed to assess the coparenting alliance in formation.

A systems consultation takes part in two sessions. During the first session, the family interactions are observed and recorded in the LTP and in other family tasks, such as diaper changing, feeding, and separation-reunion. The parents are aware that the consultant receives little information regarding their problems before the observation. In this way, the consultant remains to some extent blind to the issues at hand, to prevent any bias on his side. After a period of rapport building, the parents and infant are seated in chairs in a triangular formation for the LTP portion of the consultation. If the family has experienced problems in performing the task, the consultant may join the family in the LTP setting and make a direct intervention aimed at triggering changes in the interactive patterns.[6] Then the consultant asks the parents whether they consider that the video is representative of their style of interaction. It is at the end of the observation session that the therapist and the family formulate the motive of the consultation. A second session is scheduled with the therapist and the family for the video feedback. In the meantime, the videos are examined from a clinical perspective as well as micro-analyzed to detect the interactive pattern sequences that best illustrate the family resources and the family problems. Thus, the therapist will use the video feedback to strengthen positive interactive patterns and, if possible, to work on family negative interactive patterns.

The integrative, communication-centered, parent-infant counseling and psychotherapy developed by the Papoušeks, generally called the Munich Model, is also a systemic model based on interdisciplinary research on infant regulation, preverbal learning, and preverbal communication conducted by Hanus and Mechthild Papoušek.[5,27] This approach, developed in the early 1990s, focuses on early communication with regard to joint regulation of adaptative developmental tasks, and particularly on the interplay between the infant's integrative and self-regulatory capacities and the parents' intuitive competencies. Therapeutic elements and techniques from various schools were integrated into this model. It can be conducted with a large diversity of infant behavioral syndromes and psychological problems in parents. The age range includes the first 3 years of life. This model directly addresses patterns of communication at the interface between observable interaction and the parent's conscious and unconscious affects and representations.

This intervention starts with an interdisciplinary diagnostic analysis of the behavioral manifestations, and the immediate and distant conditions of their origin. The assessment includes infant regulatory capacities (eg, developmental level, strengths and difficulties, temperament, quality of solitary play), amount and quality of parental distress (eg, physical and emotional well-being, resources and stress factors, the couple's relationship, family, and social network), and parent-infant communication and relationships (eg, patterns of communication in disorder-related interactional contexts, and attachment behavior). The goal of the treatment is discussed with the parents beforehand and it is always threefold, resolving the behavioral problem, unburdening the parents, and supporting positive relational experiences. Three main interrelated modules are considered to be important: developmental counseling, supportive psychotherapy, and video-supported guidance in communication. These are complemented if needed by psychodynamic communication-centered relational therapy.

Video-supported guidance is used at the level of parent-infant communication. It is mainly directed at observable parent-infant interactions or those described by the parents, and particularly at the patterns of communication in contexts in which the behavioral problems are the most evident (eg, feeding interactions or limit setting). The therapist draws the parents' attention to observable communication patterns during the session and regularly uses videotaped observations. The goal is to replace dysfunctional communication patterns marked by negative contingency between the infant's and the parents' behavior with functional patterns. Specific interactional sequences are selected and analyzed together with the parents. Video feedback, with its technical potential for repetition and pausing, still-framing, slow motion, and time-lapse replay of selected sequences, allows the parents to become aware of particular interactional patterns. However, Mechthild Papoušek considers that this procedure should be used with caution because each video image intrudes into the most intimate sphere of the parent. Therefore, in this model, a secure and protective therapeutic relationship is an indispensable precondition for any video-supported intervention. Special attention is given to the parents' experience and feelings after an observed situation has been recorded or just before viewing it with the parent to help them to deal with any potential vulnerability. As in most of the treatments discussed in this article, the therapist is expected to have thoroughly reviewed and analyzed the contents of the video. It is also easier for the parents to become involved in the emotional processes elicited by the video feedback if the child is not present at the session.

At the beginning, the parents and therapist look at the positive segments repeatedly, which allows the parents to identify the moments of attunement and to experience them emotionally. The therapist carefully probes for the parents' feelings and associations. Even subtle feelings of relaxation, joy, or pride may be reinforced by the therapist's affective attunement. Later in the session, the parents are encouraged to identify with their infant, and to experience how their own behavior is perceived from the infant's perspective. This initial focus on positive sequences is followed by a joint analysis of difficult interaction sequences that are directly related to the behavioral problems.

Papoušek considers that when viewing a short segment of a dysfunctional interaction pattern, it is advantageous to first address the parents' representational level of associated feelings and to find out which specific behaviors on the part of the infant trigger which affects in the parent. The parents are also encouraged to identify with the baby, and to reflect closely from the baby's perspective at a behavioral and emotional level. The parents and the therapist then look for negatively contingent relations at the behavioral and representational level, and for the psychodynamic mechanisms that may trigger or resolve the dysfunctional communication pattern. The therapist uses microanalysis during video feedback to decode the sequences of parent-infant communications, and to identify the positive and negative interactions. Papoušek observes that it is often difficult to determine whether and to what extent the infant's temperament (eg, irritability or low arousal threshold) or parental factors (eg, depressive inhibition of intuitive competencies or distorted perception) are the cause of the derailment of parent-infant communication. Most often, both sides contribute to maintaining maladaptive interaction patterns by their behavior. Papoušek observes that parents are often able to recognize the mechanisms of negative reciprocity, or the signs of over- or understimulation in their own responses. Attempts are then made to find ways to break this vicious circle of negative reciprocities, and to practice alternative behaviors within the therapeutic context.

TRANSACTIONAL MODEL INTERVENTIONS

Interaction Guidance treatment is a therapeutic model developed by McDonough[1] and created specifically to meet the needs of infants and their families who previously refused treatment referral or were unsuccessfully engaged in mental health treatment.[28] Many of these families could be described as being overburdened by risk factors such as poverty, poor education, family mental illness, substance abuse, lack of parenting partner, and inadequate social support.[1,29–31]

As a transactional model, Interaction Guidance treatment incorporates principles of the family system theory into a multigenerational transactional intervention and considers the multiple relational contexts of the infant, such as the baby's caregivers, the extended family members, and the broader social and cultural networks in which the family lives. Because many of these overburdened families are preoccupied with everyday life challenges, observable interactions between baby and caregiver serve as the therapeutic intervention focus.

The key process features of interaction guidance are (1) encouraging the family to define the problem or issue of concern as they see it, (2) working hard and quickly to establish a positive working alliance, (3) emphasizing a family's strengths and recognizing their vulnerabilities and limitations, (4) using an egalitarian and cooperative approach in the engagement and treatment of the families. Families are generally seen weekly for 10 to 12 one-hour treatment sessions. The therapist monitors treatment progress weekly with the family and he jointly decides with the parents the definition of treatment success.

Treatment structure includes (1) clinical assessment of family functioning, social support, and interaction style to acquire clear understanding of the family's view of the problem or situation; (2) involving family members in the treatment planning and choosing who comes to the treatment, and (3) delivering the treatment.

The treatment sessions are usually held in a specially designed playroom equipped with developmentally appropriate toys selected by the therapist. Toys and play material are chosen because they invite use by more than one person. Each session involves two main phases: videotaping the family play sequence, and viewing the videotape. The sequence of activities during each session remains fairly consistent throughout treatment. Once the family is welcomed into the playroom, the therapist inquires about what has occurred in the family's life since the last visit. If the therapist considers that family members are satisfied that their concerns have been addressed, he invites the family to play with their infant the way they would do if they were at home. The therapist videotapes approximately 6 minutes of the play sequence, remaining in the treatment room but trying not to interact with family members. He makes particular note of behaviors that need to be modified or altered because of their critical importance. Content and style can provide important clinical information to the therapist. Content refers to *what* the dyad or family is doing. Are they playing, talking, negotiating, or fighting? Style addresses *how* the family goes about interacting. For example, when the parent plays with the infant, does the parent follow the infant's lead or does the parent try to have the baby do what he wants? By observing family members together, the therapist can draw attention to the pleasurable feelings derived from family interactions and nurture and coach these behaviors from reluctant or insensitive interaction partners.

After recording the play interaction sequence, the family and the therapist view the videotape. Initially, the clinician attempts to solicit comments from the parent(s) concerning their perception of the play sequence, and their thoughts and feelings regarding their infant and their role as parents. A series of systematic probes are posed to the family, such as "was this play session typical of what happens at home?" or "were you surprised by anything that happened during the session?" Following the caregiver's comments, the therapist highlights specific examples of positive parenting behavior and parental sensitivity in reading and interpreting their infant's behavior. He uses what is positive in the parent as the foundation for improving and building a more satisfying relationship with the baby before attempting to intervene in areas of family concern. During these repeated occasions, most families begin to realize that the focus of treatment is positive in nature and that the therapist will address family-identified problems through the use of competence and strength. This video feedback intervention can thus be a powerful therapeutic experience for parents overburdened by guilt and disappointment.

The use of videotape in treatment allows for immediate feedback to parent(s) or family regarding their own behavior and its effect on the infant's behavior. However, the viewing and feedback aspect of the sessions seem especially meaningful to the family at the beginning of the treatment. As families become more comfortable verbalizing their thoughts and concerns spontaneously with the therapist, they seem to view the videotape feedback as an opportunity to reflect on what the televised event represents to them or stirs up in a broader context, such as events of the past week or experiences from years past and the feelings associated with these memories. At the end of the treatment, the clinician edits a videotape documenting the changes that occurred in parent-child interactions and family transactions over the course of the treatment. He gives it to the family as a record and an example of their sensitive and positive parenting.

This treatment has proved to be successful for families caring for infants with growth failure, regulation disorders (sleeping, feeding or excessive crying), biologic vulnerabilities (substance-exposed), and genetic disorders.[1,32] It also proved to be efficient in the treatment of feeding disorders in an adapted version of Interaction Guidance,[33] which included an individually tailored educational component (eg, information about regulatory difficulties or other specific problems exhibited by the infant) and the traditional phases of videotaping the family play sequence and video feedback.

The Interaction Guidance-Geneva Model was developed in Geneva (Switzerland) in the late 1980s by a small group trained by McDonough.[34–36] It was implemented in the context of several outcome and process studies on brief mother-infant psychotherapies with infants presenting functional troubles[21,37] and early behavior problems.[38,39] The disorders targeted in these studies determined an initial restrictive use of this treatment for disorders such as sleep and eating problems, separation difficulties, inconsolable and fussy babies, tantrums and early conflicting relationships. This intervention proved to decrease significantly the rate of behavioral symptoms (such as sleeping or feeding problems) and to improve the quality of mother-child interaction. Mothers came to view their children as well as their own childrearing competencies considerably more positively.[40]

For more than 15 years, this model has been used in a great variety of situations and proved to be particularly useful with depressed or anxious mothers, and with mothers lacking insight or too much intellectualizing. Several adaptations of the initial model were introduced to promote an optimally adjusted therapeutic setting. These adaptations mainly concern the observation context (game or other interactive behavior occurring during the session) and the timing and setting of video feedback (immediate, deferred, with or without the child).

Interaction Guidance was also adapted to the treatment of language delays as well as communication and autistic spectrum disorders by one of the first practitioners of Interaction Guidance in Geneva.[41] In these treatments, the refined observation of the interactions aims to help the parents to better understand their child's special needs and to propose more adjusted and mutually gratifying responses. In the treatments of language delays, the video feedback specifically targets the components of interactions that correspond to the prerequisites of the language emergence (eg, joint attention, pace of exchanges, turn taking, and so forth). The treatment of children with autistic spectrum disorders required a modification of the therapeutic setting to propose a supportive context allowing the parents to experiment with more harmonious interactions with their troubled child. During the parent-child game, the therapist may use two types of interventions: *modeling* (participation in a parent-child game and proposition of an interactive model to the parent) and *prompting* (suggestions or instructions whispered to the parent). Interaction Guidance has been demonstrated to be successful in allowing the parents to rapidly develop a deeper empathy toward their child's difficulties and a better acceptance of the diagnosis and of further therapeutic measures.[42]

Professionals of different disciplines (speech therapists, psychomotor therapists, social workers, educationists, specialized teachers, psychiatrists, and pediatricians), working in different clinical contexts (neonatology unit, kindergarten, residential treatment centers for adolescents, private practice, and so forth), have been successfully trained with the Geneva Model. They applied this model according to their therapeutic aims and in their specific intervention contexts (such as observations of parent-premature baby around the incubator, feeding moments at home, and so forth).

An illustration of the Interaction Guidance-Geneva Model is presented in the following section. The case was referred to our service by the kindergarten and was included in our study on behavior problems. The treatment was conducted by the first author.

THE CASE OF SAMUEL

Samuel is a 35-month-old boy who was described by his mother as "nervous and agitated since he was a baby." His mother said that he was strong-willed, stubborn, and never forgets his aim. After the parents' separation, 6 months earlier, he became defiant and sometimes aggressive with his mother, laughing if she became angry with him. At home, Samuel frequently refused to eat and the mother let him eat whatever he liked whenever he wanted. His mother did not want his father to participate in the sessions due to severe marital conflict. As a child, she remained in her own country and was brought up by her grandparents when her parents came to work in Switzerland. She herself had behavior problems and was thrown out of two schools before her father decided to bring her to Switzerland when she was 13 years old. Her behavior problems stopped when she joined her parents. Despite this, mother did not see any relationship between her own childhood and her son's actual difficulties.

During the evaluation before treatment, Samuel was extremely agitated and defiant with the examiner, and aggressive with his mother. After he broke several pieces of the assessment materials, his mother smiled at him in a tender way and said to the examiner: "You see, he is not frightened! Even with you!"

During the first session, after a brief exploration of the toys available to him, Samuel interrupted the interview with a remote-control car. Despite this, his mother paid no attention to him. This rapidly worsening disturbance made it impossible to complete the interview and the therapist was obliged to remove the noisy toy. In response, Samuel fell to the floor in tears. Even then, his mother remained distant and showed no emotion. The therapist explained to Samuel why he had not been allowed to play with that toy, and reassured him that he would get it back later. She said that she recognized that this was a difficult moment for him; she then explored with the mother *her* feelings about the therapist's having forcefully set limits. The therapist encouraged the mother to get closer to her child and try to comfort him.

These interactions addressed three problems that had been identified in the course of the treatment: (1) the child's need for support; (2) the mother's difficulties in frustrating her child and setting limits; and (3) the disturbance of mutual emotional regulation that was linked, in part, to the mother's difficulty in identifying and responding to her child's distress. The videotaping and the analysis of the mother-child game allowed engagement in the therapeutic process.

During the mother-child game, Samuel snuggled close to his mother, who led the interactions at a quick pace. He carefully observed her and followed her propositions. The emotional climate was tense but warm. Suddenly, during a doll's tea-party, Samuel put a piece of plastic fruit in his mouth. His mother burst out laughing and then abruptly ordered him to remove it, simultaneously yanking it out of his mouth. Mother and child were in a control battle until Samuel ran around the play room frantically such that his mother was unable to catch him.

At the video feedback of mother-child play, excerpts from the first part of the play session were selected to illustrate Samuel's motivation, cooperation, and pleasure. His mother was guided to observe how he was seeking physical proximity with her, paying close attention to her, imitating her, and responding positively to her bids. This video feedback aimed, as a first step, to help the mother to identify Samuel's needs for security and support.

To facilitate the mother's ability to see for herself the possible trigger of the vicious circle of disorganizing mother-child interactions that were observed on video, the therapist selected the key moment during which the mother laughed at Samuel as he was putting the piece of plastic fruit in his mouth. At first, the mother believed that her response to Samuel's behavior was a clear and firm "no!" and that Samuel had persisted because he was strong-willed and stubborn. She had to see this video sequence several times with the positive encouragement of the therapist to consider what she had seen on the tape, to recognize her own behavior. She finally did realize that her first response to Samuel had been a mocking roar of laughter and that this affective response had reinforced the difficult behavior of the child.

During the second session, the emotional climate was notably more harmonious. Samuel was less disruptive with and more affectionate toward his mother. His bids for her attention alternated between provocation from a distance and seeking physical proximity and comfort.

The treatment was completed in seven sessions. By the time of termination, Samuel's mother had succeeded in firmly setting limits with Samuel whether or not he mounted a protest. She noticed, with relief, that he always came back to her after his bouts of disorganized aggressive behavior, as if he had "calmed down." Follow-up after the treatment's termination showed that Samuel had become more autonomous and had presented significantly less disruptive behavior at home and in his preschool.

DISCUSSION

Video feedback techniques are thus potentially important tools that can facilitate and accelerate intrapsychic and behavioral change as either the mainstay of treatment or as a supplement to an ongoing psychotherapy. Video feedback aides the development of the therapeutic alliance, and a feeling of shared intersubjective experience between parent and therapist and parent and child. Video feedback interventions have an increase in positive parenting as a common goal. But they often use different mechanisms and techniques. Whereas some approaches specifically teach and focus on parenting behaviors like, for example, maintaining focused attention on the child or using frequent praise, others, such as nondirective psychodynamic therapies, provide parents with the opportunity to view and reflect on their own psychic functioning and that of their children during their daily interactions. The therapeutic target in this latter example will often be the parent's mental representations of herself, her relationship with her child, and of her child as she imagines his subsequent growth and increasing autonomy. It is ultimately up to the therapist and parents to figure out which type of intervention might be indicated and best suited to a given, particular dyad. Early research on these techniques is promising, although the field will be strengthened by future systematic examination of the outcomes associated with these clinically valuable tools.

REFERENCES

1. McDonough SC. Promoting positive early parent-infant relationships through interaction guidance. Child Adolesc Psychiatr Clin N Am 1995;4(3):661–72.
2. Beebe B. Brief mother-infant treatment: psychoanalytically informed video feedback. Infant Ment Health J 2003;24(1):24–52.
3. Zelenko M, Benham A. Videotaping as a therapeutic tool in psychodynamic infant-parent therapy. Infant Ment Health J 2000;21(3):192–203.
4. Schechter D, Coots T, Zeanah CH, et al. Maternal mental representations of the child in an inner-city clinical sample: violence-related posttraumatic stress and reflective functioning. Attach Hum Dev 2005;7(3):313–31.
5. Papousek M. Vom ersten Schrei zum ersten Wort. Anfaenge der Sprachentwicklung in der vorsprachlichen Kommunikation. Bern: Huber; 1994.
6. Fivaz-Depeursinge E, Corboz-Warnery A, Keren M. The primary triangle, treating infants in their families. In: Sameroff AJ, McDonough SC, Rosenblum KL, editors. Treating parent-infant relationship problems, strategies for intervention. New York: The Guilford Press; 2005. p. 123–51.
7. Marvin R, Cooper G, Hoffman K, et al. The Circle of Security project: attachment-based intervention with caregiver-pre-school child dyads. Attach Hum Dev 2002; 4(1):107–24.
8. Bakermans-Kranenburg MJ, van Ijzendoorn MH. Gene-environment interaction of the dopamine D4 receptor (DRD4) and observed maternal insensitivity predicting externalizing behavior in preschoolers. Dev Psychobiol 2006;48(5):406–9.
9. Bakermans-Kranenburg MJ, Van Ijzendoorn MH, Mesman J, et al. Effects of an attachment-based intervention on daily cortisol moderated by dopamine receptor D4: a randomized control trial on 1- to 3-year-olds screened for externalizing behavior. Dev Psychopathol 2008;20(3):805–20.
10. Van Zeijl J, Mesman J, Van Ijzendoorn MH, et al. Attachment-based intervention for enhancing sensitive discipline in mothers of 1- to 3-year-old children at risk for externalizing behavior problems: a randomized controlled trial. J Consult Clin Psychol 2006;74(6):994–1005.
11. Juffer F, Bakermans-Kranenburg MJ, van Ijzendoorn MH. The importance of parenting in the development of disorganized attachment: evidence from a preventive intervention study in adoptive families. J Child Psychol Psychiatry 2005;46(3):263–74.
12. Juffer F, Bakermans-Kranenburg MJ, van Ijzendoorn MH. Promoting positive parenting: an attachment-based intervention. Mahwah (NJ): Lawrence Erlbaum; 2007.
13. Velderman MK, Bakermans-Kranenburg MJ, Juffer F, et al. Effects of attachment-based interventions on maternal sensitivity and infant attachment: differential susceptibility of highly reactive infants. J Fam Psychol 2006;20(2):266–74.
14. Stein A, Wooley H, Senior R, et al. Treating disturbances in the relationship between mothers with bulimic eating disorders and their infants: a randomized, controlled trial of video feedback. Am J Psychiatry 2006;163(5):899–906.
15. Bakermans-Kranenburg MJ, van Ijzendoorn MH. Research review: genetic vulnerability or differential susceptibility in child development: the case of attachment. J Child Psychol Psychiatry 2007;48(12):1160–73.
16. Ainsworth MDS, Blehar MC, Waters E, et al. Patterns of attachment: a psychological study of the strange situation. Hillsdale (NJ): Lawrence Erlbaum; 1978.
17. Brisch KH, Bechinger D, Betzler S, et al. Early preventive attachment-oriented psychotherapeutic intervention program with parents of a very low birthweight

premature infant: results of attachment and neurological development. Attach Hum Dev 2003;5(2):120–35.

18. Egeland B, Farrell Erikson M. Lessons from steep, linking theory, research, and practice for the well-being of infants and parents. In: Sameroff AJ, McDonough SC, Rosenblum KL, editors. Treating parent-infant relationship problems, strategies for intervention. New York: The Guilford Press; 2004. p. 213–42.

19. Fraiberg S. Clinical studies in infant mental health: the first year of life. New York: Basic Books; 1980.

20. Cramer B. Short-term dynamic psychotherapy for infant and their parents. Child Adolesc Psychiatr Clin N Am 1995;4:649–59.

21. Cramer B, Robert-Tissot C, Stern D, et al. Outcome evaluation in brief mother-infant psychotherapy: a preliminary report. Infant Ment Health J 1990;11(3):278–300.

22. Cramer B. Mother-infant psychotherapies: a widening scope in technique. Infant Ment Health J 1998;19(2):151–67.

23. Schechter DS, Myers M, Brunelli S, et al. Traumatized mothers can change their minds about their toddlers: understanding how a novel use of videofeedback supports positive change of maternal attributions. Infant Ment Health J 2006; 27(5):429–47.

24. Cummings J, Wittenberg JV. Supportive expressive therapy—parent child version: an exploratory study. Psychotherapy Theory, Research, Practice, Training 2008;45(2):148–64.

25. Fivaz-Depeursinge E, Corboz-Warnery A. The primary triangle: a developmental systems view of fathers, mothers and infants. New York: Basic Books; 1999.

26. Keren M, Fivaz-Depeursinge E, Tyrano S. Using the Lausanne family model in training: an Israeli experience. Signal 2001;9(3):5–10.

27. Papousek H, Papousek M. Intuitive parenting: a dialectic counterpart to the infant's integrative competence. In: Osofsky J, editor. Handbook of infant development. New York: Blackwell; 1987. p. 669–720.

28. McDonough SC. Interaction guidance: an approach for difficult-to-engage families. In: Zeanah C, editor. Handbook of infant mental health. New York: The Guilford Press; 2000. p. 485–93.

29. Zeanah CMS. Clinical approaches to families in early intervention. Semin Perinatol 1989;13(6):513–22.

30. McDonough SC. Treating early relationship disturbances with interaction guidance. In: Fava V, Stern G, editors. Models and techniques of psychotherapeutic interventions in the first years of life. Milan (Italy): Raffaello Cortina Editora; 1991. p. 221–33.

31. McDonough S. Interaction guidance, promoting and nurturing the caregiving relationship. In: Sameroff AJ, McDonough SC, Rosenblum KL, editors. Treating parent-infant relationship problems, strategies for intervention. New York: The Guilford Press; 2004. p. 79–96.

32. McDonough SC. Models of interaction for parents and children. In: Gomes-Pedro JFP, Folque Patricio M, editors. Bébé XXI: infants and families in the next century. Lisbon (Portugal): Fundação Calouste Gulbenkian; 1996. p. 221–33.

33. Benoit D, Madigan S, Lecce S, et al. Atypical maternal behavior toward feeding-disordered infants before and after intervention. Infant Ment Health J 2001;22(6): 611–26.

34. Berney C. Guidance interactive et logopédie: liens et apports. Parole d'Or 1992; 11:25–7 [in French].

35. Rusconi Serpa S. La guidance interactive: les points essentiels du traitement. Psychoscope 1992;10:7–10 [in French].

36. Robert-Tissot C. La guidance interactive: une thérapie des interactions. Langage & pratiques 2003;32:18–28 [in French].
37. Robert-Tissot C, Cramer B. When patients contribute to the choice of their treatment. Infant Ment Health J 1998;19(2):245–59.
38. Lüthi Faivre F, Sancho Rossignol A, Rusconi Serpa S, et al. Troubles du comportement entre 18 et 36 mois: symptomatologie et psychopathologie associées. Neuropsychiatr Enfance Adolesc 2005;53:176–85 [in French].
39. Sancho Rossignol A, Knauer D, Rusconi Serpa S, et al. Les troubles précoces du comportement sont-ils l'expression d'une psychopathologie spécifique? Psychiatr Enfant 2005;48(1):157–98 [in French].
40. Robert-Tissot C, Cramer B, Stern DN, et al. Outcome evaluation in brief mother-infant psychotherapies: report on 75 cases. Infant Ment Health J 1996;17:97–114.
41. Berney C. Guidance interactive en logopédie. Langage & pratiques 2003;32: 2–17 [in French].
42. Lacroix M. Troubles de la relation et de la communication: formulation des commentaires en guidance interactive. Langage & pratiques 2003;32:41–53 [in German].

Psychopharmacology and Preschoolers: A Critical Review of Current Conditions

John Fanton, MD[a], Mary Margaret Gleason, MD[b,c],*

KEYWORDS

• Preschool • Psychopharmacology • Treatment
• ADHD • Infant mental health

Researchers and clinicians increasingly recognize the early childhood origins of impairing psychiatric conditions and the disruption to normal functioning that these disorders cause in children and families. The need to develop and demonstrate how evidence-based treatments[1] (see also the articles by Lieberman and Horn and Dickstein and Shepard, elsewhere in this issue) can reduce suffering and alter negative developmental trajectories is quite compelling.

Research focused on psychopharmacological interventions for preschoolers with severe psychiatric disorders lags behind clinical practice, even though evidence of biological abnormalities has been demonstrated in some psychiatric disorders.[2–5] Thus, clinicians and families face complex dilemmas. They must weigh identified and unknown risks, benefits, and alternatives of psychopharmacological interventions to treat children for whom psychotherapy has been ineffective, unavailable, or not tried.

Overall, epidemiological samples of prescription rates document a pattern of increasing medication use for very young children; although the specific patterns vary for individual medications and in different populations. For example, in the 1990s, rates of prescriptions for psychopharmacological agents increased two- to three-fold in some preschool populations,[6,7] whereas the latter half of that decade found rates of stimulant prescriptions in a nationally representative sample to have stabilized.[8] However, during the same period, antipsychotic prescription rates for

[a] Department of Psychiatry, Tufts University School of Medicine, Western Campus at Baystate Medical Center, 759 Chestnut Street, Springfield, MA 01199, USA
[b] Department of Pediatrics, Tulane University School of Medicine, 1440 Canal Street, TB 52, New Orleans, LA 70112, USA
[c] Department of Psychiatry & Neurology, Tulane University School of Medicine, 1440 Canal Street, TB 52, New Orleans, LA 70112, USA
* Corresponding author. Department of Pediatrics, Tulane University School of Medicine, 1440 Canal Street, TB 52, New Orleans, LA 70112.
E-mail address: mgleason@tulane.edu (M.M. Gleason).

Child Adolesc Psychiatric Clin N Am 18 (2009) 753–771
doi:10.1016/j.chc.2009.02.005
1056-4993/09/$ – see front matter © 2009 Elsevier Inc. All rights reserved.

childpsych.theclinics.com

preschoolers with Medicaid more than doubled.[9] A number of factors may explain these trends, including increased awareness of severe mental health problems in young children,[10] development of medications considered safer than their older counterparts,[9] increased experience of practicing providers treating younger populations, as well as increased behavioral expectations of very young children in structured settings, such as childcare or preschool.[11]

This article describes the factors that make preschool psychopharmacological treatment more complex than that for older children, reviews the evidence for and against its use for the treatment of specific disorders, and recommends future directions for clinical practice guidelines and research.

For clinicians considering treatment approaches for very young children diagnosed with psychiatric disorders, a number of factors warrant special consideration and have recently been addressed by a panel of national experts. In 2007, a group funded by the American Academy of Child and Adolescent Psychiatry (AACAP) published recommendations for using psychopharmacological treatment in very young children (>36 months) with severe psychiatric disorders.[12] The group not only provided recommendations about specific diagnoses but also presented general principles for assessment and treatment. More specifically, these principles emphasize the importance of (1) a multi-informant, comprehensive assessment, (2) the use of psychotherapeutic interventions, especially evidence-based therapies, before considering medications, and (3) the conscientious use of medications for children with moderate to severe symptoms and functional impairment for which there is reasonable expectation that psychiatric medications may help. Finally, the group recommended that providers use a clinical case trial "n of 1" model when treating very young children with medications—including a structured assessment that includes attention to symptoms as well as functional impairment, a system for ongoing monitoring of treatment effects, and a plan for discontinuation of the medication after a specified period of successful treatment to reassess the child's underlying psychopathology and maturation. The group also advocated for increased federally funded research to guide psychopharmacological treatment of very young children, given many of the treatment concerns and public health priorities addressed here.

Although research catches up to clinical practice, there are numerous caveats to keep in mind, even beyond those known to be specific to an individual child, disorder, or medication, for the practicing provider. First, and perhaps most striking, is the poorly understood interaction between the rapid, normal neurodevelopmental changes that occur in very young children and what acute or chronic exposure to psychotropic medication does to developing brains. The early years of life is a period during which the most rapid synaptogenesis and pruning of neural networks take place, thereby beginning the process of establishing higher cognitive functions.[13] This development is sensitive to both environmental and chemical influences, and can be influenced in positive as well as adverse directions. For example, lead exposure, maternal depression, and child maltreatment are all associated with abnormal CNS findings in young children.[14–16] Similarly, it has been shown that therapeutic interventions can affect CNS development and function, enhancing cognitive development and the hypothalamic-pituitary-adrenal activity in positive ways.[17,18] Currently, it is not known whether exposure to psychopharmacological agents in the early years has a harmful influence on CNS maturation or whether early medication exposure and normalization of functioning may be protective against later psychopathologies and measurable CNS dynamics.

Second, as described in this issue, the evidence that supports the validity of the currently used diagnostic nosologies (Diagnostic and Statistical Manual of Mental

Disorders, fourth edition [DSM-IV][19] and the Diagnostic Criteria:0-3R[20]) is growing but still limited.[21–23] The long-term prospective validity of psychiatric diagnoses in very young children is not well documented, with the exception of attention-deficit/hyperactivity disorder (ADHD) and posttraumatic stress disorder (PTSD), which appear to demonstrate "homotypic continuity", meaning that the disorder continues to be present at follow-up.[24–26] New data suggest that the more severe the condition in early childhood, the more likely it demonstrates homotypic continuity or persists as is.[27] Prospective studies show that the majority of children with mental health problems as toddlers and preschoolers will continue to have a psychiatric diagnosis in their school-age years, though not necessarily the same condition, suggesting that heterotypic continuity has valid clinical implications since some children will continue to have a disorder in their school-age years, albeit transformed from its preschool presentation.[28–30] The question of diagnostic continuity of preschool disorders is particularly relevant in the discussion of psychopharmacological treatment, since medications are typically used to treat specific disorders. If a preschool disorder does not demonstrate homotypic continuity, it is not clear that the medication used for the school-age presentation of a disorder is the best choice for preschool intervention.

Additionally, children have been described as "therapeutic orphans" in the US drug regulatory system.[31] Preschool populations have been neglected more than their school-aged peers as evidenced by the fact that there are only four medications approved for psychiatric indications in children younger than 6 years of age: haloperidol, chlorpromazine, d-amphetamine, and risperidone (in children 5 years and older).[32] Thus, nearly all prescribing for preschoolers is off-label, including methylphenidate (MPH), which is the most studied and commonly used.[33] It is important to note that "off-label" is not equivalent to "contraindicated", and leaders in the field have argued that off-label does not necessarily indicate lack of demonstrable efficacy.[34] Off-label indicates only that efficacy for a specific indication in a specific population has not been adequately demonstrated to the Food and Drug Administration (FDA) by any manufacturer or institution. As is true for children in general, there are unique challenges to conducting large clinical trials in preschoolers even with recent financial incentives for manufacturers to seek FDA approval for specific indications,[35] including significant safety and ethical considerations discussed here.[36]

Practical challenges in using psychopharmacological agents to treat preschoolers are abundant, including the administration of medication and its dosing. Many preschoolers have difficulties swallowing pills.[37,38] Some medications come in liquid formulations (**Table 1**), although it is not unusual for children to be selective about tastes and textures, especially alcohol-based formulations. Liquid preparations allow the use of very low doses and small incremental titrations and can be useful for treating very young children in whom large dose changes are not optimal or tolerable. Transdermal administration, as with clonidine (Catapres) or MPH (Daytrana), similarly eliminates the difficulties with swallowing pills and provides some flexibility with dosing.[39] For a fee, medications may be compounded, creating suspensions and specific flavors to improve compliance.

Although the oft-quoted mantra "start low and go slow" is important as applied to preschoolers and psychiatric populations generally, it is particularly true with psychiatric medications, since they are not dosed by weight, unlike other pediatric medications. This fact, combined with the lack of systematic studies focused on dosing in preschoolers, increases the challenge of determining initial doses of medication, with the exception of MPH, which is described in the following section. For example, there are limited systematic studies of atypical antipsychotic agents, used largely in autistic populations, but there are reports of risperidone use starting at a dose of

Table 1
Nontablet formulations of psychiatric medications used for preschoolers

Medication	Brand Name	Formulation	Lowest Dose Available
Methylphenidate	Daytrana	Transdermal patch	10 mg
	Metadate CD	Capsule—contents can be sprinkled on food	10 mg
	Ritalin LA	Capsule—contents can be sprinkled on food	20 mg
	Methylin	Liquid—grape	10 mg/5 mL
Mixed amphetamine salts	Vyvanse	Capsule—contents can be dissolved in water and smaller doses given	20 mg
	Adderall XR	Capsule—contents can be sprinkled on food	5 mg
Clonidine	Catapres-TTS	Transdermal patch	0.1 mg
Risperidone	Risperdal-M tab	Oral disintegrating tablet	0.5 mg
Fluoxetine	Prozac	Solution—mint flavor	20 mg/5 mL
Sertraline	Zoloft	Alcohol-based	20 mg/mL
Citalopram	Celexa	Liquid—mint	10 mg/5 mL

0.25 mg/d.[40] Preschoolers metabolize most medications more rapidly due to enhanced hepatic activity particular to this developmental period, though the pharmacokinetics and dynamics of most major psychiatric drugs are poorly understood in preschool populations.[41] For medications that are available only in pill form, 1/4 pill is the smallest realistic dose possible, recognizing that the dosing becomes less exact when parents or pharmacists cut the pill. A very low dose can be used as a test dose to identify adverse effects (eg, with stimulants) or for medications that have not been formulated with a focus on children's doses, such as selective serotonin reuptake inhibitors (SSRIs). The lowest-dose preparations of stimulants are often small, although for 3- and 4-year-olds, half of the lowest dose of immediate release forms may be the most reasonable first dose.

Although there is increasing attention to the psychiatric needs of very young children, a recent search of the National Institutes of Health website (http://crisp.cit.nih.gov, accessed November 12, 2008) revealed only five federally funded studies investigating the use of medications for preschoolers, all of them focused on ADHD and three that are follow-up studies related to the Preschool ADHD Treatment Study (PATS). Search terms included "preschool" and the following terms: "psychiatry," "psychopharmacology," "mental health," and "medications," and results did not vary when the same searches were performed with "young child" replacing "preschool". A search in clinicaltrials.gov found only two additional studies, with only two of the seven total actively recruiting. Thus, it appears that federally funded research will continue to yield limited information to guide clinicians in the upcoming years. Nevertheless, it is important to review what is known.

ATTENTION-DEFICIT/HYPERACTIVITY DISORDER

Although ADHD is extremely prevalent and well characterized in school-aged children, it is an understudied condition among preschool youth, with a particular paucity of studies examining combination or sequential therapies.[33] Treatments for preschool ADHD are complicated, and there is a lack of specialists who have early childhood expertise.[42] Insurance regulations have discouraged clinicians from working with parents directly in the absence of the child, in spite of the evidence that play therapy and one-on-one cognitive-behavioral therapy (CBT) are not effective treatments for ADHD, although parent behavioral training (PBT) is.[43,44] Key opinion leaders in the United Kingdom have reviewed the available data and concluded that medication should not be recommended for use in children with ADHD younger than 5 years of age.[45] Citing the same lack of guidelines and controlled studies to inform clinicians who are prescribing psychotropic medications to very young children in the United States, the 2007 Preschool Psychopharmacology Working Group (PPWG) outlined recommendations for clinical decisions that follow diagnosis-specific algorithms when prescribing medications for early childhood conditions to complement the American Academy of Pediatrics and AACAP best practice parameters.[12,46,47] Experts who helped generate the latest preschool ADHD treatment data contributed to the PPWG and have also addressed the pragmatic issues of diagnosing and managing preschool ADHD in clinical terms, emphasizing the many caveats known.[48]

The primary challenge that clinicians face is an accurate diagnosis. The conventional wisdom about preschool behaviors is that transient developmental problems are not easily distinguished from those of a more persistent and diagnosable condition. However, several reports substantiate contemporary DSM and International Classification of Diseases (ICD) diagnostic criteria originally established for school-aged children with ADHD or hyperkinetic disorder, with only slight modifications (primarily school related) for preschool children.[22,49] Longitudinal data and clinical experience support the predictive validity of the diagnosis, and families and primary care providers can distinguish the normal transient variants from the more clinically impairing diagnostic conditions.[25,50,51] For families responding to a survey about their 3-year-olds' behaviors, maternal report and elevated scores on a behavioral screening test predicted clinical diagnoses several years later of ADHD and ODD.[27] In this same cohort, the more severe the initial symptom presentation the more likely that the condition was chronic and identified as early as 3 years of age by parents and pediatricians.[52] Similarly, preschool children with ADHD demonstrate measurable and significant impairment in psychosocial dysfunction.[25,53]

Although psychostimulants have often become the first line of treatment for school-aged children with ADHD, preschool children have been identified as having unique developmental, mood, and growth sensitivities to psychotropic medications, which complicates treatment considerations.[54–56] In the largest, controlled, psychiatric medication trial in preschoolers, PATS demonstrated that MPH had reasonable margins of safety and efficacy for children 3 to 5.5 years old.[57] Hyperactivity and impulsive behavioral problems were reduced in PATS, although the effect size observed was smaller than that demonstrated in the Multimodal Treatment of ADHD (MTA) study for school-aged children.[58] Design accommodations in PATS that were made for ethical considerations limited its strength and interpretability, since reconsenting procedures at each treatment decision point, although providing additional protection for children involved in the study, also increased the attrition rate of subjects completing each of the eight phases.[59] With the additional limit placed on dosing at 10 mg three times a day, these factors likely reduced the study's power and effect size of the intervention, since there was notable attrition during controlled portions of the trial, and some children may have done even better at higher dosing.[57] For children with ADHD and three or more comorbid conditions, PATS did not demonstrate an effect of stimulants at all, similar to findings in the MTA.[60] For those children with ADHD alone or with comorbidities, PATS does not help improve the understanding of how psychosocial interventions compare to or enhance the effects of medications, as it was never intended to compare the two, and the results of the PBT in PATS need to be reviewed with consideration.[59] The PBT offered in PATS was an add-on intervention to comply with requests made by the monitoring ethics and safety boards charged with approving PATS design[59] and not as a comparison intervention as had been the case in the MTA trial. Parental satisfaction with the PATS PBT may have been higher than how the primary outcome (response rate of 7% "significantly improved") has been presented, since another 7% reported "improvement," and another 13% reported no desire to pursue medications, suggesting that these families may have felt that they were better prepared to manage the behaviors without medication.[61] As such, PATS is vulnerable to a similar criticism made of the Treatment of Adolescent Depression Study in that the psychosocial intervention used in both had not been shown to be validated in the target population before recruitment.[62] Since PATS concluded recruiting, six controlled trials for preschool psychosocial therapies have been published,[43,63–68] compared with only three trials before PATS was proposed.[69–71] Yet none of them has evaluated psychosocial treatments head to head with medication or as to how they may enhance one another. With these additional established interventions, future multimodal studies should include an established and proven psychosocial intervention to understand how PBT compares and may enhance medication treatments. Despite these limitations, PATS will serve as a reference for years to come for future practice and research considerations, as it is a landmark study that demonstrates that MPH can reasonably be used with expectations of it improving the hallmark symptoms of ADHD in preschoolers.[2]

Several other issues for the prescribing clinician require special consideration. Prior to the MTA study, immediate-release stimulants were used mostly for school days, but with the introduction and popularity of long-acting preparations (eg, Concerta and Adderall XR), direct to consumer advertising, and how the MTA data have been interpreted, there has been an almost doubling of total days for children on medication from 10 years ago.[72] For preschoolers just starting a new medication during a period of robust neurodevelopment, clinicians will want to consult with the family, reevaluate response and side effects, and adjust strength and the dosing schedule, while also considering medication holidays to minimize the unknown possible detrimental impact of long-term stimulant use. Informed consent, with stimulants or other medications, is important to provide for all treatments, but especially for conditions where even the best-studied medication is off-label. Though it is unknown how the long-term use of stimulants affects CNS maturation,[73,74] it has been well established in PATS and pre-PATS trials that preschoolers have more mood, sleep, appetite, and growth side effects in response to stimulants compared with older children.[54,55,57,75–77] Chronic stimulant use in older children with ADHD does not induce intracellular cytogenetic damage or sudden cardiac events, though this again is an understudied area of research for preschoolers.[78,79] Yet dangers of psychotropic use are still present. The highly publicized tragic death of a preschool-aged girl prescribed several psychopharmacological agents reminds us of the ever-present safety, medical, and legal issues of using medications[80] and to be vigilant for comorbidities, confounding variables influencing diagnosis and treatment, and for issues of parental competence. It is important to document consent obtained from guardians for treatment with medications, including awareness of off-label use; but it is also crucial to inform families that the number of comorbidities present could neutralize the effectiveness of interventions proposed. For this purpose, clinicians might intentionally curb the expectations of families for what somatic therapies can offer.[60] The confusing regulatory issues of stimulant medications for children younger than 6 years of age, as noted above, do not help clinicians or families either. MPH is the best-studied medicine for preschool ADHD, but it does not have FDA approval, whereas dextroamphetamine is approved down to age 3 despite a complete lack of reasonable evidence for this indication.[32]

Although much may be said for the case of establishing FDA approval for MPH in preschool ADHD, to date the same cannot be said for non-MPH stimulants or nonstimulant ADHD medications as to their demonstration of efficacy in preschool ADHD. Atomoxetine (ATX) has been shown to decrease measures of hyperactivity, inattentiveness, and impulsivity in a small sample (n = 22) of 5- and 6-year-olds,[81] and an active trial is recruiting 3- to 5-year-olds to investigate if it has similar efficacy (versus placebo) as shown in older children.[82] As with older children, preliminary results show a smaller effect size for ATX compared with that typically found with MPH.[83]

The responsible use of medication, most specifically MPH, has an acceptable level of evidence to support its use as part of a comprehensive care plan, although there are a number of complicating circumstances surrounding the diagnosis and treatment of preschool ADHD.[84] Controlled trials involving multimodal combination or sequencing treatments involving stimulants and established psychosocial interventions are needed in preschool populations, since there are more safety and efficacy issues found in the very young relative to their older peers. Additionally, there are no controlled, head-to-head comparison studies at all of MPH to other stimulants or nonstimulants for reference to treat preschool children with ADHD who may or may not have other disruptive behavioral and communication disorders or ineffective response to MPH, so there remains much unknown.[33]

DISRUPTIVE BEHAVIOR DISORDERS

For disruptive behavior disorder, the weight of evidence for psychotherapy far outweighs that which supports psychopharmacological treatment. A strong empirical base supports "parent-management training" and other behavioral interventions to treat oppositional defiant disorder (ODD) and conduct disorder in preschoolers.[85,86] These treatments are effective and are associated with persistent improvement in child disruptive behavior disorders. However, the evidence-based treatments are not available in all settings, and some children may not have access to them. For these children, a traditional behavioral intervention is recommended, with attention to positive reinforcement for positive or prosocial behaviors and safe, predictable consequences for unsafe or otherwise unacceptable behaviors. Additionally, evidence-based interventions, such as Parent Child Interaction Therapy have reported dropout rates as high as 33%,[87] indicating that some families may not be a good fit for this intervention.

Medication may be considered for preschoolers who do not improve with behavioral treatment, for those who cannot participate in psychotherapeutic interventions, and for those who continue to demonstrate severe, unsafe behaviors and/or notable impairment related to disruptive behavior disorders (such as risk of expulsion from child care). However, there are no published studies examining psychopharmacological treatment of systematically diagnosed ODD. For disruptive behavior disorders, ongoing behavioral management in the home and other settings, including school or childcare, is strongly recommended.[88] For children with comorbid ADHD or impulsivity, stimulant treatment should be considered before treating ODD specifically. Of the nonstimulant medications used to treat aggression in older children, risperidone is the medication for which the most preschool published data exist[89] and which may be considered to treat severe, unsafe disruptive behavior disorders in conjunction with behavioral and family-focused treatments. One case series examined the treatment outcomes of eight preschoolers with aggression who received risperidone.[90] The treatment was associated with a decrease in symptom severity over variable duration as well as an average weight gain of 5.5 kg. Most published studies of risperidone in preschoolers use starting doses of 0.25 mg/d, with high doses of up to 3.0 mg/d. Monitoring of metabolic, motor, and growth parameter adverse effects should be done as per the AACAP practice parameters.[91]

ANXIETY

Anxiety disorders are the most common category of preschool psychiatric disorders. Nearly 10% of preschoolers meet the criteria for an anxiety disorder.[92] Rates of specific phobia, separation anxiety disorder (SAD), generalized anxiety disorder (GAD), and social phobia (SP) each cluster around 2%. Fewer preschoolers meet criteria for PTSD (approximately 0.6%),[93] and the prevalence of obsessive compulsive disorder (OCD) has not been described in preschoolers. Although most prescriptions for preschoolers are written for stimulants, prescriptions for antidepressants represent about 12% to 20%, and likely some of these are intended to treat anxiety disorders.[94,95]

Tandon and colleagues have presented a review of the nonpharmacological interventions for preschool anxiety disorders, in an article elsewhere in this issue. Despite the prevalence of these disorders, there are limited data to guide treatment recommendations for children with anxiety disorders, either pharmacologically or psychotherapeutically. For preschoolers as with their school-age peers, psychotherapy is the first-line treatment for anxiety, because it is less likely to be accompanied by risk of adverse effects as with medication. CBT in very young children presents challenges related to language development and must be adapted for the developmental needs of very young children.[96]

Anxiety disorders can be separated into three distinct clinical clusters for the purpose of discussing psychopharmacological treatment. SAD, GAD, SP, selective mutism (SM), and specific phobias can be considered together, as research in older children suggests that they are responsive to similar pharmacological treatments (eg,[97]). The literature focused on OCD and posttraumatic stress disorder must be considered separately.

Few studies have examined the use of antianxiety medications in preschoolers. The published literature focused on children younger than 6 years of age includes 16 children whose treatment outcomes for anxiety are described (**Table 2**). Of these, three children had anxiety disorders that included SM, specific phobias, comorbid SP, posttraumatic feeding disorder, and SAD. Two were successfully treated with fluoxetine, one for SM (in combination with nonpharmacological treatments)[98] and the other for what was described as specific phobias and panic attacks.[99] One case report also described failed trials of hydroxyzine (which has an FDA indication to treat anxiety) and alprazolam.

In this context, SSRIs may be considered to treat severe GAD, SAD, SM, and specific phobia in preschoolers after a failure of CBT or other psychotherapeutic intervention. For such cases requiring medication treatment, studies in older children suggest that fluoxetine, sertraline, and fluvoxamine may be effective.[100–102] However, research focused on safety suggests that fluoxetine should be the first choice unless there are compelling clinical reasons to choose sertraline or fluvoxamine.[103,104] Doses as low as 2.5 to 5 mg/d of fluoxetine or 5 to 10 mg/d sertraline are appropriate starting points to allow monitoring of adverse effects. When discussing SSRI use with parents, it is important to discuss all known side effects, including the FDA black box warning about potential suicidal ideation in depressed children and adolescents.

Table 2
Published studies of psychopharmacological treatment of anxiety disorders

Medication	Disorder	Study Design	Ages(y.mo)	Outcome
Fluoxetine[98]	Selective mutism	Case report	4.1	Freely speaking, CBCL T score 68–>60 (internalizing)
Fluoxetine[99]	Multiple anxiety disorders	Case report	2.5	Decreased anxiety
Sertraline[105]	OCD	3 case reports	4.0–5.0	Reduced symptoms on CYBOCS, hyperarousal requiring intervention (risperidone)
Clonidine[106]	PTSD plus aggression	Open trial (n=7)	3.0–6.0	Decreased arousal, aggression, and anxiety
Buspirone[121]	SAD + social phobia + feeding disorder	Case report	4.0	Decreased anxiety, increased eating, symptoms recurred with discontinuation
Risperidone[122]	Acute stress disorder	Case series	1.1, 3.2, 3.9	Improved sleeping, decreased ASD symptoms

Abbreviations: ASD, autism spectrum disorder; CYBOCS, Child Yale-Brown Obsessive Compulsive Scale.

Oner and Oner described three case reports of preschoolers with OCD.[105] All 3 children were started on 25 mg/d of sertraline. Of these, two developed activation, which was treated with risperidone. The authors reported resolution of symptoms in all three, with two patients achieving a score of zero on the Child Yale-Brown Obsessive Compulsive Scale (CYBOCS). These three case reports serve as the beginning of a literature focused on psychopharmacological treatment of OCD in preschoolers, but because of methodological issues, caution must be used in generalizing the findings to other children. With the stronger evidence base supporting CBT, it is recommended that CBT be used as a first-line treatment for preschoolers with OCD, but SSRIs may be considered for children whose symptoms persist at a high level and impair functioning after CBT or for those who do not have access to appropriate psychotherapies. These case reports highlight not only the potential for treating preschool OCD with an SSRI but also the high rates of adverse effects and may suggest the value of lower doses. Although the authors report resolution of symptoms with the addition of an atypical antipsychotic agent, the use of pharmacological interventions to treat adverse effects is generally not recommended because of the total lack of data regarding the safety of concurrent administration of more than 1 psychopharmacologic agent in very young children.

The case reports and clinical experience provide anecdotal information regarding SSRI dosing. The OCD case report suggests that dosing as high as 25 mg of sertraline, which is the adult starting dose for PTSD, may increase the risk of adverse effects. Thus, doses as small as 2.5 mg of fluoxetine or 5 mg of sertraline may be appropriate starting doses for very young children with OCD.

Psychopharmacological interventions for PTSD are also understudied. One case series of seven children focused on PTSD and disruptive behaviors. The children received clonidine after intensive treatment in a therapeutic nursery.[106] Clonidine was associated with a reduction in hyperarousal, aggression, and sleep in most children. Doses ranged from 0.05 to 0.15 mg/d, administered by transdermal patches. Although helpful in contributing to our understanding of treatment of disorganized, trauma-exposed preschoolers, the lack of diagnostic specificity limits the study's generalizability to PTSD. There is only one randomized, controlled study of the psychopharmacological treatment of pediatric PTSD, and it did not demonstrate a benefit of sertraline compared to CBT.[107] To date, although SSRIs are recommended for the treatment of school-age and adolescent PTSD, recommending them for preschoolers would require extrapolation from adult systematic studies down to very young children. Thus, medications are not recommended to treat preschool PTSD, although the comorbid conditions may respond to psychopharmacological interventions.

MOOD DISORDERS

Preschool depression has been well studied and characterized as a valid diagnosis, as described by Tandon and colleagues in this issue. It is interesting that for this well-defined disorder, there are no published studies focused on controlled, treatment trials, either psychotherapeutic or psychopharmacological. Experts in preschool major depression recommend dyadic therapy with attention to emotional regulation as the first-line treatment in the absence of any systematic treatment studies. It is very unusual for psychotherapy not to reduce symptoms and improve functioning (J. Luby personal communication, 2007). When a child continues to meet criteria for major depressive disorder and has significant impairment in spite of psychotherapy, psychopharmacological intervention can be considered.

For school-age children and adolescents, there is a stronger empirical base to recommend the use of SSRIs, fluoxetine in particular, than in preschool children to treat major depressive disorder (as reviewed in[108]). Consequently, in rare situations in which psychotherapy does not improve a preschooler's symptoms and impairment to a functional level, fluoxetine can be considered. It is recommended because it is the only SSRI that has been shown to be superior to placebo in school-age children, although sertraline, citalopram, and paroxetine have demonstrated efficacy compared with placebo in adolescents.[103] Therefore, it is the only SSRI with a demonstrable beneficial efficacy-to-safety ratio in school children.[104,108] Extrapolating benefits and safety data from adolescents to preschool children is more problematic than that for school-aged children, and so sertraline, citalopram, and paroxetine would not be recommended for use in preschoolers. A trial of fluoxetine should last 4 to 6 weeks, and doses can be increased every 4 weeks. Treatment effects can be monitored with the Preschool Feelings Checklist.[109] As with children and adolescents, tricyclic antidepressants have not been shown to be effective in treating pediatric depression and have the risk of significant adverse effects including death,[110] and, therefore, they are not recommended in preschoolers.

The issue of a valid diagnosis in preschool populations is fraught with controversy, and no more so than with bipolar disorder.[111] Only one study has systematically addressed the application of the diagnostic criteria for mania in preschoolers.[112] However, rates of prescriptions for atypical antipsychotic agents were increasing rapidly even before the 2006 FDA approval of risperidone for autism-related agitation.[9] Published reports describe the use of medications alone and in combination (up to four medications concomitantly) for children who have been clinically diagnosed with bipolar disorder (**Table 3**).[113,114] When a clinician is considering the diagnosis of bipolar, it is important to apply the diagnostic criteria, with attention to grandiosity, hypersexuality, and elation, which differentiate a group of very impaired children from preschoolers with other disorders.[112] The symptoms of irritability and aggressive

Table 3
Published studies of psychopharmacological treatment of children diagnosed with bipolar disorder

Medication	Study Design	N	Ages (y.mo)	Outcome
Risperidone[117]	Open trial (8 wk)	16	4.0–6.0	18 point decrease on YMRS, 2.2 kg weight gain
Olanzapine[117]	Open trial (8 wk)	15	4.0–6.0	12 point decrease on YMRS 3.2 kg weight gain
Multiple medications (valproate, stimulants, atypical antipsychotic agents)[114]	Retrospective chart review	31	4.0–6.0	20 point decrease on YMRS Not presented
Valproate[123]	Retrospective chart review	9	1.9–5.0	Clinical description of decreased aggression, improved sleeping, decreased oppositional behaviors Not presented
Lithium and carbamazepine[124]	Retrospective chart review	6	3.0–5.11	"Stable", "successfully treated", decreased mood lability Not presented
Carbamazepine[125]	Case report	1	5.2	Improved Not presented
Risperidone, lithium, Topiramate[118]	Case report	1	4.6	On risperidone monotherapy: decreased irritability; with added topiramate: improved sleep, mood stability 15.4 kg weight gain on risperidone

Abbreviation: YMRS, Young Mania Rating Scale.

behaviors alone should not be treated as bipolar disorder.[115] As with other disorders, psychotherapeutic interventions are recommended before considering psychopharmacological interventions for bipolar disorder.[12] To date, there are no systematic studies of psychotherapeutic interventions in preschoolers diagnosed with bipolar disorder, although a trial of a modified parent management training program with a focus on enhancing emotional regulation is underway.[116] Published case reports and retrospective chart reviews describe reductions in symptoms (see review in[12]) when children diagnosed with bipolar disorder are treated with mood stabilizers (eg, valproic acid) or atypical antipsychotic agents (eg, risperidone). One prospective, open trial described the reductions in scores on the Young Mania Rating Scale (YMRS) in children on either risperidone or olanzapine.[117] These reports, as well as other reports focused on risperidone in preschoolers, also highlight the risk of adverse effects with atypical antipsychotic agents, especially prolactin level changes of unclear clinical significance and weight gain (ranging from 2 to 15 kg in 2 months).[40,117,118] The current state of controversy about diagnostic validity, challenges of clinical care, risk of adverse effects from medication, and need for invasive laboratory monitoring all make psychotherapy a safer and preferred treatment for children with extreme emotional and behavioral dysregulation. If psychotherapy fails after a reasonable trial period, expert consultation should be sought to examine the course of treatment and determine if a child continues to have severe impairment and might benefit from a trial of medication.

Only 2 medications have FDA approval for use in juvenile bipolar disorder: lithium, which was approved based on lower standards than prospective FDA evaluations require, and aripiprazole, which was recently approved for pediatric bipolar disorder in children as young as 10 years of age.[111] One randomized, placebo-controlled trial, not listed by the National Library of Medicine's PubMed, demonstrated the superiority of aripiprazole over placebo in children and adolescents with acute mania.[119] In preschoolers, there are more reports using risperidone than aripiprazole, although not necessarily with superior outcomes. Until more evidence is available, risperidone would be recommended as first line, because there is more information about its use in preschoolers. Given the numerous and ominous side effects for atypical antipsychotic agents, including the need for vigilant monitoring of potential adverse effects, such as weight gain, dyslipidemia, and insulin resistance, providers are cautioned about using this class of medications as mere "antiagitation" interventions without strong, clinically supported diagnoses and comprehensive treatment plans addressing contributing psychosocial stressors.[91] Lithium, which has been studied using randomized, controlled trials in children and adolescents, requires frequent laboratory tests and may interfere with toilet training, and so it is not recommended in very young children.[120]

SUMMARY

The assessment and treatment of very young children with severe psychiatric disorders symbolizes the best and worst that child psychiatry has to offer the public: it is an opportunity to improve and alter the development of a number of chronic maladies, but it may be simultaneously creating other, equally serious problems in so doing when relying on pharmacologic interventions alone. Preschool children are incontrovertibly influenced by biological, relational, and environmental etiologic factors, and understudied psychopharmacological interventions should neither be first line nor the exclusive treatment given the relative weight of evidence for safety and efficacy supporting psychotherapeutic interventions for nearly every disorder. In real-world clinical practice, an increasing number of children receive prescriptions as part of their psychiatric treatment. An evidence-informed, judicious approach to psychopharmacological treatment may add to a multimodal psychiatric treatment plan for the severely impaired child left with few other options. Clinicians are encouraged to use a systematic approach to measuring treatment outcomes and to sharing these outcomes through publication of "n of 1" trials, which will add to the knowledge base about early childhood psychiatric disorders.

REFERENCES

1. Smyke AT, Dumitrescu A, Zeanah CH. Attachment disturbances in young children I: the caretaking casualty continuum. J Am Acad Child Adolesc Psychiatry 2002;41(8):972–82.
2. Vitiello BMD. Recent NIMH clinical trials and implications for practice. J Am Acad Child Adolesc Psychiatry 2008;47(12):1369–74.
3. Greenhill LL, Jensen PS, Abikoff H, et al. Developing strategies for psychopharmacological studies in preschool children. J Am Acad Child Adolesc Psychiatry 2003;42(4):406–14.
4. Luby JL, Heffelfinger A, Mrakotsky C, et al. Alterations in stress cortisol reactivity in depressed preschoolers relative to psychiatric and no-disorder comparison groups. Arch Gen Psychiatry 2003;60(12):1248–55.
5. Scheeringa MS, Zeanah CH, Myers L, et al. Heart period and variability findings in preschool children with posttraumatic stress symptoms. Biol Psychiatry 2004;55(7):685–91.
6. Zito JM, Safer DJ, Valluri S, et al. Psychotherapeutic medication prevalence in medicaid-insured preschoolers. J Child Adolesc Psychopharmacol 2007;17(2):195–203.
7. Zito JM, Safer DJ, dosReis S, et al. Trends in the prescribing of psychotropic medications to preschoolers. Journal of the American Medical Association 2000;283(8):1025–30.
8. Zuvekas SH, Vitiello B, Norquist GS. Recent trends in stimulant medication use among U.S. children. Am J Psychiatry 2006;163(4):579–85.
9. Patel NC, Crismon ML, Hoagwood K, et al. Trends in the use of typical and atypical antipsychotics in children and adolescents. J Am Acad Child Adolesc Psychiatry 2005;44(6):548–56.
10. Connor DF. Preschool attention deficit hyperactivity disorder: a review of prevalence, diagnosis, neurobiology, and stimulant treatment. J Dev Behav Pediatr 2002;23:S1–9.
11. Keenan K, Wakschlag LS. More than the terrible twos: the nature and severity of behavior problems in clinic-referred preschool children. J Abnorm Child Psychol 2000;28(1):33–46.
12. Gleason MM, Egger HL, Emslie GJ, et al. Psychopharmacological treatment for very young children: contexts and guidelines. J Am Acad Child Adolesc Psychiatry 2007;46(12):1532–72.
13. Shonkoff JP, Phillips DA. From neurons to neighborhoods: the science of early childhood development committee on integrating the science of early childhood development. Washington, DC: National Academy Press; 2000.
14. Mendelsohn AL, Dreyer BP, Fierman AH, et al. Low-level lead exposure and behavior in early childhood. Pediatrics 1998;101(3):e10.
15. Dawson G, Ashman SB, Panagiotides H, et al. Preschool outcomes of children of depressed mothers: role of maternal behavior, contextual risk, and children's brain activity. Child Dev 2003;74(4):1158–75.

16. Dozier M, Manni M, Gordon M. Foster children's diurnal production of cortisol: an exploratory study. Child Maltreat 2006;11(2):189–97.

17. Dozier M, Peloso E, Lewis E, et al. Effects of an attachment-based intervention on the cortisol production of infants and toddlers in foster care. Dev Psychopathol 2008;20(3):833–49.

18. Nelson CA, Zeanah CH, Fox NA, et al. Cognitive recovery in socially deprived young children: the Bucharest Early Intervention Project. Science 2007; 38(5858):1937–40.

19. APA. Diagnostic and statistical manual of mental disorders IV-TR. 4th edition. Washington, DC: American Psychiatric Association; 2000.

20. Zero to Three Diagnostic Classification Task Force. Diagnostic classification of mental health and development disorders of infancy and early childhood: DC:0-3R. Washington, DC: Zero to Three Press; 2005.

21. Luby JL, Mrakotsky C, Heffelfinger A, et al. Characteristics of depressed preschoolers with and without anhedonia: evidence for a melancholic depressive subtype in young children. Am J Psychiatry 2004;161(11):1998–2004.

22. Lahey BB, Pelham WE, Stein MA, et al. Validity of DSM-IV attention-deficit/hyperactivity disorder for younger children. J Am Acad Child Adolesc Psychiatry 1998;37(7):695–702.

23. Scheeringa MS, Peebles CD, Cook CA, et al. Toward establishing procedural, criterion, and discriminant validity for PTSD in early childhood. J Am Acad Child Adolesc Psychiatry 2001;40(1):52–60.

24. Keenan K, Wakschlag LS. Can a valid diagnosis of disruptive behavior disorder be made in preschool children? Am J Psychiatry 2002;159(3):351–8.

25. Lahey BB, Pelham WE, Loney J, et al. Three-year predictive validity of DSM-IV attention deficit hyperactivity disorder in children diagnosed at 4-6 years of age. Am J Psychiatry 2004;161(11):2014–20.

26. Scheeringa MS, Zeanah CH, Myers L, et al. Predictive validity in a prospective follow-up of PTSD in preschool children. J Am Acad Child Adolesc Psychiatry 2005;44(9):899–906.

27. Harvey E, Youngwirth S, Thakar D, et al. Predicting school-aged ADHD and ODD from preschool diagnostic assessments. J Consult Clin Psychol, in press.

28. Briggs-Gowan MJ, Carter A. Social-emotional screening status in early childhood predicts elementary school outcomes. Pediatrics 2008;121:957–62.

29. Lavigne JV, Arend R, Rosenbaum D, et al. Psychiatric diagnoses with onset in the preschool years: I stability of diagnoses. J Am Acad Child Adolesc Psychiatry 1998;37(12):1246–54.

30. Egger HL. Longitudinal studies in preschool psychopathology (Symposium 11). Paper presented at: 55th Annual Meeting of the American Academy of Child and Adolescent Psychiatry; Chicago (IL); October 20, 2008.

31. Assael BM. Therapeutic orphans: European perspective. Pediatrics 1999; 104(3):591–2.

32. Greenhill LL. The use of psychotropic medication in preschoolers: indications, safety and efficacy. Can J Psychiatry 1998;43:576–81.

33. Ghuman JK, Arnold LE, Anthony BJ. Psychopharmacological and other treatments in preschool children with attention-deficit/hyperactivity disorder: current evidence and practice. J Child Adolesc Psychopharmacol 2008;18(5):413–47.

34. Nasrallah H. Diagnosis 2.0: are mental illnesses diseases, disorders, or syndromes? Curr Psychiatr 2009;8(1):14–6.

35. Kauffman RE. Clinical trials in children: problems and pitfalls. Paediatr Drugs 2000;2(6):411–8.

36. Sharav VH. The impact of the Food and Drug Administration Modernization Act on the recruitment of children for research. Ethical Hum Sci Serv 2003;5(2): 83–108.

37. Beck MH, Cataldo M, Slifer KJ, et al. Teaching children with attention deficit hyperactivity disorder (ADHD) and autistic disorder (AD) how to swallow pills. Clin Pediatr (Phila) 2005;44(6):515–26.

38. Ghuman JK, Cataldo MD, Beck MH, et al. Behavioral training for pill-swallowing difficulties in young children with autistic disorder. J Child Adolesc Psychopharmacol 2004;14(4):601–11.

39. Arnold LE, Lindsay RL, Lopez FA, et al. Treating attention-deficit/hyperactivity disorder with a stimulant transdermal patch: the clinical art. Pediatrics 2007; 120(5):1100–6.

40. Luby J, Mrakotsky C, Stalets MM, et al. Risperidone in preschool children with autistic spectrum disorders: an investigation of safety and efficacy. J Child Adolesc Psychopharmacol 2006;16(5):575–87.

41. Coté CJ. Pediatric anesthesia. In: Miller RD, editor. Miller's anesthesia. 6th edition. Philadelphia: Elsevier; 2005.

42. Barkley RA, Shelton TL. Multi-method Psycho-educational Intervention for Preschool Children with Disruptive Behavior: Preliminary Results at Post-treatment. J Child Psychol Psychiatry 2000;41(3):319–32.

43. Bor W, Sanders MR, Markie-Dadds C. The effects of the Triple P-Positive Parenting Program on preschool children with cooccurring disruptive behavior and attentional/hyperactive difficulties. J Abnorm Child Psychol 2002;30:571.

44. Pelham WE, Fabiano GA. Evidence-based psychosocial treatment for attention-deficit/hyperactivity disorder: an update. J Clin Child Adolesc Psychol 2008;37: 184–214.

45. Taylor EC, Kendall T. In: Attention deficit hyperactivity disorder: diagnosis and management of ADHD in children, young people and adults, vol. 072. National Institute for Health and Clinical Excellence; 2008. p. 1–59.

46. Pliszka S. Practice parameter for the assessment and treatment of children and adolescents with attention-deficit/hyperactivity disorder. J Am Acad Child Adolesc Psychiatry 2007;46(7):894–921.

47. Clinical practice guideline: treatment of the school-aged child with attention-deficit/hyperactivity disorder. J Am Acad Child Adolesc Psychiatry 2002;41(5): 537.

48. Kratochvil CJ, Egger H, Greenhill LL, et al. Pharmacological management of preschool ADHD. J Am Acad Child Adolesc Psychiatry 2006;45(1):115–8.

49. Lahey BB, Applegate B. Validity of DSM-IV ADHD. J Am Acad Child Adolesc Psychiatry 2001;40(5):502–3.

50. Lavigne JV, Binns HJ, Christoffel KK, et al. Behavioral and emotional problems among preschool children in pediatric primary care: prevalence and pediatricians' recognition. Pediatric Practice Research Group. Pediatrics 1993;91(3): 649–55.

51. Wolraich ML. Attention-deficit/hyperactivity disorder: can it be recognized and treated in children younger than 5 years? Infants Young Child 2006;19(2):86–93.

52. Fanton JH, Macdonald B, Harvey EA. Preschool parent-pediatrician consultations and predictive referral patterns for problematic behaviors. J Dev Behav Pediatr 2008.

53. Healey DM, Miller CJ, Castelli KL, et al. The impact of impairment criteria on rates of ADHD diagnoses in preschoolers. J Abnorm Child Psychol 2008; 36(5):771–8.

54. Swanson J, Greenhill L, Wigal T, et al. Stimulant-related reductions of growth rates in the PATS. J Am Acad Child Adolesc Psychiatry 2006;45:1304.

55. Wigal T, Greenhill L, Chuang S, et al. Safety and tolerability of methylphenidate in preschool children with ADHD. J Am Acad Child Adolesc Psychiatry 2006;45:1294.

56. Greenhill LL, Posner K, Vaughan BS, et al. Attention deficit hyperactivity disorder in preschool children. Child Adolesc Psychiatr Clin N Am 2008;17(2):347–66.

57. Greenhill L, Kollins S, Abikoff H, et al. Efficacy and safety of immediate-release methylphenidate treatment for preschoolers with ADHD. J Am Acad Child Adolesc Psychiatry 2006;45(11):1284–93.

58. Vitiello B, Abikoff HB, Chuang SZ, et al. Effectiveness of methylphenidate in the 10-month continuation phase of the Preschoolers with attention-deficit/hyperactivity disorders treatment study (PATS). J Child Adolesc Psychopharmacol 2007;17:593.

59. Kollins S, Greenhill L, Swanson J, et al. Rationale, design, and methods of the Preschool ADHD Treatment Study (PATS). J Am Acad Child Adolesc Psychiatry 2006;45(11):1275–83.

60. Ghuman JK, Riddle MA, Vitiello B, et al. Comorbidity moderates response to methylphenidate in the Preschoolers with Attention-Deficit/Hyperactivity Disorder Treatment Study (PATS). J Child Adolesc Psychopharmacol 2007;17(5):563–79.

61. Kollins S. Outcome results from NIMH, multi-site preschool ADHD treatment study. Paper presented at: Proceedings of the 51st AACAP Annual Meeting, 2004; Washington, DC.

62. Hollon SD, Garber J, Shelton RC. Treatment of depression in adolescents with cognitive behavior therapy and medications: a commentary on the TADS Project. Cogn Behav Pract 2005;12(2):149–55.

63. Barkley RA, Shelton TL, Crosswait C, et al. Multi-method psycho-educational intervention for preschool children with disruptive behavior: preliminary results at post-treatment. J Child Psychol Psychiatry 2000;41:319.

64. Shelton TL, Barkley RA, Crosswait C, et al. Multimethod psychoeducational intervention for preschool children with disruptive behavior: two-year post-treatment follow-up. J Abnorm Child Psychol 2000;28:253.

65. Sonuga-Barke EJ, Daley D, Thompson M, et al. Parent-based therapies for preschool attention-deficit/hyperactivity disorder: a randomized, controlled trial with a community sample. J Am Acad Child Adolesc Psychiatry 2001;40:402.

66. Corrin EG. Child group training versus parent and child group training for young children with ADHD. In: Fairleigh Dickinson U, editor. ProQuest information & learning. p. 3516.

67. McGoey K, DuPaul G, Eckert T, et al. Outcomes of a multi-component intervention for preschool children at-risk for attention-deficit/hyperactivity disorder. Child Fam Behav Ther 2005;27:33.

68. Jones K, Daley D, Hutchings J, et al. Efficacy of the Incredible Years basic parent training programme as an early intervention for children with conduct problems and ADHD. Child Care Health Dev 2007;33:749.

69. Strayhorn JM, Weidman CS. Reduction of attention deficit and internalizing symptoms in preschoolers through parent-child interaction training. J Am Acad Child Adolesc Psychiatry 1989;28:888.

70. Strayhorn JM, Weidman CS. Follow-up one year after parent child interaction training: Effects on behavior of preschool children. J Am Acad Child Adolesc Psychiatry 1991;30:138.

71. Pisterman S, McGrath P, Firestone P, et al. Outcome of parent-mediated treatment of preschoolers with attention deficit disorder with hyperactivity. J Consult Clin Psychol 1989;57:628.

72. Pelham WE. Multimodal Treatment for ADHD: Choosing, Sequencing, and Combining Treatments. Paper presented at: The Fifth Biennial Niagara Conference on Evidence-Based Treatments for Childhood and Adolescent Mental Health Problems, 2007; Niagara-on-the-Lake, Ontario, Canada.

73. Brandon CL, Steiner H. Repeated methylphenidate treatment in adolescent rats alters gene regulation in the striatum. Eur J Neurosci 2003;18(6):1584–92.

74. Kratochvil CJ, Greenhill LL, March JS, et al. The role of stimulants in the treatment of preschool children with attention-deficit hyperactivity disorder. CNS Drugs 2004;18(14):957–66.

75. Firestone P, Musten LM, Pisterman S, et al. Short-term side effects of stimulant medication are increased in preschool children with attention-deficit/hyperactivity disorder: a double-blind placebo-controlled study. J Child Adolesc Psychopharmacol 1998;8:13.

76. Schleifer M, Weiss G, Cohen N, et al. Hyperactivity in preschoolers and effect of methylphenidate. Am J Orthop 1975;45:38.

77. Barkley RA, Karlsson J, Strzelecki E, et al. Effects of age and ritalin dosage on the mother-child interactions of hyperactive children. J Consult Clin Psychol 1984;52:750.

78. Witt KL, Shelby MD, Itchon-Ramos N, et al. Methylphenidate and amphetamine do not induce cytogenetic damage in lymphocytes of children with ADHD. J Am Acad Child Adolesc Psychiatry 2008;47(12):1375–83.

79. Biederman J, Spencer TJ, Wilens TE, et al. Treatment of ADHD with stimulant medications: response to nissen perspective in the New England Journal of Medicine. J Am Acad Child Adolesc Psychiatry 2006;45(10):1147–50.

80. Couric K. What killed Rebecca Riley? Katie Couric Reports on the Diagnosis of Bipolar Disorder In Kids. 60 Minutes; September 20, 2007.

81. Kratochvil CJ, Vaughan BS, Mayfield-Jorgensen ML, et al. A pilot study of atomoxetine in young children with attention-deficit/hyperactivity disorder. J Child Adolesc Psychopharmacol 2007;17:175.

82. Ghuman J. Atomoxetine Pilot Study in Preschoolers with ADHD. Available at: clinicaltrials.gov. 2008.

83. Newcorn JH, Kratochvil CJ, Allen AJ, et al. Atomoxetine and osmotically released methylphenidate for the treatment of attention deficit hyperactivity disorder: acute comparison and differential response. Am J Psychiatry 2008; 165(6):721–30.

84. Luby JL. Psychopharmacology of psychiatric disorders in the preschool period. J Child Adolesc Psychopharmacol 2007;17(2):149–52.

85. Kaminski JW, Valle LA, Filene JH, et al. A meta-analytic review of components associated with parent training program effectiveness. J Abnorm Child Psychol 2008;36(4):567–89.

86. Thomas R, Zimmer-Gembeck MJ. Behavioral outcomes of Parent-Child Interaction Therapy and Triple P-Positive Parenting Program: a review and meta-analysis. J Abnorm Child Psychol 2007;35(3):475–95.

87. Hood KK, Eyberg SM. Outcomes of parent-child interaction therapy: mothers' reports of maintenance three to six years after treatment. J Clin Child Adolesc Psychol 2003;32(3):419–30.

88. Hamilton SS, Armando J. Oppositional defiant disorder. Am Fam Physician 2008;78(7):861–6.

89. Connor DF, Boone RT, Steingard RJ. Psychopharmacology and aggression: II. A meta-analysis of nonstimulant medication effects on overt aggression-related behaviors in youth with SED. J Emot Behav Disord 2003;11(3):157–68.

90. Cesena M, Gonzalez-Heydrich J, Szigethy E, et al. A case series of eight aggressive young children treated with risperidone. J Child Adolesc Psychopharmacol 2002;12(4):337–45.

91. AACAP. Practice parameters for use of atypical antipsychotic agents. J Am Acad Child Adolesc Psychiatry, in press.

92. Egger HL. Diagnostic assessment of a young child presenting with anxiety symptoms. Paper presented at: 55th Meeting of the American Academy of Child and Adolescent Psychiatry; Chicago, IL; October 28, 2008.

93. Egger HL, Angold A. Common emotional and behavioral disorders in preschool children: presentation, nosology, and epidemiology. J Child Psychol Psychiatry 2006;47(3–4):313–37.

94. DeBar LL, Lynch F, Powell J, et al. Use of psychotropic agents in preschool children: associated symptoms, diagnoses, and health care services in a health maintenance organization. Arch Pediatr Adolesc Med 2003;157(2):150–7.

95. Luby JL, Stalets M, Belden A. Psychotropic prescriptions in a sample including both healthy and mood and disruptive disordered preschoolers: relationships to diagnosis, impairment, prescriber type, and assessment methods. J Child Adolesc Psychopharmacol 2007;17(2):205–15.

96. Scheeringa MS, Salloum A, Arnberger RA, et al. Feasibility and effectiveness of cognitive-behavioral therapy for posttraumatic stress disorder in preschool children: two case reports. J Trauma Stress 2007;20(4):631–6.

97. RUPP Anxiety Study. Fluvoxamine for the treatment of anxiety disorders in children and adolescents. N Engl J Med 2001;344:1279–85.

98. Wright HH, Cuccaro ML, Leonhardt TV, et al. Case study: fluoxetine in the multimodal treatment of a preschool child with selective mutism. J Am Acad Child Adolesc Psychiatry 1995;34(7):857–62.

99. Avci A, Diler RS, Tamam L. Fluoxetine treatment in a 2.5-year-old girl. J Am Acad Child Adolesc Psychiatry 1988;37(9):901–2.

100. Walkup JT, Albano AM, Piacentini J, et al. Cognitive behavioral therapy, sertraline, or a combination in childhood anxiety. N Engl J Med 2008;359(26): 2835–6.

101. Walkup JT, Labellarte MJ, Riddle MA, et al. Fluvoxamine for the treatment of anxiety disorders in children and adolescents. N Engl J Med 2001;344(17): 1279–85.

102. Birmaher BM, Axelson DA, Monk KR, et al. Fluoxetine for the treatment of childhood anxiety disorders. J Am Acad Child Adolesc Psychiatry 2003;42(4): 415–23.

103. Bridge JA, Iyengar S, Salary CB, et al. Clinical response and risk for reported suicidal ideation and suicide attempts in pediatric antidepressant treatment: a meta-analysis of randomized controlled trials. JAMA 2007; 297(15):1683–96.

104. Whittington C, Kendall T, Fonagy P, et al. Selective serotonin reuptake inhibitors in childhood depression: a systematic review of published and non-published data. Lancet 2004;363:1341–5.

105. Oner O, Oner P. Psychopharmacology of pediatric obsessive-compulsive disorder: three case reports. J Psychopharmacol 2008;22(7):809–11.

106. Harmon RJ, Riggs PD. Clonidine for posttraumatic stress disorder in preschool children. J Am Acad Child Adolesc Psychiatry 1999;35(9):1247–9.

107. Cohen JA, Mannarino AP, Perel J, et al. A pilot randomized controlled trial of combined trauma-focused CBT and sertraline for childhood PTSD symptoms. J Am Acad Child Adolesc Psychiatry 2007;46(7):811–9.

108. AACAP. Practice parameter for the assessment and treatment of children and adolescents with depressive disorders. J Am Acad Child Adolesc Psychiatry 2007;46(11):1504–26.
109. Luby JL, Heffelfinger A, Koenig-McNaught AL, et al. The Preschool Feelings Checklist: a brief and sensitive screening measure for depression in young children. J Am Acad Child Adolesc Psychiatry 2004;43(6):708–16.
110. Caksen H, Akbayram S, Odabas D, et al. Acute amitriptyline intoxication: an analysis of 44 children. Hum Exp Toxicol 2006;25(3):107–10.
111. AACAP. Practice parameter for the assessment and treatment of children and adolescents with bipolar disorder. J Am Acad Child Adolesc Psychiatry 2007; 46(1):107–25.
112. Luby JL, Belden A. Defining and validating bipolar disorder in the preschool period. Dev Psychopathol 2006;18(4):971–88.
113. Danielyan A, Pathak S, Kowatch RA, et al. Clinical characteristics of bipolar disorder in very young children. J Affect Disord 2007;97(1–3):51.
114. Scheffer RE, Niskala, Apps JA. The diagnosis of preschool bipolar disorder presenting with mania: open pharmacological treatment. J Affect Disord 2004; 82(Suppl 1):S25–34.
115. Quinn CA, Fristad MA. Defining and identifying early onset bipolar spectrum disorder. Curr Psychiatry Rep 2004;6(2):101–7.
116. Luby JL, Stalets M, Blankenship S, et al. Treatment of preschool bipolar disorder: A novel parent-child interaction therapy and review of data on psychopharmacology. In: Geller B, Delbello MP, editors. Treatment of Childhood Bipolar Disorder; in press.
117. Biederman J, Mick E, Hammerness P, et al. Open-Label, 8-Week trial of olanzapine and risperidone for the treatment of bipolar disorder in preschool-age children. Biol Psychiatry 2005;58(7):589.
118. Pavuluri MN, Janicak PG, Carbray JA. Topiramate plus risperidone for controlling weight gain and symptoms in preschool mania. J Child Adolesc Psychopharmacol 2002;12(3):271–3.
119. Bristol-Meyers Squibb. Abilify prescribing information. Tokyo 2008.
120. Hagino OR, Weller EB, Weller RA, et al. Untoward effects of lithium treatment in children aged four through six years. J Am Acad Child Adolesc Psychiatry 1995; 34(12):1584–90.
121. Hanna GL, Feibusch EL, Albright KJ. Buspirone treatment of anxiety associated with pharyngeal dysphagia in a four-year-old. Pediatr Crit Care Med 2005;6(6): 676–81.
122. Meighen KB, Hines LA, Lagges AM. Risperidone treatment of preschool children with thermal burns and acute stress disorder. J Child Adolesc Psychopharmacol 2007;17(2):223–32.
123. Mota-Castillo M, Torruella A, Engels B, et al. Valproate in very young children: an open case series with a brief follow-up. J Affect Disord 2001;67:193–7.
124. Tumuluru RV, Weller EB, Fristad MA, et al. Mania in six preschool children. J Child Adolesc Psychopharmacol 2003;4:489–94.
125. Tuzun U, Zoroglu SS, Savas HA. A 5-year-old boy with recurrent mania successfully treated with carbamazepine. Psychiatry Clin Neurosci 2002;56(5):589.

Infant Mental Health and the "Real World"-Opportunities for Interface and Impact

Paula D. Zeanah, PhD, MSN[a],*, Letia O. Bailey, MSW[a], Susan Berry, MD, MPH[b]

KEYWORDS

- Infant mental health • Preventive interventions
- Evidence-based practices

The term "infant mental health" (IMH) may conjure up the image of an infant on a couch "talking" to a therapist, but the relatively new field of IMH is notable for its strong interdisciplinary integration of clinical and research activities. A well-established and growing literature recognizes the importance of early childhood experience not only to later health and development[1–4] but also to alleviation of current distress or suffering[5–7] and to the quality of significant relationships throughout life. Although nationally representative epidemiologic studies regarding the prevalence of early childhood disorders are not yet available, recent data suggest that even toddlers and preschoolers can experience internalizing and externalizing disorders at rates comparable to older children.[8]

Perhaps the most important aspect of infant and early childhood mental health is the contribution of the parent-child relationship context to social, emotional, behavioral, cognitive, and even physical development. Symptom presentation is often closely tied to parents' and children's experiences of being with the other. The parent's ability to be nurturing, responsive, consistent, and to provide a physically and emotionally safe environment is a factor that shapes the infant's external and internal experience. Parental experience is affected not only by the physical characteristics and needs of the child and the child's responsiveness to the parent but also by the immediate circumstances that affect parental functioning. Poverty and lack of basic resources,[9,10] domestic violence or previous trauma history,[11] maternal depression and other mental health issues,[12,13] and the parent's own history of being parented all can affect, directly or indirectly, the relationship quality of the infant and parent.

[a] Department of Psychiatry and Neurology, Tulane University School of Medicine, Tulane University Institute of Infant and Early Childhood Mental Health, 1440 Canal Street, TB 52, New Orleans, LA 70112, USA
[b] Louisiana State University Health Sciences Center, 200 Henry Clay Avenue, LA 70118, USA
* Corresponding author. 1440 Canal Street, TB 52, New Orleans, LA 70112.
E-mail address: pzeanah@tulane.edu (P.D. Zeanah).

Child Adolesc Psychiatric Clin N Am 18 (2009) 773–787
doi:10.1016/j.chc.2009.03.006
1056-4993/09/$ – see front matter © 2009 Elsevier Inc. All rights reserved.

The opportunity for prevention and early intervention is appealing and motivating for many professionals who enter the field of IMH. Yet the vast majority of infants and their caregivers never encounter a child mental health professional, much less one trained and skilled in IMH assessments and interventions. Children presenting with symptoms are most likely to be seen in pediatric health care, child care, or early education settings; caregivers who have social or mental health needs that affect caregiving are most likely to be seen in adult health, adult mental health, or social service settings. With some exceptions, these settings typically do not interface with one another. Because these settings have different priorities and approaches to services and service delivery, the opportunity to understand and "work with" the parent-infant relationship as part of interventions is likely to be missed. Thus, one of the great challenges for the field of IMH is the need for an array of integrated services that can meet the varied needs of infants and their caregivers and that can support healthy, nurturing relationships.

In this issue, investigators have presented a number of approaches to assessment and treatment of disorders in infancy and early childhood. In this article, we begin with a definition and brief discussion of the scope of IMH. We provide a framework that guides our perspective on IMH services, which occur for the most part outside of traditional psychiatric settings. Examples of general and specific models of care that hold promise for expanding access to services and support to our youngest children and their families are presented, including detailed descriptions of one preventive and two IMH treatment programs that developed in community settings. These mostly nontraditional approaches provide great opportunities not only to impact a larger number of individuals of infants and their families but also to provide opportunities from "lessons learned." Finally, implications for policy and future service development are discussed.

DEFINITION AND SCOPE OF IMH

As implied in the opening statement, there is often discomfort with the idea that infants and young children may have "mental health problems." This in part is the result of stigma associated with mental illness as well as lack of knowledge about how infants know and experience their world.[3] In this article, we use the terms "IMH" and "early childhood mental health" interchangeably and consider the target age range for this field to begin during pregnancy and continue until the child is 5 to 6 years of age.[1,4]

Infant mental health is defined as "the young child's capacity to experience, regulate, and express emotions, form close and secure relationships, and explore the environment and learn... in the context of the caregiving environment that includes family, community, and cultural expectations for young children."[14]

Several points need to be highlighted here. First, the purview of IMH is both the promotion of healthy development (prevention and early intervention) as well as interventions that seek to minimize or eliminate emerging or actual problems in social, emotional, cognitive, and behavioral development. Second, the importance of infant experience in context, especially the context of the infant-caregiver relationship, is emphasized. It is through the infant's relationship with his or her caregiver that the infant begins to understand himself, himself with others, and the world around him. Finally, the focus on family, community, and cultural influences on IMH underscores the importance of understanding intergenerational influences on parenting as well as risk and protective factors that can be identified and modified to ensure the most positive long-term outcomes.

The overarching goals of IMH are to reduce or eliminate suffering in a child with mental health problems, to prevent adverse outcomes, and to promote healthy outcomes by enhancing social competence and resilience. Extrapolating from those overarching goals, we believe all services serving very young children and their families must (1) enhance the ability of caregivers to effectively care for and nurture young children; (2) ensure that families in need of additional services and/or instrumental resources can obtain them; and (3) increase the ability of all those who work with infants, young children, and their families to identify, address, and prevent social-emotional problems in early childhood.[15]

FRAMEWORK FOR IMH SERVICES

Models of IMH in nontraditional mental health settings draw on the experiences of integrating mental health services for older patients into medical or educational settings. We present one example of a traditional approach before discussing newer innovations of providing IMH services. A commonly used traditional approach to incorporating mental health services into nonmental health settings is psychiatric consultation liaison. Typically associated with school and hospital settings, this problem-focused approach includes a limited assessment thorough enough to determine pertinent issues and a short-term intervention or set of recommendations for the primary providers. If additional or comprehensive care is required, the consultant may make recommendations back to the consultee to carry out, make referrals to other providers as necessary, or provide the ongoing care. A significant role for the consultant is providing liaison services, including guidance, education, and support to the consultee. To be successful, the consultant needs to understand the "question behind the (referral) question." This requires being familiar with the "cultural context" of the consultee, including the language, goals, priorities, and needs of the service or agency. Sometimes the clinical question is intertwined with transference or counter-transference, boundary, or other interpersonal issues, which also must be addressed. Thus, the consultant must take the time to develop relationships with the consultee and to develop a meta-understanding of the context in which services take place. In IMH consultations, clinicians attend to the many levels of relationships—their own relationship with the consultee, with the patient, and the caregiver-infant relationship.

Specifically in IMH, the emphasis in intervention focuses on altering infant and parent behaviors and family functioning to preserve (prevention) or restore (treatment) infants to more normative developmental trajectories. In many cases, an IMH program may include all levels of intervention, including universal interventions, targeted preventive interventions, and specific treatment. In IMH, the distinction between prevention and treatment is often muddied, as treatment may in fact prevent later problems.[16] Next, we provide examples of specific IMH services within each "level of care" and describe one preventive intervention and two treatment models in greater detail.

Universal Interventions

Universal services seek to avert or prevent onset of problems and to enhance social-emotional development. Examples in IMH include education regarding normal infant health and development and healthy parent-infant relationships and providing access or referral to additional services as needed. They are considered to be important for all infants and families, with or without risk, and can be generated in a variety of settings.

Medical homes are one potential avenue for providing preventive mental health care. The American Academy of Pediatrics (AAP) defines the medical home model of delivering primary care as accessible, continuous, comprehensive, family-centered, coordinated, compassionate, and culturally effective care.[17] The specifics of implementation of the medical model vary and are described on the AAP Web site (www. aap.org). Strategies for addressing mental health issues are not well described yet, but screening and referral and coordination with educational, developmental, and other supportive services are part of this model.[18]

An example of universal prevention that incorporates features of early childhood mental health in health care is the Bright Futures program.[19] Bright Futures is "a set of principles, strategies, and tools that are theory based and systems oriented that can be used to improve health and well-being of all children." Bright Futures was initiated in 1990 with federal funding, including Health Resources and Services Administration, Maternal Child Health Bureau with later support from the Department of Health and Human Services, and Centers for Medicare and Medicaid Services.[19] Currently, the implementation of the project is under the auspices of the AAP, and the tools can be accessed at www.brightfutures.aap.org.

The Bright Futures Health Supervision Guidelines for well-child care focus on factors that increase attention to and quality of IMH using a developmentally based, family-centered, strength-based approach. In addition to incorporating family community and social-cultural issues, Bright Futures also directly addresses the child's psychosocial functioning by recommending screening, brief interventions such as counseling or education, and referral as necessary.[20] The Bright Futures program provides practical tools, including handouts for parents, guidelines for clinicians, and office-management approaches that support the integration of mental health care attention in primary care settings.

A more specific approach to addressing social-emotional development is the ABCD II initiative, supported by the Commonwealth Fund (Utah, California, Illinois, Iowa, and Minnesota).[21] This model focused on low-income children via well-child visits. Goals of the initiative included training primary care providers, improving screening of social-emotional development, improving referrals, and increasing links to and collaboration with community partners. Pediatricians used validated, standardized screening tools, but they were less likely to use them if referral sources were not available. A number of strategies aimed at improving referral networks and developing work groups and partnerships to improve practice and strengthen policy strategies were identified. All 5 states made progress toward the goals of developing state-specific programs, which included training for providers on specific screening techniques, toolkits for beginning screening projects, support in identifying referral agencies, networking among primary care providers, and policy initiatives to address reimbursement barriers to care.[21] Future research should examine the impact of screening and identification of early childhood mental health problems on improved mental health outcomes for these young children.

High-quality child care, defined more than a decade ago by Scarr,[22] includes supportive, responsively contingent, and developmentally appropriate interactions with adults in a safe, healthy, and stimulating environment. Quality child care for all children is another example of a universal intervention that can promote IMH. In a large, multisite, prospective, longitudinal study by the National Institute of Child Health and Development, investigators found that quality of care was related to cognitive and language outcomes as well as social and behavioral outcomes in young children.[23] Interventions to enhance early child care quality are underway (eg,[24]), and early data demonstrate positive effects of these interventions on teachers and children.[25] Mental health consultation programs for child care setting are among the few factors that may be protective against child care expulsions.

These examples highlight some of the efforts that have potential to improve the early development of all children. It is important to point out, however, that universal early childhood mental health interventions must be accompanied by the availability of basic needs, such as safe housing, appropriate nutrition, and general health and human services. If these are not available, a broad community effort may be needed to establish such services.

Selective Interventions

Selective interventions are provided to families and their young children who are "at risk" for poorer social and emotional outcomes. Within the "at-risk" group, some individuals may have no evidence of problems; for others, difficulties may be emerging or apparent. The type, structure, intensity and place of service, strategies, and targeted outcomes are variable, but usually outcomes are monitored or measured.

One selective intervention that has received national and international attention is the Nurse Family Partnership (NFP). Developed by David Olds and his colleagues, this home visitation program targets first-time, low-income mothers. Highly trained, experienced registered nurses begin working with mothers before the 28th week of pregnancy and meet with the mother, and then mother and infant, on an approximately weekly or biweekly basis until the infant turns age 2 years. Based on attachment, human ecology, and social learning theories, NFP has three major goals: to improve pregnancy health outcomes, to improve infant health and development outcomes, and to improve maternal life course development. Actual and potential problems are addressed, but specific goals are client driven, and the approach is to identify and build upon client strengths to garner personal and family/community resources. The development of a trusting, dependable, positive nurse-client relationship is crucial to the success of the intervention. For each visit, the nurses use manualized guidelines to address personal health, environmental health, quality of caregiving for the infant, maternal life course development, and use of family and community support systems. Nurses provide guidance and psychosocial support as well as appropriate medical and mental health referrals and assistance with navigating complicated health and social systems. Interventions and outcomes are tracked over time to monitor fidelity to the model as well as selected outcomes. Through a series of randomized, controlled trials, NFP has demonstrated significant impact across a variety of maternal and infant health and social outcomes, including reduction in child maltreatment, serious accidental injuries in children, delays in subsequent pregnancies, and increased maternal employment, as well as reductions in child and maternal criminal and antisocial behaviors as long as 15 years after program completion.[26–30] In addition, some studies have shown that the NFP is highly cost beneficial.[31,32] A strength of this program is that the research has demonstrated effectiveness in "real-world" settings rather than highly controlled research environments.

In our experience in Louisiana, many of the families served by NFP have significant psychosocial and mental health issues, including, but not limited to, family and community violence, trauma, personality and family issues, as well as depression and other diagnosed (and undiagnosed) mental health disorders. Because of inadequate community mental health services available, we developed a mental health model that includes two major components. First, all NFP nurses in Louisiana receive an in-depth (30 hour) training in IMH, which includes social-emotional development, attachment theory and classifications, cultural and ethnic aspects of parenting, infant psychopathology, general assessment of perinatal and IMH problems, brief interventions, and attention to transference and countertransference issues. In addition, a licensed mental health professional with IMH training provides consultation, education, support, and guidance to the nurses via case conferences, team meetings, and individual consultation. The consultant also provides direct services to families, in the home, including assessment, intervention, and referrals as needed. The mental health consultant is considered part of the NFP "team," and the nurses and consultant work closely together to coordinate activities. More systematic research is needed, but the model is well-accepted and valued among the teams who have the consultation available.[33,34]

Indicated Preventive Interventions

Indicated preventive interventions are those that target young children or parents who are already displaying symptoms but have not yet reached the level of a diagnosable disorder. Thus, the emphasis is on preventing the symptoms from becoming clinical disorders.

A number of studies have shown that perinatal depression is related to significant negative effects on caregiver functioning as well as infant outcomes in the cognitive, behavioral, developmental, and medical domains.[35] Even when depressive symptoms do not meet diagnostic criteria for major depression, they can be associated with negative infant outcomes. Thus, pregnant and postpartum women with symptoms of depression are an important group for indicated preventive interventions. For these parents, interventions that include infant massage, music, and interaction coaching are associated with improved parent-infant interactions.[36,37] Despite the growing evidence base supporting interventions for depressed mothers,[35] more studies are needed on impact of early intervention on women with symptoms of depression during the perinatal period.

Another example of an indicated intervention is the work of van den Boom.[38] She designed an intervention for children at risk for insecure attachment because of irritable temperament. Using a randomized, controlled trial targeting low-income Dutch mothers with 6- 9-month-old infants, the intervention included three home visits designed to increase maternal sensitivity to infant cues. By the end of the program, intervention mothers were significantly more responsive, stimulating, and visually attentive to their infants, and by age 12 months, their infants were more likely to be securely attached compared with control infants.[38,39] Follow-up studies have shown similar promising results.[40]

As can be seen from the above examples, successful preventive interventions can take many forms and can be implemented in a variety of early childhood settings, including the home, and are often implemented by nonmental health providers with support from mental health professionals.

TREATMENT: DEVELOPMENT OF INTERVENTION PROGRAMS IN THE "REAL WORLD"

Even in early childhood, some children experience mental health problems that require interventions. For these children, developing a successful treatment model requires collaborative planning, coordination, and often, funding across federal, state, and local entities and availability of services in multiple early childhood settings (eg, child's medical home, community mental health centers, educational settings, and family environments). In this section, we describe two treatment models developed to treat very young children in Louisiana, where poor child health outcomes have spurred the development of innovative preventive and early intervention programs at both the state and local levels. We discuss program development as well as program implementation and outcomes to highlight the many "real-world" factors that can influence IMH program development.

INFANT MENTAL HEALTH IN A COMMUNITY HEALTH CLINIC: HEALTHY BEGINNINGS

Healthy Beginnings, an IMH services program colocated in a city health department clinic, was developed in response to a needs assessment that highlighted the need for early childhood mental health services. The New Orleans City Health Department clinic leaders recognized that the city health system addressed preventive maternal and pediatric health care needs well, but behavioral and mental health needs were largely undetected and unaddressed (S. Berry, personal communication, 2001). Community mental health centers available for older children and adolescents did not provide services for infants and young children. In response to the needs assessment, the Health Department partnered with Tulane University and the Louisiana Office of Public Health to create Healthy Beginnings, a clinically sound, ecologically valid, and integrated system of medical and mental health care. The purpose of this government-academic collaborative project was three-fold: to enhance the mental health of infants and young children of New Orleans through prevention and treatment; to train and educate health and mental health professionals about mental health issues in infants, children, and their families; and to contribute to the IMH knowledge base through clinical research.

Healthy Beginnings targeted children, ages birth to 5 years, and their families who received their health care through the New Orleans City Health Department. The clinic served a very low-income, urban population that was more than 90% African American. By providing mental health services in the City Health Department Clinics, patients in need of IMH services could be identified and referred seamlessly to the IMH clinic on-site by the nurse or primary care physician during regular health care visits. This colocated model allowed the IMH team, the physicians, and the nurses to develop an integrated service delivery model of physical and mental health in an environment that was familiar and accessible to families.

Funding was secured through a private local foundation, and the project represented a collaborative effort among five partners, including Tulane University School of Medicine's Section of Child Psychiatry, the New Orleans City Health Department, the Louisiana State Office of Public Health, the Louisiana State Office of Mental Health, and the Children's Bureau of New Orleans, a nonprofit United Way partner agency. Each collaborator contributed important components of the project, including in-kind services, such as office space to house the project, staff to manage referrals and scheduling of clients, and funding and staff for training, clinical, and administrative supervision. All collaborators participated in the guidance and oversight for the project.

Services included IMH assessment and therapeutic interventions, including psychiatric treatment and case management intended to optimize family functioning (eg, housing, food, clothing, transportation). Clinical services included a range of evidence-based therapies, including parent-child psychotherapies, individual insight-oriented psychotherapy, play therapy, and psychopharmacological intervention. A unique aspect of Healthy Beginnings was the ability to address maternal mental health issues, including mild-moderate depression, in the context of the program, using psychotherapeutic as well as psychopharmacological interventions.

All Healthy Beginnings clinicians received training in IMH and supervision by a clinician with extensive IMH experience. In addition, the health clinic staff, including nurses, physicians, and key administrators for the project, received a 30-hour training in IMH during the first year of the project to enhance identification and referral of infants and young children. The IMH and clinic staff, as well as collaboration partners, participated in additional formal training to heighten recognition of racial and class differences within and between providers and those served and begin to bridge differences that could arise from culture-based misunderstandings.

Because Healthy Beginnings represented an innovative approach to infant mental services, it included a research component to evaluate the program systematically. One research question compared the feasibility and effectiveness of clinic versus home-based clinical assessment and intervention. The initial clinical assessment protocol included at least one home visit and at least one health clinic visit for each family, standardized interviews and a parent-child interaction procedure, and standardized symptom checklists addressing infant/child behavior problems and competencies, maternal depression, and partner violence. Clients were to be randomly assigned to either home or clinic-based care after the assessment period.

Early on, it became clear that families would not accept randomization to clinic or home-based services for a variety of reasons. Many families maintained strong opinions about where they preferred to receive services. There were practical barriers to providing clinic-based services, including lack of reliable transportation and the costs and difficulties of using public transportation with young children. Though transportation vouchers were provided for cab fare, the majority of families (about two-thirds) preferred home-based services. On the other hand, barriers to providing home-based services included risks and/or safety concerns associated with a client's home (eg, domestic violence and active substance abuse) or neighborhood and families' discomfort with having clinicians enter their homes due to privacy or cultural issues. Individualizing location of service provision became the program approach.

Also, there was disagreement among the multidisciplinary IMH staff regarding the assessment battery that was developed to address research questions, including baseline data, presenting problems, and use and impact of services. It became apparent that varied training both across and within disciplines translated into a range of viewpoints about how to begin working with clients. Some clinicians felt that the approximate 3-hour battery was too long for clients who experienced numerous chronic life stressors and had inconsistent follow through with keeping IMH appointments. They felt that a long assessment process would delay treatment, interfere with developing a therapeutic alliance, and would interrupt a psychotherapeutic principle of "beginning where the client is." Other clinicians felt that it was important to obtain a baseline assessment to clarify and understand the issues before beginning formal treatment and that the systematic assessment process could be carried out without interfering with developing an alliance with the family. Ultimately, the team administered structured measures within a time frame that met the needs of each specific family and allowed the clinician to develop a positive therapeutic relationship with the family. This compromise allowed effective data gathering and service delivery to this high-risk population.

In addition, Healthy Beginnings faced a number of challenges both during the initial phases of development and in ongoing implementation of the program. Even with well-received formal and informal cross-system training and improvement in IMH knowledge, many of the health clinic staff seemed uncomfortable talking about relevant mental health issues, and they sometimes avoided telling clients why they were being referred to the "program down the hall." Consequently, the IMH team often did not receive completed referrals and often were at a loss to understand the nature of the presenting concern during the initial interview with the family. Additionally, given the stigma of mental health clinics within the community, many families initially declined to participate in IMH services when they learned more about the nature of the services. Thus, the IMH team made it a practice to include the clinic nurse supervisor and/or the pediatrician into weekly IMH case conferences to increase communication, reduce traditional disciplinary boundaries, allow the Healthy Beginnings team to gain better understanding of the presenting problem, and to involve the health clinic staff in developing a sensitive plan for discussing mental health services with the family.

Another clinical challenge in implementing Health Beginnings was the rate of maternal mental health problems, in particular depression, which was nearly 60% of those served based on screening measures[41] (Bellow S, Zeanah P, Larrieu J, et al: Healthy Beginnings Annual Summary, Tulane University, unpublished report, 2004). Because of the significant impact of maternal depression on early child development[35,36] and recent findings that improvement in maternal depression is associated with decreases in child symptoms[41] and may facilitate treatment engagement, treatment for mothers was considered a priority. However, access to local public mental health resources was extremely limited due to the requirements of high acuity (typically serving only the chronically and severely mental ill) and long waiting lists. Thus, the program began to include treatment of caregiver depression as 1 important avenue to optimize interventions to young children.

Healthy Beginnings became a successful partner in the community. All agency partners and health clinic staff supported the program from the outset enthusiastically. Everyone agreed that such services were needed, and there was a synergy among the partners and a strong commitment to the success of the program. The ability to provide services at the point of entry in the health care system enabled families and staff to become more familiar with early childhood behavioral and emotional issues and improved coordination with and access to other services. In addition, the flexibility to offer services in the home or the clinic increased the ability to provide individualized, safe, and salient services to clients. The importance of a strong relationship context between parents and infants, within the program, and across services, and between collaborative partners, was repeatedly reinforced. Finally, the program was re-funded for a second 2-year period, allowing adequate time for the program to develop further and adapt to administrative challenges, such as some staff turnover and moving from one health clinic to another.[41]

When the funding period for Healthy Beginnings ended, the IMH-trained clinicians, case managers, and leadership team were uniquely poised to continue providing IMH services. Because an existing state-funded early childhood initiative had selected New Orleans as a new site for serving low-income families, the Healthy Beginnings team was able to join this program and continue working with the same population of clients. Thus, this new initiative gave the Healthy Beginnings team the opportunity to grow and evolve into a larger program that could serve more individuals and families.

INFANT MENTAL HEALTH IN A COMMUNITY NETWORK: EARLY CHILDHOOD SUPPORTS AND SERVICES

Recognizing the need for early identification and intervention of social, emotional, and behavioral problems, the Louisiana Office of Mental Health developed Early Childhood Supports and Services (ECSS), a model of care specifically targeting high-risk, low-income families with children ages birth through 5 years. The Office of Mental Health partnered with the Department of Social Services to fund ECSS, and currently nine ECSS teams operate across the state of Louisiana.

The ECSS model strives to identify and mitigate conditions for young children who are affected by psychosocial risk factors (eg, abuse, neglect, exposure to violence, parental mental illness, parental substance abuse, poverty, and/or developmental disability). Major goals of the program include (1) establishing local multiagency networks that serve high-risk families with young children to enable identification, screening, and referral for potential services; (2) supporting families by addressing basic needs through case management and referral (eg, assistance in finding adequate housing, obtaining suitable childcare, providing emergency funds for unanticipated financial crises, and so on); and (3) providing mental health services to children and families in need. A hallmark of the ECSS model is the partnership of local community agencies to develop and integrate a comprehensive system of care for young children and their families. ECSS's partners may include any local agencies and service providers who interact with families who have young children, such as Head Start and Early Head Start, Education, Mental Health, Public Health, Addictive Disorders, Community Services and child protection, Family Support, and Developmental Disabilities[42] (Louisiana Office of Mental Health: Early Childhood Supports and Services, unpublished report, 2002).

Children and families enter the ECSS system through a Network partner, from whom they often receive services. Families meet with representatives from participating agencies for an interagency staffing and a comprehensive service plan is developed to address problems that may interfere with family functioning. The process is family driven, and families may decline to participate in any ECSS service that is recommended to them; they may consent to case management services only, IMH services only, or to both.

The IMH service component includes evaluation, care coordination, and treatment. Each child referred for IMH services receives an initial evaluation by a child psychiatrist. Standardized parent report and observational assessments focused on the child and the parent-child interactions are conducted with the family before initiating treatment. Home and clinic-based services include parent support, evidence-based parent-management training, play therapy, and parent-child dyadic therapies. Children may also be followed by a child psychiatrist, and a small proportion may receive pharmacotherapy. All professionals and paraprofessionals on the IMH team receive specialized training in the field of IMH. When treatment of one or more caregivers or a noneligible older sibling is indicated, that person is referred for services to one of the participating ECSS Network Agencies. In the event that urgent family needs cannot be met through the community partners, ECSS also has access to "Emergency Intervention" Temporary Assistance for Needy Families funds, which are allocated for emergencies to meet nonrecurrent, short-term financial needs (eg, childcare expenses, rent, utilities, food, furniture, appliances, and so on) to address basic needs as well as factors that interfere with the child's mental health.

In sum, families referred to ECSS can receive one or a combination of services, including case management and coordination of social services, use of emergency intervention funds as necessary, IMH screening and assessment, and intervention and treatment. In a preliminary evaluation of the program that included a small subset of the participants, families who participated in ECSS reported significantly decreased parenting stress during the time of ECSS involvement, with larger decreases in stress associated with more treatment services and longer duration of treatment. Additionally, parents reported having fewer barriers to employment as a result of their involvement in ECSS. Anecdotally, families reported that they appreciated the "one-stop shopping" format of the interagency approach. Given the lack of reliable transportation and limited integrated services by community professionals, creating a plan of intervention together with multiple agencies has proved to be invaluable to families entering the program. The program has served children with a wide variety of behavioral, social, emotional, and cognitive issues and is viewed in communities as an important resource for at-risk families. ECSS represents a well-accepted model of family-driven, community-based IMH delivery that is both consistent across the state and tailored to local practices[42] (Center for Educational Accountability: ECSS executive summary: Louisiana early childhood supports and services infant mental health program: 5 year program evaluation report 2002–2007, University of Alabama at Birmingham, unpublished report, 2007).

SUMMARY AND IMPLICATIONS

The implementation of Healthy Beginnings and ECSS shares some common lessons learned that may be beneficial to the development of similar programs. First, even though there may be agreement about the need for and general goals of such programs, both programs took more time than anticipated to integrate and coordinate new services into well-established systems of care. Complex health care, mental health, and social service systems each have their own culture, language, and goals, and all must have at least a working knowledge of the other. Second, mental health stigma is prevalent, and even with training, nonmental health professionals need support to feel comfortable talking with families and making effective referrals. Integrating early childhood mental health services into other health, educational, or social services may increase access, and flexibility to provide services both in the home and clinic settings may improve the acceptability and salience of programs for families. Community outreach, education for parents and other professionals, and multiagency coordination may increase the access and acceptability of IMH services. Furthermore, in our experience, there are important reasons to be able to address maternal mental health as well as child and relationship issues within the same program, rather than referring to adult mental health services. Clinically salient interventions that not only address the caregiver's specific mental health issues but also focus on caregiving abilities are crucial to early childhood outcomes. The overwhelming community, agency, and professional support of these programs, as well as parental acceptance, suggests that IMH programs that are integrated into other community programs are worthy of further study and development.

Finally, development of such programs also shares a number of other challenges. Work force development has been identified as an urgent issue for the development of infant and early childhood mental health services.[42–44] The examples in this article show how a variety of professionals who provide IMH services increase access and extend services to those who otherwise may not be served. However, there is a need to improve basic knowledge and skill across and within disciplines.[42] Furthermore, there is uneven exposure to perinatal and early childhood mental health in traditional mental health training programs (adult and child psychiatry, psychology, and social work), and IMH is typically not taught in primary care disciplines and public health programs, even though they are increasingly taking on responsibility for mental health screening and early intervention services.[43,44]

A number of states are adopting IMH credentialing to enhance workforce development, but there is no nationally recognized credentialing process. A challenge for the field is clarification of roles, skills and knowledge base, and responsibilities of the various professionals, paraprofessionals, and others involved in direct and supportive IMH services.[44]

In addition to work force issues, there are a number of payor issues that limit services. For example, Medicaid policies limit the type and scope of mental health services and do not provide coverage for "alternative" mental health services, such as the use of case managers and/or collaborative practice, telepsychiatry, and mental health consultative services to primary care professionals.[45] Multiple funding streams have been recommended as a way to leverage funding for mental health services to young children and families, and there are some positive efforts at maximizing federal, state, and local resources for early childhood mental health services.[46–48]

Finally, as we noted at the beginning of this article, infant and early childhood mental health is a field characterized by strong interdisciplinary integration. The hope, and emerging evidence, is that early preventive and intervention approaches will decrease the likelihood of longer-term, and perhaps more intractable, problems from occurring. It is clear that the development of quality early childhood mental health services depends on the availability of a range of integrated services across mental health, health, social, and educational systems. Thus, it is imperative that clinicians, program developers, and policy makers recognize the intricate interplay between health, social, emotional, and cognitive development that occur in the earliest years.

ACKNOWLEDGMENTS

The authors are grateful to the agencies and individuals involved in the Healthy Beginnings program, including the New Orleans City Department of Health, Children's Bureau of New Orleans, the Institute of Mental Hygiene, and Tulane University School of Medicine, as well as the Louisiana Office of Mental Health and Louisiana Department of Social Services who direct ECSS. In addition, we are grateful to the families with whom we work in the service of very young children's mental health.

REFERENCES

1. Dube SR, Felitti VJ, Dong M, et al. The impact of adverse childhood experiences on health problems: evidence from four birth cohorts dating back to 1900. Prev Med 2003;37:268–77.
2. Felitti VJ, Anda RF, Nordenberg D, et al. Relationship of childhood abuse and household dysfunction to many of the leading causes of death in adults: The Adverse Childhood Experiences (ACE) Study. Am J Prev Med 1998;14:245–58.
3. Robinson M, Oddy WH, Li J, et al. Pre-and postnatal influences on preschool mental health: a large-scale cohort study. J Child Psychol Psychiatry 2008;49: 1118–28.
4. Shonkoff JP, Phillips D. From neurons to neighborhoods: the science of early childhood development. Washington, D.C.: National Academy Press; 2000.
5. Rusconi-Serpa. Video feedback in parent-infant therapy. Child Adolesc Psychiatr Clin N Am in this issue, 2009.
6. Smyke AT, Zeanah CH, Fox NA, et al. Psychosocial interventions: Bucharest Early Intervention Project. Child Adolesc Psychiatr Clin N Am in this issue, 2009.
7. Lieberman AF, Horn P. Giving voice to the unsayable: Repairing the effects of trauma in infancy and early childhood. Child Adolesc Psychiatr Clin N Am in this issue, 2009.
8. Egger HL, Angold A. Common emotional and behavioral disorders in preschool children: presentation, nosology, and epidemiology. J Child Psychol Psychiatry 2006;47:313–37.
9. Aber LJ, Jones S, Cohen J. The impact of poverty on the mental health of very young children. In: Zeanah CH, editor. Handbook of infant mental health. New York: Guilford Press; 2000. p. 113–20.
10. Evans GW. The environment of childhood poverty. Am Psychol 2004;50:77–92.

11. Lieberman AF, Amaya-Jackson L. Reciprocal Influences of attachment and trauma: using a dual lens in the assessment and treatment of infants, toddlers, and preschoolers. In: Berlin L, Amaya-Jackson L, Ziv Y, editors. Enhancing early attachment: theory, research and intervention. New York: Guilford Press; 2003. p. 100–24.

12. Carter AS, Garrity-Rokous FE, Chazan-Cohen R, et al. Maternal depression and comorbidity: predicting early parenting, attachment security, and toddler social-emotional problems and competencies. J Am Acad Child Adolesc Psychiatry 2001;40:18–26.

13. Zeanah CH, Zeanah PD. Towards a definition of infant mental health. Zero to Three 22:13, 2001. p. 13–20.

14. Zero to Three Infant Mental Health Steering Committee. Definition of infant mental health. Washington, D.C.: Zero To Three; 2001.

15. Zeanah CH, Zeanah PD. The scope of infant mental health. In: Zeanah CH, editor. Handbook of Infant Mental Health. 3rd edition. New York: Guilford Press, in press.

16. Zeanah CH, Larrieu JA, Heller SS, et al. Evaluation of a preventive intervention for maltreated infants and toddlers in foster care. J Am Acad Child Adolesc Psychiatry 2001;40:214–21.

17. AAP. Policy statement: the medical home. Pediatrics 2002;110:184 reaffirmed 2008.

18. Available at: www.aap.org. Accessed December 19, 2008.

19. Green M, Palfrey MS, editors. In: National Center for Education in Maternal and Child Health. Bright futures: guidelines for health supervision of infants, children, and adolescents. Washington, DC: Georgetown University; 2000.

20. Hagan JF, Shaw JS, Duncan PM. Bright futures: guidelines for health supervision of infants, children, and adolescents. 3rd Edition. Elk Grove, IL: American Academy of Pediatrics; 2008.

21. Kaye NP. Improving the delivery of health care that supports young children's healthy mental development: early accomplishments and lessons learned from a five-state consortium. New York City: National Academy for State Health Policy and The Commonwealth Fund; 2006.

22. Scarr S. American child care today. Am Psychol 1998;53:95–108.

23. NICHD Early Child Care Research Network. Child care and child dev. New York: Guilford Press; 2005.

24. Shepard S, Dickstein S. Preventive Intervention for early childhood behavioral problems: An ecological perspective. Child and Adolescent Psychiatric Clinics of North America in press.

25. Webster-Stratton C, Hammond M. Treating children with early-onset conduct problems: a comparison of child and parent training interventions. J Consult Clin Psychol 1997;35:93–109.

26. Olds D, Henderson C, Cole R, et al. Long-term effects of nurse home visitation on children's criminal and antisocial behavior: 15-year follow-up of a randomized controlled trial. JAMA 1998;280:1238–44.

27. Kitzman H, Olds DL, Henderson CR Jr, et al. Effects of prenatal and infancy home visitation by nurses on pregnancy outcomes, childhood injuries, and repeated childbearing: a randomized controlled trial. JAMA 1997;278:644–52.

28. Olds DL, Eckenrode J, Henderson CR Jr, et al. Long-term effects of home visitation on maternal life course and child abuse and neglect: fifteen-year follow-up of a randomized trial. JAMA 1997;278:637–43.

29. Olds DL, Kitzman H, Cole R, et al. Effects of nurse home visiting on maternal lifecourse and child development: age-six follow-up of a randomized trial. Pediatrics 2004;114:1550–9.

30. Olds DL, Sadler L, Kitzman H, et al. Programs for parents of infants and toddlers: recent evidence from randomized trials. J Child Psychol Psychiatry 2007;48:221–3.
31. Aos S, Lieb R, Mayfield J, et al. Benefits and costs of prevention and early intervention programs for youth. Olympia Washington Institute for Public Policy; 2004.
32. Karoly LA, Kilburn MR, Cannon JS. Early childhood interventions: proven results, future promise. In: RAND, editor. Santa Monica, CA: Rand Corporation; 2005.
33. Boris N, Larrieu J, Zeanah PD, et al. The process and promise of mental health augmentation of nurse home visiting programs: data from the Louisiana nurse-family partnership program. Infant Ment Health J 2006;27:26–40.
34. Zeanah PD, Larrieu JA, Boris NW, et al. Nurse home visiting: perspectives from nurses. Infant Ment Health J 2006;26:41–54.
35. Knitzer J, Thebarge S, Johnson K. Reducing maternal depression and its impact on young children: toward a responsive early childhood policy framework. New York City: Columbia University; 2008.
36. Field T. Maternal depression effects on infants and early interventions. Prev Med 1998;27:2000–3.
37. Field T. The amazing infant. Oxford: Blackwell Publishing; 2007.
38. van den Boom DC. The influence of temperament and mothering on attachment and exploration: an experimental manipulation of sensitive responsiveness among lower-class mothers with irritable infants. Child Development 1994;65:1457–77.
39. van den Boom DC. Do first-year intervention effects endure? Follow-up during toddlerhood of a sample of Dutch irritable infants. Child Development 1995;66:1798–816.
40. Juffer F, Bakerman-Krakenburg MJ, Van Ijzendoorn MH. Promoting positive parenting: an attachment-based intervention. Mahway, NJ: Lawrence Erlbaum; 2007.
41. Weissman MM, Pilowsky DJ, Wickramaratne PJ, et al. Remissions in maternal depression and child psychopathology: a STAR*D-child report. JAMA 2006; 295:1389.
42. Zeanah PD, Stafford B, Nagle G, et al. In: Addressing social emotional development and infant mental health. Building early childhood comprehensive systems series, vol. 12. Los Angeles, CA: National Center for Infant and Early Childhood Health Policy; 2005.
43. Zeanah PD, Gleason MM. Infant Mental Health in Primary Health Care. In: Zeanah CH, editor. Handbook of infant mental health. 3rd edition. New York City: Guildford Press, in press.
44. Hinshaw-Fuselier S, Zeanah PD, Larrieu JA. Training in infant mental health. In: Zeanah CHJ, editor. Handbook of infant mental health. 3rd edition. New York, NY: Guilford Press, in press.
45. Kautz C, Mauch D, Smith SA. Reimbursement of mental health services in primary care settings. Rockville, MD: Substance Abuse and Mental Health Services; 2008.
46. Knitzer J. Building services and systems to support the healthy emotional development of young children: an action guide for policymakers, national center for children in poverty. New York: Columbia University Mailman School of Public Health; 2002.
47. Johnson K, Knitzer J, Kaufmann R. Making dollars follow sense: financing early childhood mental health services to promote healthy social and emotional

development in young children, National Center for Children in Poverty. New York: Columbia University Mailman School of Public Health; 2002.

48. Rosenthal J, Kaye N. State approaches to promoting young children's healthy mental development: a survey of medicaid, maternal and child health, and mental health agencies. Portland, ME: National Academy for State Health Policy; 2005.

Index

Note: Page numbers of article titles are in **boldface** type.

A

Activity level, in preschoolers, 635–636
ADHD. See *Attention-deficit/hyperactivity disorder (ADHD)*.
ADOS. See *Autism Diagnostic Observational Assessment (ADOS)*.
Aggression, in preschoolers, 634
American Academy of Child and Adolescent Psychiatry, 596
    Work Group on Research of, 594
American Psychological Association Task Force, 690
Anxiety, in preschoolers, psychopharmacology and, 760–762
Anxiety disorders, in early childhood, 600–601
    case example, 603
    comorbidity with, 601
    diagnosing discrete DSM-IV disorders, 600–601
    diagnostic continuity in, 601
    distinguishing between normative and pathologic fears, 600
    family history in, 601–602
    prognosis of, 602
    risk factors for, 601–602
    treatment of, 602
Anxious/depressed preschooler, case example, 603
Attachment
    correlates of, 667–668
    development of, 542–543
    disturbances of
        caregiver self-regulation disturbances effects on, 674
        in early childhood, **665–672**
            attachment-based interventions for, 672
            clinical implications of, 677–678
            disrupted attachment disorder, 671
            emotionally withdrawn/inhibited, 669–670
            historical background of, 668–669
            indiscriminate/disinhibited, 670
            reactive attachment disorder, 669
                course and amelioration of, 670–671
            secure-base distortions, 671
    organization and disorganization related to, 666–667
Attachment theory, origins of, 665–666
Attachment-based interventions, in parent-infant treatments, 736–744

Child Adolesc Psychiatric Clin N Am 18 (2009) 789–797
doi:10.1016/S1056-4993(09)00052-2
1056-4993/09/$ – see front matter © 2009 Elsevier Inc. All rights reserved.

childpsych.theclinics.com

Attention-deficit/hyperactivity disorder (ADHD), in preschoolers
    current knowledge of, 628–629
    described, 627–628
    developmental analysis of, 632
    developmentally refined nosology for, charting of, 636–637
    prevalence of, 631
    psychopharmacology and, 756–759
    treatment of, 637–638
    validity of, 631–632
    viewing through developmental lens, **627–643**
Autism Diagnostic Interview Schedule, 568
Autism Diagnostic Observational Assessment (ADOS), 568
Autism spectrum disorders
    diagnostic criteria for, 646
    in young children, **645–663**
        diagnostic assessment of, 651–652
        family considerations related to, 652–654
        interventions for, 654–656
        prevalence of, 645
        screening and early detection, 649–651
        signs of, 647–649
Avoidance, in early childhood event trauma, 613–614

B

Behavioral problems, early childhood, preventive intervention for, **687–706**
    described, 687–688
    parenting-focused early prevention interventions, importance of, 688
    parent-management training in, 688–701. See also *Parent-management training, in preventive intervention for early childhood behavioral problems.*
Berkeley Puppet Interview (BPI), 568
Birth, premature. See *Premature birth.*
BPI. See *Berkeley Puppet Interview (BPI).*
Bucharest, foster care in, context of, 722
Bucharest Early Intervention Project (BEIP), **721–734**
    challenges of caring for young, postinstitutionalized children, 724–726
    described, 721–722
    disseminating intervention with Romania and beyond, 729
    foster care network of, 722–729
    foster parent recruitment and training in, 723–724
    outcomes of, 730–732
    parallel processes, 729–730
    social work team of, 723
    social workers support from, 726–729

C

Caregiver(s)
    in children with attachment disturbances, 672–677
        role of, 672–674
    self-regulation of, disturbances in, 674
Caregiver-child relationship, effects on event trauma in early childhood, 617–618
CAVES (Clinician-Assisted Video Feedback Exposure Sessions), 740

CBCL. See *Child Behavior Checklist (CBCL)*.
CCRT. See *Core Conflictual Relationship Theme (CCRT)*.
Child Behavior Checklist (CBCL), 5694
Child internal representations, formal assessments, in clinical practice, 587–588
Child-parent psychotherapy (CPP), in early trauma treatment, 710–713
    clinical example, 711–713
    described, 710–711
    empirical evidence of efficacy of, 716–717
Children, young. See *Young children*.
Circle of Security (COS), 737–738
Clinical practice, relationship assessment in, **581–591.** See also *Relationship assessment, in clinical practice*.
Clinician-Assisted Video Feedback Exposure Sessions (CAVES), 740
Cognitive immaturity, event trauma in early childhood and, 615–616
Community health clinic, infant mental health in, 779–781
Community network, infant mental health in, 781–783
Community Parent Education (COPE) Program, 690
Comprehensive, evidence-based psychiatric assessment, of young children, 565–572. See also *Psychiatric assessment, of young children, comprehensive, evidence-based*.
COPE Program, 690
Core Conflictual Relationship Theme (CCRT), 741
COS. See *Circle of Security (COS)*.
CPP. See *Child-parent psychotherapy (CPP)*.

D

Depressive disorders, in early childhood, 595–598
    case example, 603
    dysthymic disorder, 598
    family history in, 598–599
    major depressive disorder, 595–597
    prognosis of, 599–600
    risk factors for, 598–599
Developmental derailment, event trauma in early childhood and, 616–617
Diagnostic and Statistical Manual of Mental Disorders (DSM), 594, 627, 645, 668, 708
"Diagnostic Classification of Mental Health and Development Disorders in Infancy and Early Childhood–Revised," 596
Diagnostic Interview Schedule for Children, IV–Young Child (DISC-IV-YC), 596
DISC-IV-YC. See *Diagnostic Interview Schedule for Children, IV–Young Child (DISC-IV-YC)*.
Disrupted attachment disorder, in early childhood, 671
Disruptive behavior disorders
    current knowledge of, 628–629
    in preschoolers
        aggression, 634
        described, 627–628
        developmental analysis of, 632
        developmentally imprecise, impossible, improbable, and inappropriate, 633–634
        developmentally refined nosology for, charting of, 636–637
        impulsivity and activity level, 635–636
        noncompliance, 634–635
        prevalence of, 629

Disruptive (*continued*)
 psychopharmacology and, 759–760
 temper loss, 634
 treatment of, 637–638
 validity of, 629–631
 viewing through developmental lens, **627–643**
DSM. See *Diagnostic and Statistical Manual of Mental Disorders* (DSM).
Dysthymic disorder, in early childhood, 598

E

Early childhood
 behavioral problems in, preventive intervention for, **687–706**. See also *Behavioral problems, early childhood, preventive intervention for.*
 disturbances of attachment and parental psychopathology of, **665–686**. See also *Attachment, disturbances of, in early childhood; Parental psychopathology.*
 event trauma in, **611–626**
  described, 611–612
 internalizing disorders in, **593–610**. See also *Internalizing disorders, in early childhood.*
 trauma in, repairing effects of, **707–720**. See also *Trauma, in infancy and early childhood.*
Early childhood psychiatric disorders
 developmentally appropriate classification of, 560–562
 limitations of current understanding of, 575
Early Childhood Supports and Services (ECSS), 781–783
ECSS. See *Early Childhood Supports and Services (ECSS).*
Emotionally withdrawn/inhibited child, 669–670
Event trauma, in early childhood, **611–626**
 assessment of, 618–619
 caregiver-child relationship and, 617–618
 cognitive immaturity and, 615–616
 developmental derailment and, 616–617
 differences in experiencing of, 615–618
 symptomatic manifestations of, 612–615
  avoidance, 613–614
  hyperarousal, 614
  overview, 612–613
  re-experiencing, 613
 treatment of, 619–622

F

Formal assessments, in clinical practice, 584–588
Foster care, for young children, new model of, **721–734**. See also *Bucharest Early Intervention Project (BEIP).*

H

Healthy Beginnings, 779–781
Hyperarousal, in early childhood event trauma, 614

I

Immaturity, cognitive, event trauma in early childhood and, 615–616
Impulsivity, in preschoolers, 635–636
Incredible Years Parent and Children Series, 690–692
Indiscriminate/disinhibited child, 670
Infant(s)
    premature. See *Premature infant.*
    trauma in, repairing effects of, **707–720.** See also *Trauma, in infancy and early childhood.*
Infant, parents, and parent-infant relationship, perinatal assessment of, **545–557**
Infant mental health
    defined, 774–775
    described, 773–774
    in community health clinic, 779–781
    in community network, 781–783
    "real world" and, **773–787**
    scope of, 774–775
    services for
        framework for, 775–778
        implications of, 783–784
        in "real world," development of, 778
        indicated preventive interventions, 778
        selective interventions, 777–778
        universal interventions, 775–777
Informal assessments, in clinical practice, 583–584
Internalizing disorders, in early childhood, **593–610.** See also Depressive disorders; *specific disorders e.g.,* Anxiety disorders.
    anxiety disorders, 600–601
    broad dimension of, 595
    case example, 603
    depressive disorders, 595–598
International Classification of Diseases, 10th revision (ICD-10), 668
Intersubjectivity, emergence of, 542–543

M

MacArthur Story-Stem Battery (MSSB), 568
Major depressive disorder, 595–597
Mental health, infant, **773–787.** See also *Infant mental health.*
Mental health problems, in young children, defining of, approaches to, 562–564
    descriptive, 562
    diagnostic, 563–564
    dimensional, 562–563
Mood disorders, in preschoolers, psychopharmacology and, 762–764
Mother-infant attachment process, unfolding of, steps in, 534–535
MSSB. See *MacArthur Story-Stem Battery (MSSB).*
Munich Model, 743

N

NBAS. See *Newborn Behavioral Assessment Scale (NBAS).*
Neonatal moment of meeting (NMM), **533–544**

Neonatal (*continued*)
    clinical examples of, 537–541
    determinantness of, 535–536
    development of attachment in, 542–543
    emergence of intersubjectivity in, 542–543
    functions of, 542–543
    NBAS in, 536
    steps in unfolding of mother-infant attachment process, 534–535
Neonate(s), moment of meeting, **533–544**. See also *Neonatal moment of meeting (NMM)*.
Newborn Behavioral Assessment Scale (NBAS), clinical situation using, 536
NFP. See *Nurse Family Partnership (NFP)*.
NMM. See *Neonatal moment of meeting (NMM)*.
Nonattachment, disorders of, in early childhood, 669
Noncompliance, in preschoolers, 634–635
Nurse Family Partnership (NFP), 777–778

O

Office of Juvenile Justice and Delinquency Prevention's Family Strengthening
    Project, 690

P

PAPA. See *Preschool Age Psychiatric Assessment (PAPA)*.
Parent internal representations, formal assessments, in clinical practice, 586–587
Parental psychopathology
    attachment implications from study of caregiver PTSD, 675–676
    clinical implications of, 677–678
    disturbances of, effects on young children, **665–686**
    role of, 672–677
Parental traumatization, following premature birth, 551
Parent-child interaction(s), formal assessments, in clinical practice, 584–586
Parent-Child Interaction Therapy (PCIT), 689
Parent-infant relationship, following premature birth, assessment of, 551–553
Parent-infant treatments, video feedback in, **735–751**. See also *Video feedback, in parent-infant treatments*.
Parenting-focused early prevention interventions, for early childhood behavioral
    problems, 688
Parent-management training
    in preventive intervention for early childhood behavioral problems, 688–701
        building capacity to meet need, 694–695
        described, 688–690
        Incredible Years Parent and Children Series, 690–692
        parent engagement and treatment responsiveness, 693–694
        review of evidence in, 692–693
    in real-world settings, 695–701
    with local adaptation, case example, 696–701
PCIT. See *Parent-Child Interaction Therapy (PCIT)*.
PECFAS. See *Preschool and Early Childhood Functional Assessment Scale (PECFAS)*.
Perinatal assessment, of infant, parents, and parent-infant relationship, **545–557**
    premature infant, 547–550

Perinatal period, described, 545
Positive Parenting Program (Triple P), 689
Posttraumatic stress disorder (PTSD)
    caregiver, attachment implications from study of, 675–676
    secure-base distortions related to, 676–677
Premature birth
    assessment of parent-infant relationship following, 551-553
    described, 546–547
    parental traumatization following, 551
Premature infant
    assessment of, 547–549
    assessment of parental subjective experience with, 549–550
Prematurity, perinatal assessment of, infant, parents, and parent-infant relationship in, **545–557**
Preschool Age Psychiatric Assessment (PAPA), 568
Preschool and Early Childhood Functional Assessment Scale (PECFAS), 597
Preschool disruptive behavior disorders, viewing through developmental lens, **627–643.** See also specific types and *Disruptive behavior disorders, in preschoolers.*
Preschooler(s)
    ADHD in, 756–759
        psychopharmacology and, 756–759
    anxiety in, psychopharmacology and, 760–762
    anxious/depressed, case example, 603
    disruptive behavior disorders in, psychopharmacology and, 759–760
    mood disorders in, psychopharmacology and, 762–764
    psychopharmacology and, **753–771**
        described, 753–756
Preterm infant, birth of, 546–547
Psychiatric assessment
    comprehensive, evidence-based, of young children, 565–572. See also *Psychiatric assessment, of young children, comprehensive, evidence-based.*
    of young children, **559–580**
        background of, 559–560
        challenges in, 573–574
        clinical formation and treatment planning, 572–573
        comprehensive, evidence-based, 565–572
            domains to be assessed in, 571
            multiaxial, 569–572
            multicultural approach, 567
            multidisciplinary approach, 566–567
            multiple informants, 566
            multiple modes, 567–569
            multiple sessions, 565
Psychiatric disorders, early childhood
    developmentally appropriate classification of, 560–562
    limitations of current understanding of, 575
Psychoanalytically oriented interventions, in parent-infant treatments, 739–741
Psychopathology, parental. See *Parental psychopathology.*
Psychopharmacology, preschoolers and, **753–771.** See also *Preschooler(s).*
Psychotherapy, child-parent, in early trauma treatment, 710–713
PTSD. See *Posttraumatic stress disorder (PTSD).*

R

RDC-PA. See *Research Diagnostic Criteria–Preschool Age (RDC-PA)*.
Reactive attachment disorder, 669
   course and amelioration of, 670–671
Re-experiencing, in early childhood event trauma, 613
Relationship assessment, in clinical practice, **581–591**
   components of, 582–583
   formal assessments, 584–588
      child internal representations, 587–588
      parent internal representations, 586–587
      parent-child interactions, 584–586
   informal assessments, 583–584
Research Diagnostic Criteria–Preschool Age (RDC-PA), 594

S

Secure-base distortions
   in early childhood, 671
   PTSD and, 676–677
SET-PC version. See *Supportive Expressive Therapy–Parent-Child (SET-PC) version*.
SSP. See *Strange Situation Procedure (SSP)*.
STAR*D study, 675
STEEP, 738–739
Strange Situation Procedure (SSP), 666
Stress, traumatic
   in infancy and early childhood, identification of, 709–710
   relational impact of, 710
Supportive Expressive Therapy–Parent-Child (SET-PC) version, 741
Systemic interventions, in parent-infant treatments, 741–744

T

Temper loss, in preschoolers, 634
Transactional model interventions, in parent-infant treatments, 744–747
Trauma
   early exposure to, contextual framework for intervention, 708–709
   event, in early childhood, **611–626.** See also *Event trauma, in early childhood*.
   in infancy and early childhood
      contextual framework for intervention, 708–709
      CPP for, 710–713
         empirical evidence of efficacy of, 716–717
      creating shared trauma narrative between child and parent, 713–716
      repairing effects of, **707–720**
         described, 707–708
   parental, following premature birth, 551
   stress related to
      in infancy and early childhood, identification of, 709–710
      relational impact of, 710
Trauma narrative, creating of, between child and parent, 713–716
Triple P. See *Positive Parenting Program (Triple P)*.

V

Video feedback
   described, 735–736
   in parent-infant treatments, **735–751**
      attachment-based interventions, 736–744
      case example, 747–748
      discussion of, 748
      psychoanalytically oriented interventions, 739–741
      systemic interventions, 741–744
      transactional model interventions, 744–747

W

Warren's Narrative Emotional Coding system, 569
Women, Infant, and Children Nutritional Supplement Program, 695

Y

Young children
   autism spectrum disorders, **645–663.** See also *Autism spectrum disorders, in young children.*
   disturbances of attachment and parental psychopathology in, **665–686.** See also *Attachment, disturbances of, in early childhood; Parental psychopathology.*
   foster care for, new model of, **721–734.** See also *Bucharest Early Intervention Project (BEIP).*
   mental health problems in, defining of, approaches to, 562–564
   psychiatric assessment of, **559–580.** See also *Psychiatric assessment, of young children.*

Z

Zero to Three National Center for Clinical Infant Programs, 669

Moving?

Make sure your subscription moves with you!

To notify us of your new address, find your **Clinics Account Number** (located on your mailing label above your name), and contact customer service at:

E-mail: elspcs@elsevier.com

800-654-2452 (subscribers in the U.S. & Canada)
314-453-7041 (subscribers outside of the U.S. & Canada)

Fax number: 314-523-5170

Elsevier Periodicals Customer Service
11830 Westline Industrial Drive
St. Louis, MO 63146

*To ensure uninterrupted delivery of your subscription, please notify us at least 4 weeks in advance of move.

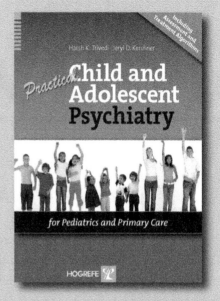
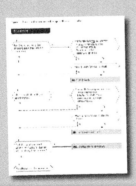
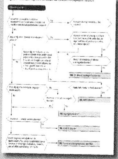
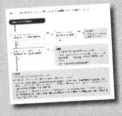
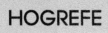

Printed and bound by CPI Group (UK) Ltd, Croydon, CR0 4YY

03/10/2024

01040465-0009